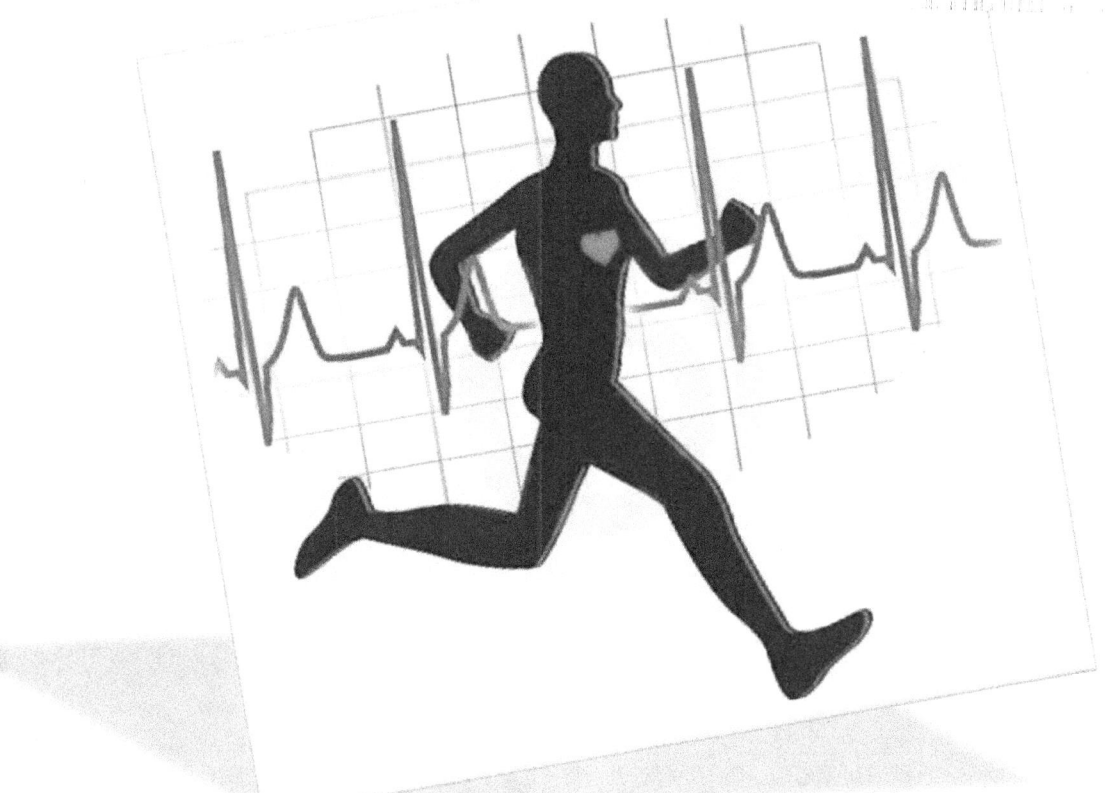

Move SomeThing!
Move Your Self into Healing, Health & Abundant Life!

Achieving and Maintaining Supreme Health and Fitness by increasing the level of Knowledge and Science of Life!

Supreme Health & Fitness by Sean Ali!

Sean Ali, BS. Health & Wellness

Move SomeThing!

Move YourSelf into Healing, Health & Abundant Life!

This book introduces the role that physical activity and fitness play in a healthy lifestyle. The number two actual cause of death is poor diet and physical inactivity (15.2%),

We know that physical activity plays a major role in the physical dimension, but it also contributes to learning, relationships, and a sense of human limitations within the broader perspective.

From the beginning of recorded history, philosophers and health professionals have observed that regular physical activity is an essential part of a healthy life.

Hippocrates wrote the following in *On Regimen in Acute Diseases,* about 400 BC: ***Eating alone will not keep a man [woman] well; he [she] must also take exercise. For food and exercise, while possessing opposite qualities, yet work together to produce health. . . .***

Regular participation in physical activity results in a reduced risk of numerous diseases and death from all causes. We now know that regular participation in physical activity **reduces** the risk of death from all causes by about 40%.

Doing physical activity on a regular basis also has been shown to have a similar impact on the following:

- **Cardiorespiratory health**: Exercise reduces the risk of heart disease and stroke, lowers blood pressure (BP), improves the blood lipid profile, and increases CRF.

- **Metabolic health**: Exercise **reduces** the risk of developing type 2 diabetes and helps to control blood glucose in those who already have type 2 diabetes.

BUILD YOUR HEALTH!

What does being healthy mean?

For some it's simpley avoidance of disease, but it is also more than that. **Health** *has been defined as a human condition possessing social, psychological, and physical dimensions.*

Positive health *is associated with a capacity to enjoy life and withstand challenges.*

Negative health *is associated with morbidity (incidence of disease) and premature mortality.*

- **Musculoskeletal health**: Exercise slows the loss of bone density that occurs with aging, and it lowers the risk of hip fractures. In addition, it improves pain management in people with arthritis. Completing progressive muscle-strengthening activities increase or preserve muscle mass, strength, and power.

- **Cancer**: Physically active people have a significantly lower risk of colon cancer and breast cancer. In addition, there is some evidence that physical activity reduces the risk of endometrial cancer and lung cancer.

- **Mental health**: Physical activity lowers the risk of depression and age-related cognitive decline, and it improves the quality of sleep.

- **Functional ability and fall prevention**: Physical activity reduces the risk of functional limitations (e.g., ability to do activities of daily living), and for those older adults at risk of falling, physical activity is safe and reduces this risk.

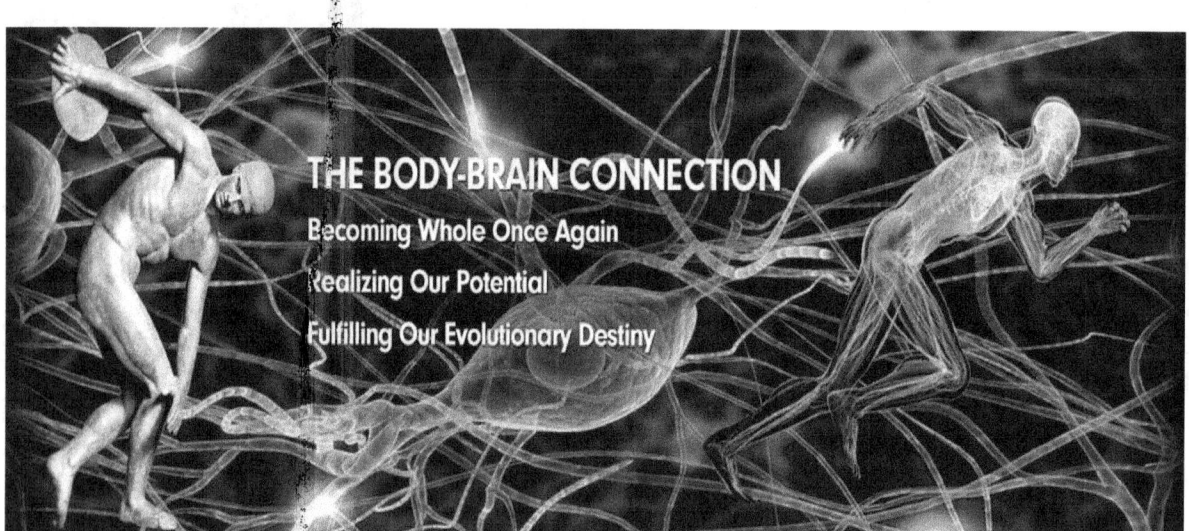

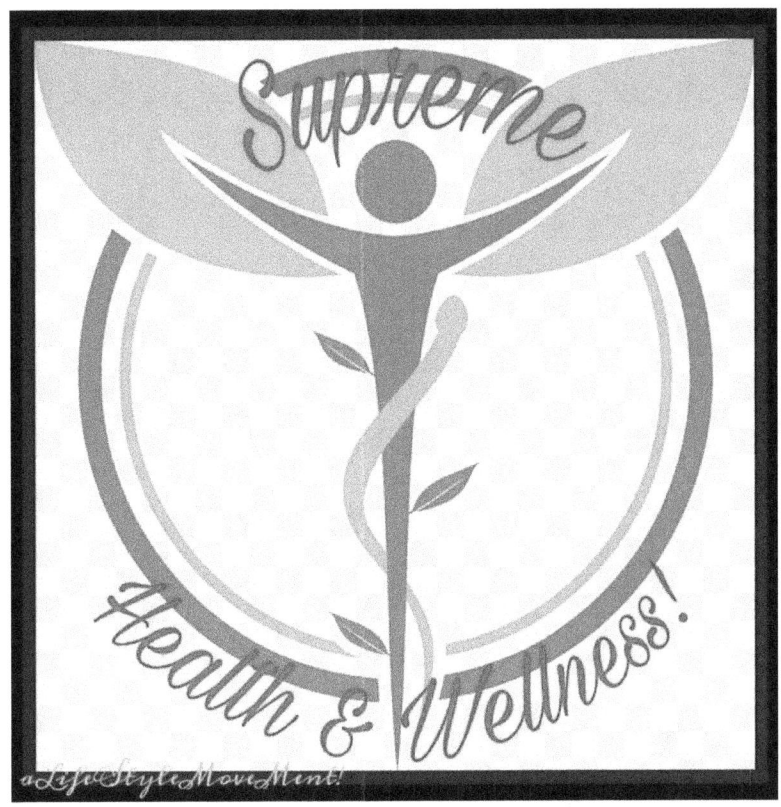

Supreme Health and Fitness by Sean Ali!

Achieving and Maintaining Supreme Health and Wellness by increasing the level of Knowledge and Science of Life!

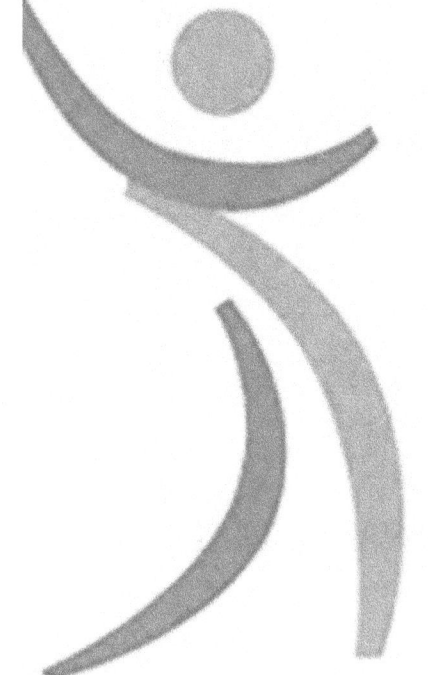

Table of Contents

*****

Introduction ...	... Page 12
Chapter One ... Move SomeThing ~ Move YourSelf! ...	... Page 22
Chapter Two ... Awesome Benefits of Moving YourSelf! ...	... Page 40
Chapter Three ... Sitting Dis-Ease ...	... Page 70
Chapter Four ... Risk Factors of Pre-Mature Death ...	... Page 86
Chapter Five ... Exercise & Brain Health ...	... Page 98
Chapter Six ... Eating 2 Live & Exercise ...	... Page 126
Chapter Seven ... Are You Fit ~ Check YourSelf ...	... Page 136
Chapter Eight ... It's Never Too Late! ...	... Page 146
Chapter Nine ... Your Energy & Work ...	... Page 160
Chapter Ten ... Your Heart-Beat & Target Heart Rate ...	... Page 186
Chapter Eleven ... Exercise & Weight Management ...	... Page 208
Chapter Twelve ... Your Musculoskeletal Health ...	... Page 220
Chapter Thirteen ... Regulating Your Body Temperature ...	... Page 232
Chapter Fourteen ... Move SomeThing Activities ...	... Page 242

Chapter Fifteen ... 5 Leading Causes of Death ...   ... Page 280

Chapter Sixteen ... Exercise & Heart Dis-Ease ...   ... Page 286

Chapter Seventeen ... Exercise & Obesity ...   ... Page 302

Chapter Eighteen ... Exercise & Diabetes ...   ... Page 318

Chapter Nineteen ... Exercise & Pulmonary Dis-Ease ...   ... Page 336

Chapter Twenty ... Bio-Mechanics of Exercise ...   ... Page 354

Chapter Twenty-One ... Life Movements & Motions ...   ... Page 380

The Cool Down and Creating Your Change ...   ... Page 402

Resources & References

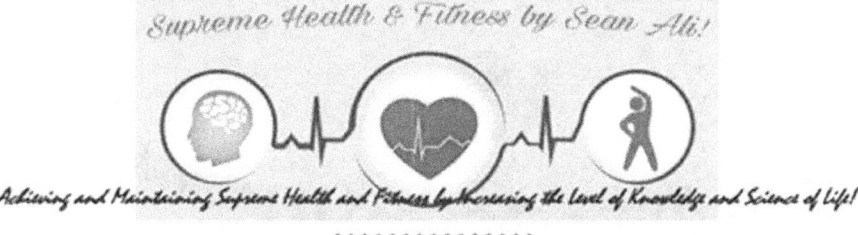

Health & Fitness Awareness!

Mission: Introduce the concepts and values of Exercise/Staying active in conjunction with the Principles of Eating to LIVE/Nutrition and how to effectively utilize them to Improve our Quality of LIFE and Increase our overall LIFE-Span.

In addition, we also aim to educate on how to convert Potential (physical, mental and spiritual) Energy into the Kinetic Energy that produces the base for Abundant LIFE.

Goal: The following 4 points underline the Core Principles needed to Successfully began to Build and Maintain Supreme Health and Fitness, which would allow us to LIVE a Full, Active and Healthy LIFE filled with endless possibilities and potential.

1. Educate on the concept of Supreme Health and Fitness.
2. Provide education on the 3 Principles of LIFE – 1. Breathing; 2. Water/Drinking; 3. Nutrition/Eating.
3. Provide education on the value of completing a Physical Health assessment; and offering an introductory survey to start the process of being Healthy!
4. Provide education on the importance of staying Active and the principles of Exercise - its value & role in disease prevention and improvement of Health.

*Are **YOU** Aware of **YOUR** health status?   If Not, get **YOUR** Assessment **TODAY**!!

*Do **YOU** want to Improve the Quality of **YOUR** Life?   If So, it's as **EASY** as a phone call!!

*For any questions, appointments or other information, please connect us at:

240-434-6959 or seanyali40@gmail.com

Supreme Health and Fitness

Sean Ali, B.S. Health and Wellness

Owner & Life Coach

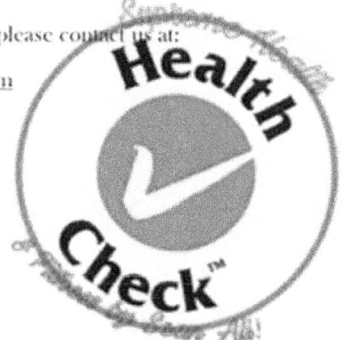

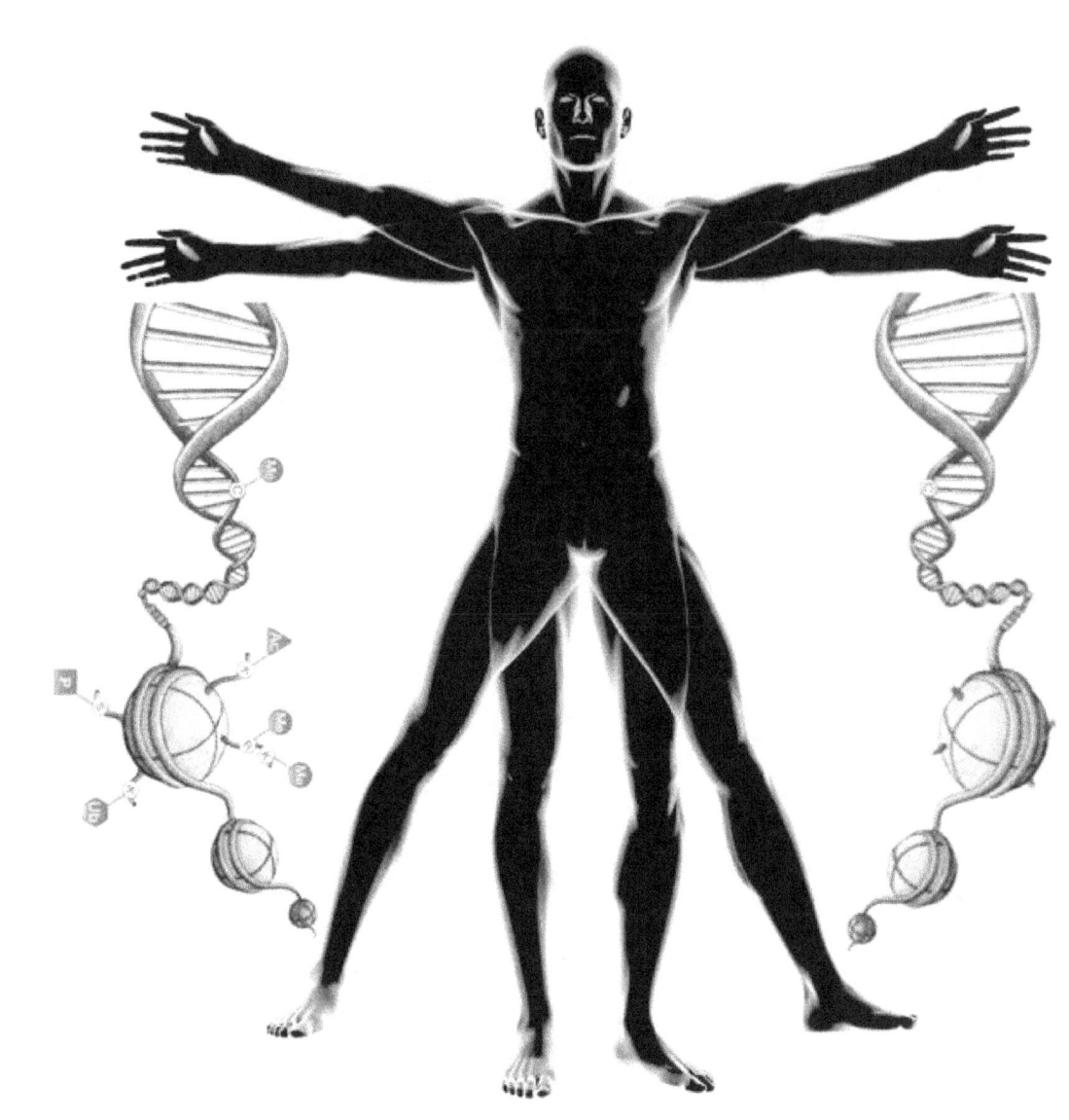

Supreme Health & Fitness! *Health & Wellness Series...Vol 3!*

Introduction

*****

In The Mighty Name Of The CREATOR ..... Peace and Blessings Of Life!

Move Something!

WHAT Are YOU Moving?

YourSelf!

WHERE Are YOU Going?

Abundant LIFE!

This is the Ground-Breaking and Exciting Volume 3 of my Self-Healing Series!

In this Volume we re-examine and re-define the Level, Intensity and Focus of performing Physical Activities or Exercises. It is my understanding that there is NO Health or Power without Exercise. This is supported by the fact that the number 2 ACTUAL Cause of premature death is BOTH Poor diet and LACK of adequate amount of Exercise.

In this book, you will be given the science of Exercise and how to Successfully apply both Exercise and Eating To Live to Build and Maintain your Supreme Health and Fitness!

Life is based on MOTION.

Your body is created of trillions of Cells that are all constantly and consistently MOVING.

Your body is created to MOVE and Sustain and Maintain perpetual MOTION.

At present, the recommended time of performing physical activities/exercises is 120-150 minutes a week or 30 – 50 minutes a day/5 days a week. I declare that this is NOT ENOUGH!

WE MUST MOVE OURSELVES AT LEAST 60 MINUTES A DAY – EVERY DAY TO BE CONSIDERED HEALTHY!!!

A Body In-Motion STAYS IN-MOTION …. A Body At-Rest STAYS AT-REST

You can Put YourSelf into the Perpetual Motion of Abundant LIFE!

Everyone should already think that "exercise" is good for them. Unfortunately, many of us only regard exercise to th0e gym or body-building.

We only seek to exercise when we want to make a 'physical' improvement – toned arms, legs, abs or getting a bigger butt or creating the beach body.

The unknown part is that most of us are not familiar with the scientific evidence that shows that physical activity provides important health benefits.

Of course, there are many reasons as to why we choose to perform a physical activity. They often include weight mangement; improving personal appearance; improving muscle strength, fitness and athletic ability for participation in sports and feeling better and being more energetic.

The Many Health Benefits of Physical Activity — Major Research Findings

1. *Regular physical activity reduces your risk of many adverse health outcomes.*

2. *Some physical activity is better than none.*

3. *For most health outcomes, additional benefits occur as the amount of physical activity increases through higher intensity, greater frequency, and/or longer duration.*

4. *Most health benefits occur with at least 250 minutes a week of moderate-intensity physical activity, such as brisk walking. Additional benefits occur with more physical activity.*

5. Both aerobic (endurance) and muscle-strengthening (resistance) physical activity is beneficial.

6. Health benefits occur for children and adolescents, young and middle-aged adults, older adults, and those in every studied racial and ethnic group.

7. The health benefits of physical activity benefits for those with disabilities.

8. The benefits of physical activity far outweigh the possibility of adverse outcomes.

The benefits from even a small amount of low-intensity physical activity are striking and almost have an immediate Positive effect on your health and fitness.

People who are physically active for about 7 hours a week have a 40 percent lower risk of dying early than those who are active for less than 30 minutes a week.

Even the **LOW** *recommended minimum of 2 hours and 30 minutes (150 minutes) a week of moderate-intensity aerobic activity (e.g. brisk walking) lowers the risk of premature death. One estimate is that as many as 250,000 deaths per year in the United States, approximately 12% of the total, are attributable to a lack of regular physical activity.*

Regular physical activity in children and adolescents not only makes them healthier and fit now, but it lowers their risk of chronic diseases and improves their chances of becoming healthy adults. It is important to encourage young people to participate in physical activities that are appropriate for their age, that are enjoyable, and that offer variety.

The Guidelines recommend that children and adolescents ages 6 to 17 do 60 minutes (1 hour) or more of physical activity each day. That includes:

Aerobic Activity: *Most of the 60 or more minutes a day should be either moderate- or vigorous-intensity aerobic physical activity (such as running, dancing, or biking), and include vigorous-intensity physical activity at least 3 days a week*

Muscle-Strengthening: *As part of the 60 or more minutes of daily physical activity, include muscle-strengthening physical activity (such as climbing trees, using playground equipment, or lifting weights) on at least 3 days of the week*

Bone-Strengthening: *As part of the 60 or more minutes of daily physical activity, include bone-strengthening physical activity (such as running or jumping rope) on at least 3 days of the week*

Finding Ways to Promote Physical Activity in Youth is very Important!

Many youth are naturally physically active and need opportunities to be active. There is an epidemic of childhood obesity. Obesity in children is a health problem because the obese children are NOT losing their weight..... they are becoming Obese Adults!

Children benefit from encouragement from parents and other adults to be active. Adults can promote youth physical activity by:

- **_Providing time for both structured and unstructured physical activity during school and outside of school.**

Children need time for active play through recess, physical activity breaks, physical education classes, after-school programs, and active time with friends and family.

- **_Providing youth with positive feedback and good role models.**

Adults should model and encourage an active lifestyle. Praise, rewards, and encouragement help youth to be active.

- **_Promoting activities that set the basis for a lifetime of activity.**

Children and adolescents should be exposed to a variety of activities: active recreation, team sports, and individual sports. In this way, they can find what they can do well in both competitive and non- competitive activities and in activities that do not require exceptional athletic skills.

Beyond Physical Activity for Health: Getting Physically Fit, guidance for Youth and Adults

Research has documented the important health benefits that youth and adults receive from at least 150 hours of moderate intensity physical activity a week ..... and they also have found that even greater benefits are gained from 300 hours a week of physical activity .... When you reach at least 420 hours a week then you set the stage for not only Healing YourSelf – BUT YOU MAY NEVER GET SICK AGAIN!

Clearly this level of physical activity contributes to fitness.

But what about getting more highly fit with the goal of improving athletic performance?

What sort, how often, how intense and what duration should physical conditioning exercises for this purpose be?

And what is the best schedule for someone who is sedentary and just embarking on a fitness program?

Unfortunately, that description fits all too many Americans.

A critical lesson from the experience of many people seeking to improve their fitness is to progress slowly. *It is a mistake to rush a conditioning program, a gradual increase in intensity and duration over at least 6 weeks to attain a minimum level of fitness is needed and gradual progression of intensity, duration and frequency over many months thereafter is advisable.*

In this book we at the following Health Benefits from completing physical activity on a regular basis also has been shown to have a similar impact on the following:

- **Cardiorespiratory health**: *Exercise reduces the risk of heart disease and stroke, lowers blood pressure (BP), improves the blood lipid profile, and increases CRF.*

- **Metabolic health**: *Exercise **reduces** the risk of developing type 2 diabetes and helps to control blood glucose in those who already have type 2 diabetes.*

- **Musculoskeletal health**: *Exercise slows the loss of bone density that occurs with aging, and it lowers the risk of hip fractures. In addition, it improves pain management in people with arthritis. Completing progressive muscle-strengthening activities increase or preserve muscle mass, strength, and power.*

- **Cancer**: *Physically active people have a significantly lower risk of colon cancer and breast cancer. In addition, there is some evidence that physical activity reduces the risk of endometrial cancer and lung cancer.*

- **Mental health**: *Physical activity lowers the risk of depression and age-related cognitive decline, and it improves the quality of sleep.*

- **Functional ability and fall prevention**: Physical activity reduces the risk of functional limitations (e.g., ability to do activities of daily living), and for those older adults at risk of falling, physical activity is safe and reduces this risk.

With this science book, I want to introduce to you just how AWESOME and POWERFUL God created you and your Body. Your body id created to Move and Do everything you Command it to do.

The Motion of Exercise generates the Energy that is the foundation and basis of the Fountain Of Youth!

You CAN Move YourSelf into your Healing!

You CAN Move YourSelf into POWER!

You CAN Move YourSelf into the Successful Enjoyment of Your Abundant Life!

Open this book and learn how Awesome and Vital Exercise is to your Health and Wellness. Learn how to Move YourSelf!

Move SomeThing!

What are you Moving?

YourSelf!

Where are You Going?

Into the Enjoyment of Your Abundant Life!

Peace and Blessings!

Sean Ali, BS. Health & Wellness

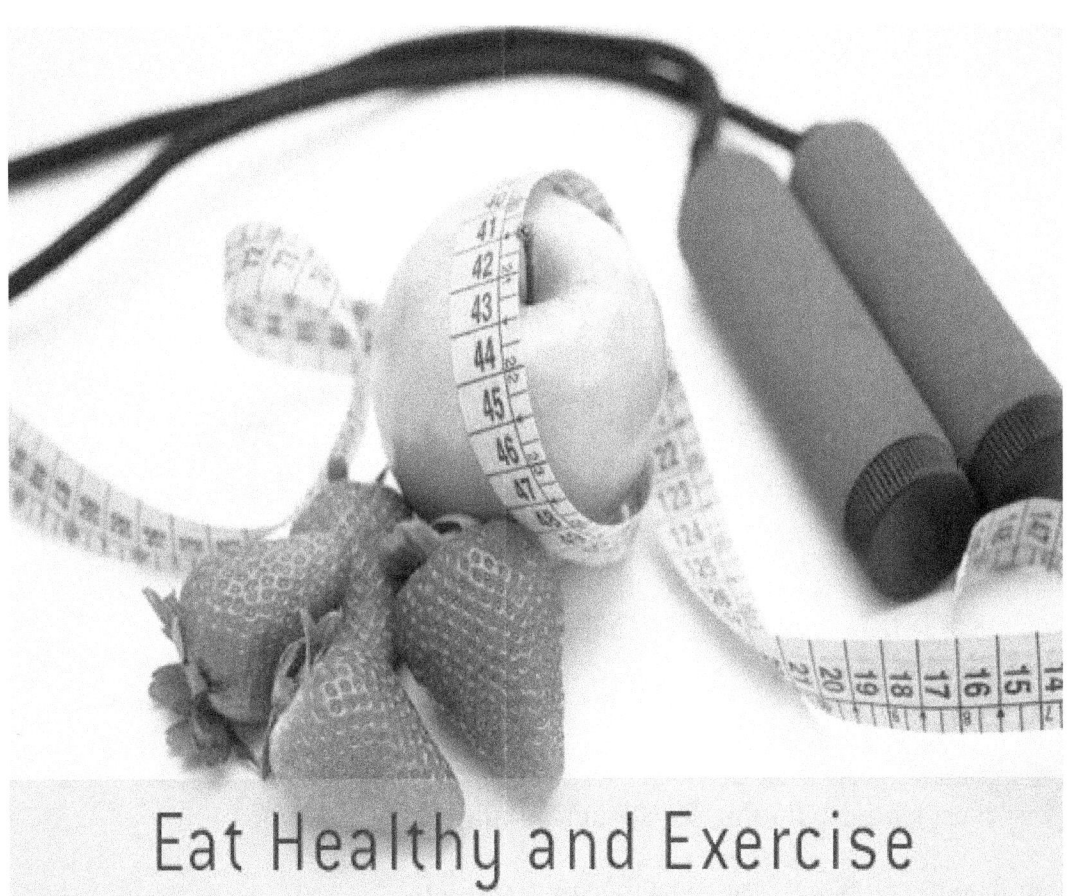

Eat Healthy and Exercise

The purpose *of a fitness program must be uppermost in the fitness professional's mind. The fitness professional is trying to help people include physical activity as a vital part of their lives.*

This assumes that the participants understand what type of physical activity is appropriate, have sufficient skills to achieve satisfaction from the activities, and have the intrinsic motivation to continue to be active for the rest of their lives.

Thus, fitness professionals help people increase their physical fitness in ways that are psychologically, mentally, and socially relevant and appealing.

Before Starting ANY Exercise Program

Check your health status.

Moderate physical activity, like walking the dog, gardening, or working around the house, is not dangerous for most people, and no medical clearance is needed for it.

People with chronic diseases, such as a heart condition, arthritis, diabetes, or high blood pressure, should talk to their physician about what types and amounts of physical activity are appropriate.

The American Heart Association suggests that you see a physician before exercising if:

- ■you have a heart condition;
- ■you take medicine for your heart and/or blood pressure;
- ■you get pains in your chest, left side of your neck, or your left shoulder or arm when you exercise;
- ■your chest has been hurting for about a month;
- ■you tend to get dizzy, lose consciousness, and fall;
- ■you get breathless with mild exertion;
- ■you have bone or joint problems that a physician told you could be worsened by exercise;
- ■you have an overweight or obesity problem;
- ■you have a medical condition, such as insulin-dependent diabetes, that requires special attention in an exercise program; or
- ■you are middle-aged or older (40 years for men; 50 years for women).

Health-Related Physical Activity Guidelines for Children/Adolescents

1. Children and adolescents should do 60 minutes (1 hour) or more of physical activity daily.

   Aerobic: Most of the 60 or more minutes a day should be either moderate- (noticeably increases breathing, sweating, and heart rate) or vigorous-intensity (substantially increases breathing, sweating, and heart rate) aerobic physical activity and should include vigorous-intensity physical activity at least three days a week. Examples of aerobic activities include running, hopping, skipping, jumping rope, swimming, dancing, and bicycling.

   Muscle-strengthening: As part of their 60 or more minutes of daily physical activity, children and adolescents should include muscle-strengthening physical activity on at least three days of the week. Muscle-strengthening activities can include resistance training or less structured activities such as playing on playground equipment, climbing trees, and playing tug-of-war.

   Bone-strengthening: As part of their 60 or more minutes of daily physical activity, children and adolescents should include bone-strengthening physical activity on at least three days of the week. Examples of bone-strengthening activities include running, jumping rope, basketball, tennis, and hopscotch.

2. It is important to encourage young people to participate in physical activities that are appropriate for their age, that are enjoyable, and that offer variety.

HEALTH

- **Health** is the level of functional or metabolic efficiency of a living organism. In humans it is the ability of individuals or communities to adapt and self-manage when facing physical, mental or social challenges.

PHYSICAL FITNESS

- **Physical fitness** is a general state of health and well-being and, more specifically, the ability to perform aspects of sports, occupations and daily activities. Physical fitness is generally achieved through proper nutrition, moderate-vigorous physical exercise, physical activity, and sufficient rest.

Physical Activity

Recommendations

- 60 minutes or more of age-appropriate moderate to vigorous-intensity
  » In 2011, only 18.5% of girls and 38.3% of boys achieved this

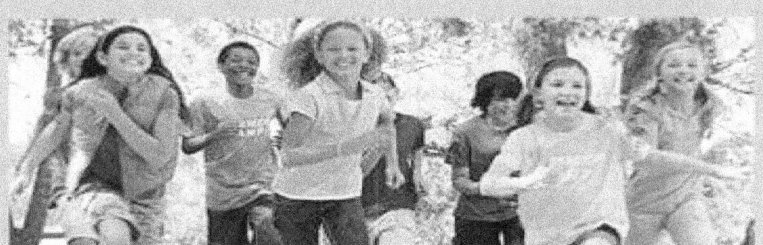

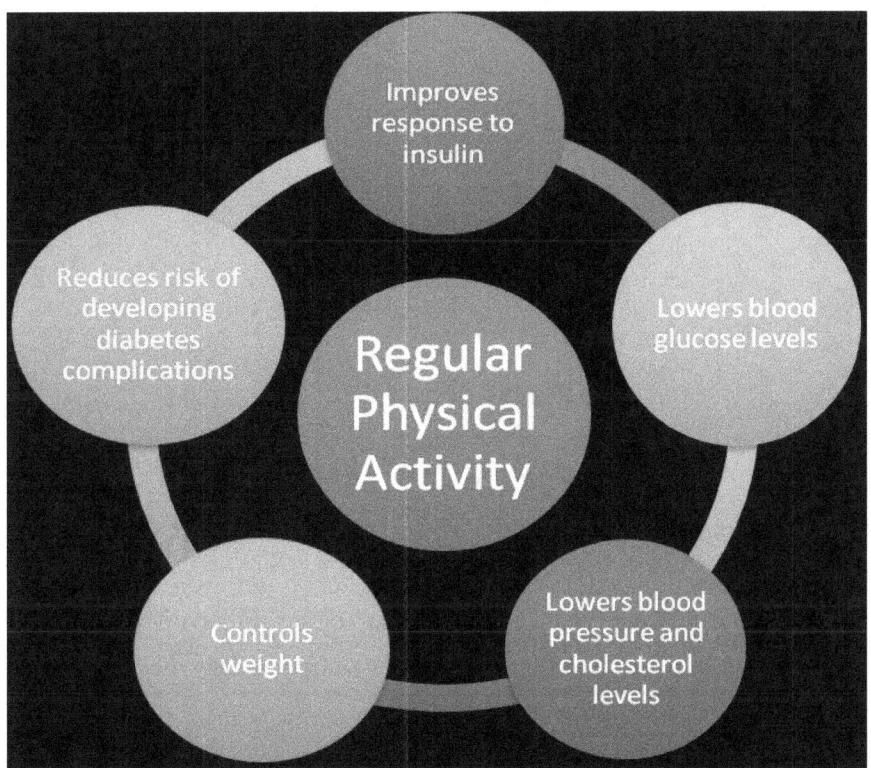

Move Something!

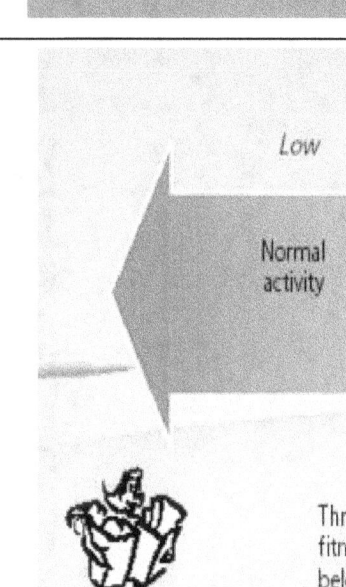
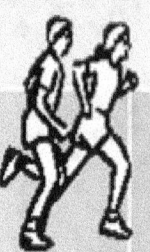

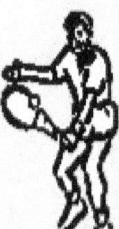
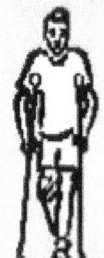

Amount of Exercise

Low — Normal activity

Moderate — Exercise zone for fitness benefits

High — Too much exercise

Threshold of training for fitness benefits (exercising below this threshold will not develop fitness but may contribute to good health)

Upper limit of safe fitness training (exercising above this threshold can lead to injury and overtraining)

Endurance
(brisk walking, jogging, swimming, etc)

Strength
(Lifting weights etc)

Types of Exercise

Balance
(Standing on one foot, heal-to-toe walk, etc.)

Flexibility
(Shoulder and upper arm stretch, calf stretch, etc.)

Chapter One

Importance of Moving YourSelf!

*****

Everyone of us should be Moving OurSelves (or striving to be), being physically active on a regular basis, completing at least 60 minutes of Cardio-Vascular Aerobics a day. Performing consistent and constant exercise is needed to maintain and improve your overall health and fitness, as well as to prevent many adverse health outcomes – including your pre-mature death.

Generally, EVERYBODY, from healthy people, people at risk of developing chronic diseases as well as people with current chronic conditions or disabilities can all benefit from regular physical activity.

We have surefire recipes for healing and good health and the formulas include regular exercise and healthy eating – Moving YourSelf and Eating To Live. Tobacco and physical inactivity, combined with unhealthy diets, are running neck-and-neck at the top of the list of actual causes of death.

It's a TRUE (and Unfortunate) fact - the average American is sitting around and eating themselves to death.

How Much Physical Activity Do You Need?

The answer to this question is intricately related to you answering the question of How Long Do You Want To LIVE?

Physical activity affects many health conditions; the specific amounts and types of activity that benefit each condition vary. One consistent finding from research studies is that once the health benefits from physical activity begin to accrue, additional amounts of activity provide additional benefits.

20 Exercise Benefits

1. Reduces body fat
2. Increases lifespan
3. Oxygenates body
4. Strengthens muscles
5. Manages chronic pain
6. Wards off viruses
7. Reduces diabetes risk
8. Strengthens heart
9. Clears arteries
10. Boosts mood
11. Maintains mobility
12. Improves memory
13. Improves coordination
14. Strengthens bones
15. Improves complexion
16. Detoxifies body
17. Decreases stress
18. Boosts immune system
19. Lowers blood pressure
20. Reduces cancer risk

Although some health benefits seem to begin with as little as 60 minutes (1 hour) a week, current modern medical advice is that the completion of at least 150 minutes (2 hours and 30 minutes) a week of moderate-intensity aerobic activity, such as brisk walking, consistently reduces the risk of many chronic diseases and other adverse health outcomes.

This is true, but these recommendations of 150 minutes a week aren't enough time of activity and it doesn't create the condition for you to exceed the current expected life-span of 82 years.

To extend your Life-Span and to Successfully Enjoy Your Abundant Life, we need to increase our level of physical activities. We have gained significant improvement on dietary, medical and other health elements.

With our Supreme Health and Fitness program, you will the level of physical activities even further and complete at least 60 Minutes of Cardiovascular Aerobics a day.

That's Right – 60 MINUTES A DAY OF CARDIOVASCULAR AEROBICS!

That's only 1 hour out of 24!

That's only 420 minutes a week out of 10,080 minutes in a week.

Increasing your amount of physical activity to 60 minutes a day increase the Energy that you Create for your body to use to Restore, Repair, Rejuvenate, Heal and manifest Power!

Physical activity is anything that gets your body moving. According to the *Physical Activity Guidelines for Americans*, you need to do two types of physical activity each week to improve your health—aerobic and muscle-strengthening.

I know 420 minutes each week sounds like a lot of time, but you do not have to do it all at once. Not only is it best to **spread your activity out during the week**, but you can **break it up into smaller chunks of time during the day.** As long as you are doing your activity at a moderate or vigorous effort for **at least 10-15 minutes at a time.**

EXCERCISE HIERARCHY

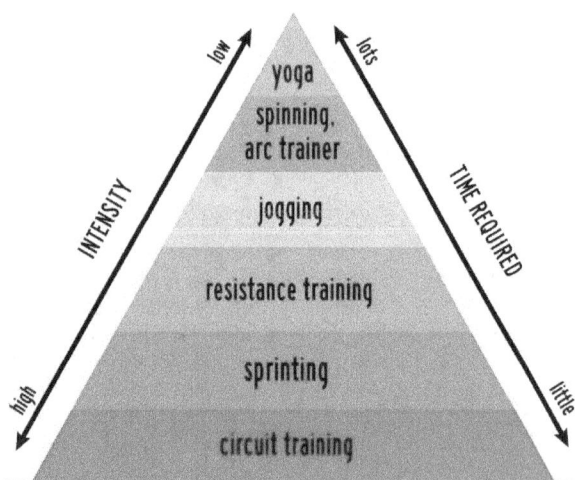

Within this 10-15 minute time frame you can have successfully create the environment for your body to create the Endorphins and Energy that you need for Mind, Body and Soul Health and Wellness!

If you go beyond 420 minutes a week of moderate-intensity activity, or 150 minutes a week of vigorous-intensity activity, you **will** gain even more health benefits

With the benefits of regular exercise or physical activity capable of doing everyone a world of good, it is mind-boggling that only a minority of Americans get enough exercise or leisure-time physical activity.

Studies that have followed the health of large groups of people for many years, as well as short-term studies, all point in the same direction: ***A sedentary (inactive) lifestyle increases the chances of becoming overweight and developing a number of chronic diseases.***

Exercise or physical activity helps many of the body's systems function better and keeps a host of diseases at bay.

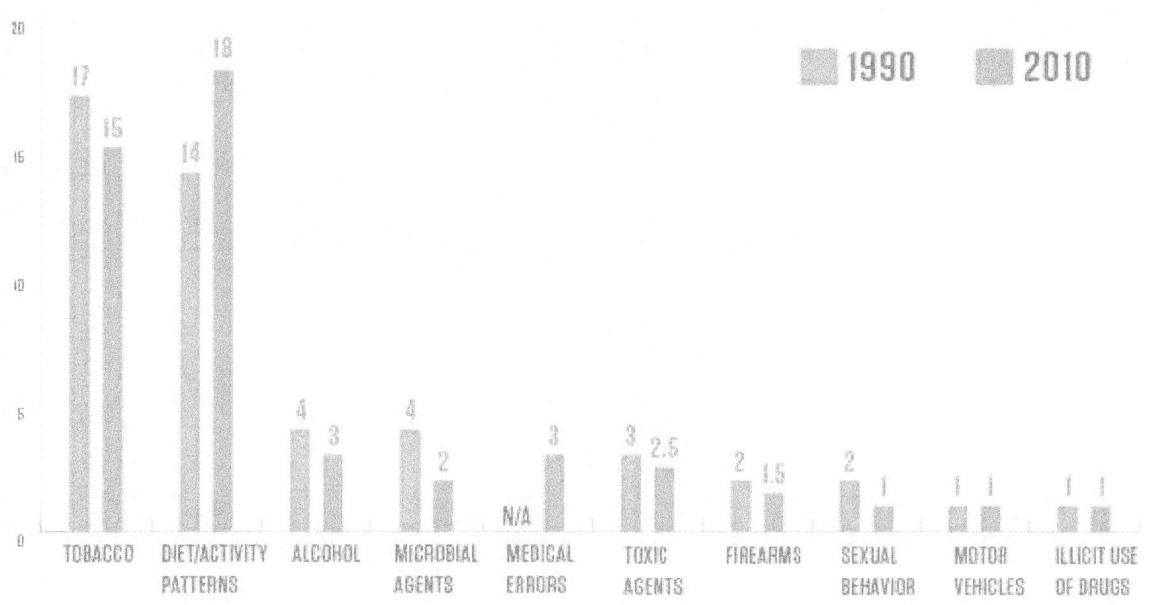

A U.S. Surgeon General's report analyzed the 10 leading causes of death and suggested that up to half of U.S. deaths were attributable to unhealthy behavior or lifestyle; 20% to environmental factors; 20% to human biological/genetic factors; and 10% to inadequacies in health care.

Behavior – your dietary and exercise choices, remains the dominant cause of premature death and disability. Today, chronic diseases—such as cardiovascular disease (primarily heart disease and stroke), cancer, and type 2 diabetes—are among the most prevalent, costly, and preventable of all health problems and account for seven out of every 10 deaths in the United States.

Chronic diseases are mostly preventable but can be difficult to change because the risk factors associated with developing chronic conditions are linked primarily to lifestyle behaviors – how you eat and your amount of motion.

(September 2015) Up to half of all premature (or early) deaths in the United States are due to behavioral and other preventable factors—including modifiable habits such as tobacco use, poor diet, and lack of exercise, according to studies reviewed in a new National Research Council and Institute of Medicine report.

While there has been progress in reducing early deaths in the United States from certain causes, such as tobacco and alcohol use, those gains are being erased by increases in deaths linked to other factors, such as poor diet and lack of physical activity.

An analysis by J. Michael McGinnis, Institute of Medicine, showed that the percent of early deaths (defined as occurring before age 80) linked to tobacco use fell from 17 percent to 15 percent between 1990 and 2010, while early deaths attributed to poor diet and lack of exercise increased from 14 percent to 18 percent during the same period

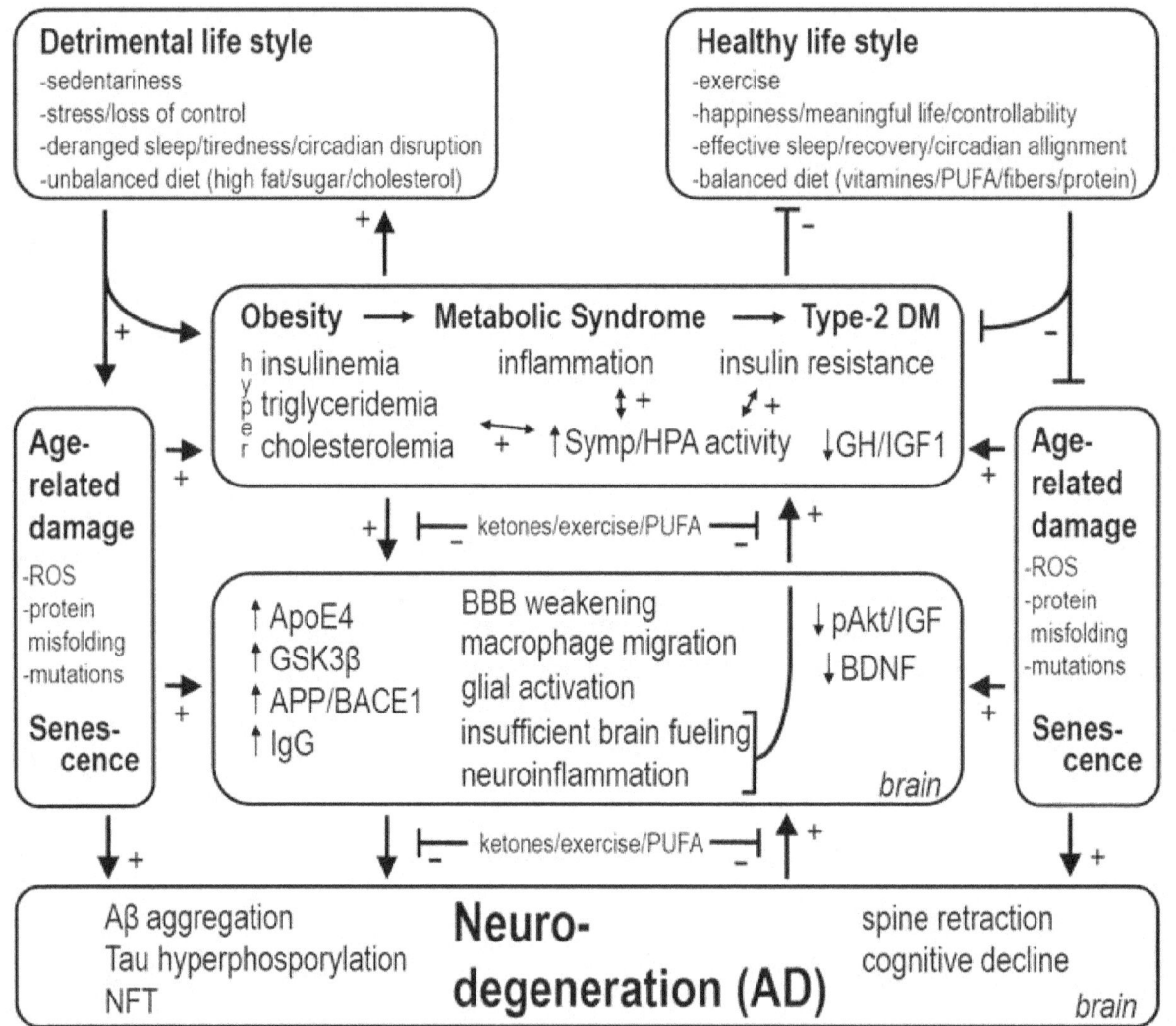

Definitions

To prepare properly for physical activity and exercise, let us start by examining two key words—"**fit**" and "**well**"—plus a few others from our everyday conversations.

Fitness, as defined by the U.S. Department of Health and Human Services (DHHS), is "the ability to carry out daily tasks with vigor and alertness, without undue fatigue, and with ample energy to enjoy leisure-time pursuits and respond to emergencies. Physical fitness includes a number of components consisting of **cardiorespiratory endurance**; **skeletal muscle endurance**, **strength** and **power**; **flexibility**; and **body composition**."

Those four components of fitness provide the basis of a balanced workout program. They are made up of structured activities aimed at increasing specific elements of fitness. Each is a health-related component of physical fitness.

The DHHS defines these components of physical fitness as follows:

- ■**Cardiorespiratory fitness (endurance)** is the ability of the circulatory and respiratory systems to supply oxygen during sustained physical activity.

- ■**Muscle-strengthening activity (strength training, resistance training, or muscular strength and endurance exercises)** is physical activity, including exercise, that increases skeletal muscle strength, power, endurance, and mass.

- ■**Flexibility** is the range of motion possible at a joint. Flexibility is specific to each joint and depends on a number of variables, including but not limited to the tightness of specific ligaments and tendons. Flexibility exercises enhance the ability of a joint to move through its full range of motion.

- ■**Body composition** refers to body weight and the relative amounts of muscle, fat, bone, and other vital tissues of the body. Most often, body composition addresses only fat and lean body mass (or fat-free mass).

The second key word is "**well**." Fitness leads to being well. **Wellness**, defined by the National Wellness Institute, is "an active process of becoming aware of and making choices toward a more successful existence."

Some have described wellness as "the constant, conscious pursuit of living life to its fullest potential." It involves the whole person and is more than physical fitness.

Wellness includes physical fitness, but it is also multidimensional.

A popular model adopted by many university, corporate, and public health programs encompasses these dimensions:

- ■**Physical:** encourages regular physical activity for cardiorespiratory, muscular, and flexibility 0fitness as well as knowledge about nutrition, and discourages the use of harmful substances.

- ■**Social:** encourages contributing to the common welfare of one's community and the pursuit of harmony in one's family.

- ■**Intellectual:** encourages creative, stimulating mental activities.

- ■**Emotional:** emphasizes an awareness and acceptance of one's feelings, enthusiasm about oneself and life, ability to deal with stress, and maintaining good relationships with others.

- ■**Spiritual:** encourages seeking meaning and purpose in human existence and developing a deep appreciation of life.

Some experts add environmental, occupational, and/or financial dimensions to the list.

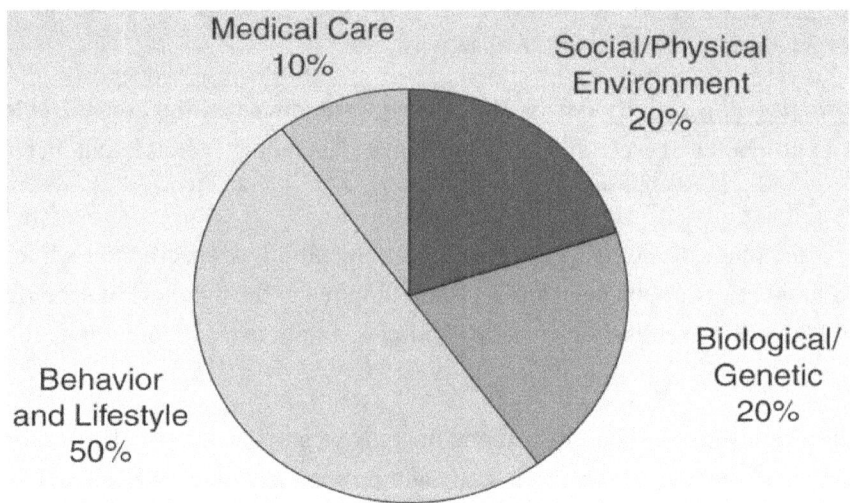

The terms "**wellness**" and "**health**" often confuse people. The DHHS defines <u>health</u> as "the human condition with physical, social and psychological dimensions, each characterized on a continuum with positive and negative poles.

Positive health is associated with a capacity to enjoy life and to withstand challenges; it is not merely the absence of disease. Negative health is associated with illness, and in the extreme, with premature death."

Finally, two other terms have been defined by DHHS: **physical activity** and **exercise**.

Physical activity is "any bodily movement produced by the contraction of skeletal muscle that increases energy expenditure above a basal level."

Physical activity includes any activity that gets you up and moving throughout the day. These activities could include grocery shopping, mowing the lawn, taking the dog for a walk, or shoveling snow from the driveway. While they may not be specifically intended to increase your muscular or cardiorespiratory endurance, daily physical activities are just as important as structured exercise.

Exercise is defined as "a subcategory of physical activity that is planned, structured, repetitive, and purposive in the sense that the improvement or maintenance of one or more components of physical fitness is the objective.

'Exercise' and 'exercise training' are used frequently in an interchangeable fashion and generally refer to physical activity performed during leisure time with the primary purpose of improving or maintaining physical fitness, physical performance, or health."

Who Are the Physically Active?

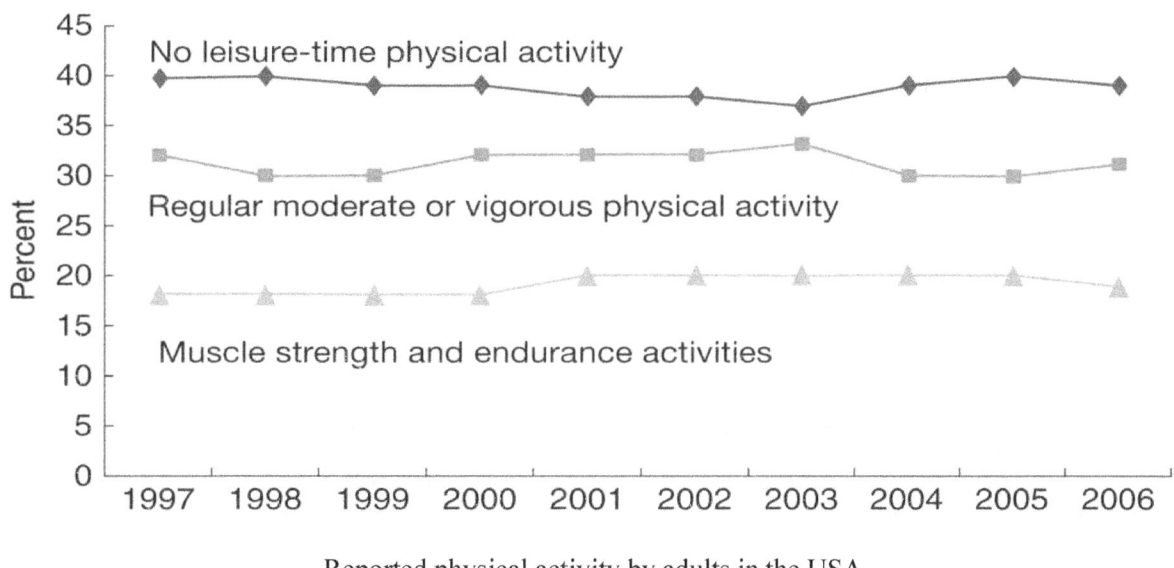

Reported physical activity by adults in the USA.

The National Center for Health Statistics (CDC 2010) reported the following (above figure - shows data for men and women combined):

- ■Four in 10 adults (39.7%) engage in no leisure-time physical activity.

- ■More than one in five adults (21.9%) engage in light-moderate leisure-time physical activity at least five times per week.

- ■From 30% to 35% of adults reported participation in moderate- or vigorous-intensity activity sufficient to meet physical activity recommendations.

- ■About one in eight adults (11.1%) engage in vigorous leisure-time physical activity five times per week.

- ■About one-fourth of adults engage in at least some leisure-time strengthening activity.

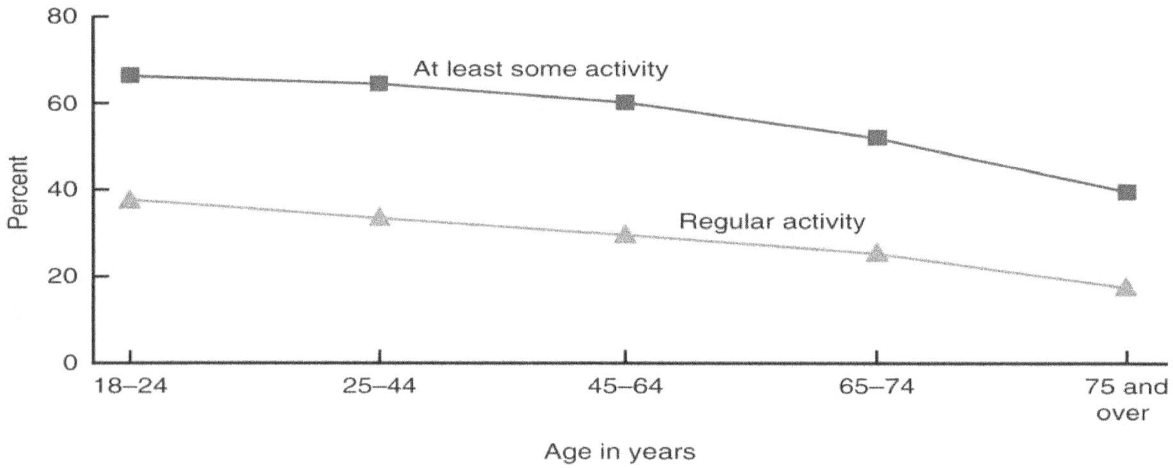

Physical Activity and Exercise

Unfortunately, more than 80% of adults do not meet the guidelines for both aerobic and muscle-strengthening activities found in *Healthy People 2020*. Out of this 80%, the poor and minorities lead in lack of exercise.

The Physical Activity objectives for *Healthy People 2020* reflect the strong state of the science supporting the health benefits of regular physical activity in moderate and vigorous physical activities and muscle-strengthening activities.

We just can't separate Daily exercise from being Healthy or as a intricate part of the Healing and Wellness process.

Nutrition and Weight Status

The Nutrition and Weight Status objectives for ***Healthy People 2020*** reflect strong science supporting the health benefits of eating a healthful diet and maintaining a healthy body weight. The objectives also emphasize that efforts to change diet and weight should address individual behaviors.

You should plan your dietary choices and your exercise activities according to your own needs or else you can risk injuring yourself or further exacerbating your present health condition.

Poor diet and physical inactivity are the most important factors contributing to an epidemic of overweight and obesity affecting men, women, and children. Even in the absence of the overweight category, poor diet and physical inactivity are associated with major causes of morbidity and mortality in the United States.

Being physically active is one of the most important steps that Americans of all ages can take to improve their health.

Examining the Relationship Between Physical Activity & Health

In many studies covering a range of issues, researchers have focused on exercise as well as on the more broadly defined concept of physical activity. Exercise is a form of physical activity that is planned, structured, repetitive, and performed with the goal of improving health or fitness.

So, although all exercise is physical activity, not all physical activity is exercise.

Studies have examined the role of physical activity in many groups — men and women, children, teens, adults, older adults, people with disabilities, and women during pregnancy and the postpartum period.

These studies focused on the role that physical activity plays in many health outcomes, including:

- ■premature (early) death;
- ■diseases such as coronary heart disease, stroke, some cancers, type 2 diabetes, osteoporosis, and depression;
- ■risk factors for disease, such as high blood pressure and high blood cholesterol;
- ■physical fitness, such as aerobic capacity, and muscle strength and endurance;
- ■functional capacity (the ability to engage in activities needed for daily living);
- ■mental health, such as depression and cognitive function; and
- ■injuries or sudden heart attacks.

THREE TYPES OF EXERCISE

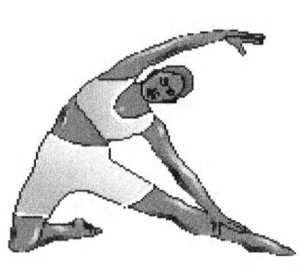

Stretching, for flexibility

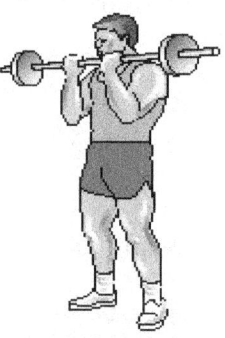

Weight-bearing, for strengthening muscles and bone mass

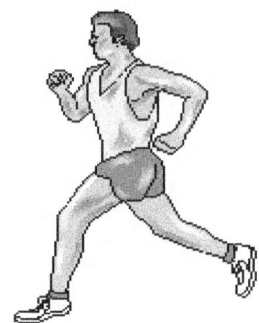

Aerobic, for the heart

These studies have also prompted questions regarding what type and how much physical activity is needed for various health benefits.

To answer this question, investigators have studied three main kinds of physical activity: **aerobic**, **muscle strengthening**, and **bone strengthening**.

- Group 1- Aerobic Activities
- Group 2- Muscle Strengthening Activities
- Group 3- Bone Strengthening Activities

Aerobic, Muscle-strengthening & Bone-strengthening Activity

Aerobic activities, also called **endurance activities**, are physical activities in which people move their **large** muscles in a rhythmic manner for a sustained period. Running, brisk walking, bicycling, playing basketball, dancing, and swimming are all examples of aerobic activities.

Aerobic activity makes a person's heart beat more rapidly to meet the demands of the body's movement.

Over time, regular aerobic activity makes the heart and cardiovascular system stronger and fitter.

Aerobic physical activity has these components:

- **Frequency**

- **Intensity,** or how hard a person works to do the activity. The intensities most often examined are moderate intensity (equivalent in effort to brisk walking) and vigorous intensity (equivalent in effort to running or jogging);

- **Duration,** or how long a person does an activity in any one session.

Although these components make up a physical activity profile, research has shown that the total amount of physical activity (minutes of moderate-intensity physical activity, for example) is more important for achieving health benefits than is any one component (frequency, intensity, or duration).

AEROBIC ACTIVITIES

- Aerobic activities are also called "cardio" exercise. Normally, these activities increase our heart and breathing rate. This cause us to sweat profusely and breathe harder. Our heart pumps blood more vigorously, causing oxygen to circulate throughout our body. This allows us to sustain aerobic exercise for a few minutes.
- Ex. jogging, running, swimming, and dancing
- Benefits: Help lower risks of cardiovascular disease, diabetes, and osteoporosis.

Examples of Different Aerobic Physical Activities and Intensities

Moderate Intensity

- Walking briskly (3 miles per hour or faster, but not race-walking)
- Water aerobics
- Bicycling slower than 10 miles per hour
- Tennis (doubles)
- Ballroom dancing
- General gardening

Vigorous Intensity

- Racewalking, jogging, or running
- Swimming laps
- Tennis (singles)
- Aerobic dancing
- Bicycling 10 miles per hour or faster
- Jumping rope
- Heavy gardening (continuous digging or hoeing, with heart rate increases)
- Hiking uphill or with a heavy backpack

Type of Physical Activity	Children	Adolescents
Examples of Moderate- and Vigorous-Intensity Aerobic, Muscle-Strengthening, and Bone-Strengthening Activities for Youth		
Aerobic Moderate–Intensity	• Active recreation such as hiking, skateboarding, rollerblading • Bicycle riding* • Brisk walking	• Active recreation, such as canoeing, hiking, cross-country skiing, skateboarding, rollerblading • Brisk walking • Bicycle riding* (stationary or road bike) • Housework and yard work such as sweeping or pushing a lawn mower • Playing games that require catching and throwing, such as baseball, softball

Muscle-Strengthening Activity

This kind of activity, which also includes **resistance training** and **lifting weights**, causes your body's muscles to work or hold against an **applied force** or **weight**. These activities often involve relatively heavy objects, such as weights, which are lifted multiple times to train various muscle groups.

Muscle-strengthening activity can also be done by using elastic bands or body weight for resistance (climbing a tree or doing push-ups, for example).

Muscle-strengthening activity also has 3 components:

- **Intensity**, or how much weight or force is used relative to how much a person is able to lift;

- **Frequency**, or how often a person does muscle strengthening activity; and

- **Repetitions**, or how many times a person lifts a weight (analogous to duration for aerobic activity). The effects of muscle-strengthening activity are limited to the muscles doing the work. It's important to work all the major muscle groups of the body: the legs, hips, back, abdomen, chest, shoulders, and arms.

Muscle-strengthening activities provide additional benefits not found with aerobic activity. The benefits of muscle-strengthening activity include increased bone strength and muscular fitness. Muscle-strengthening activities can also help you maintain muscle mass during a program of weight loss.

Muscle-strengthening activities make muscles do more work than they are accustomed to doing, which creates an overload on your muscles. Resistance training, including weight training, is a familiar example of muscle-strengthening activity. Other examples include working with resistance bands, doing calisthenics that use body weight for resistance (such as push-ups, pull-ups, and sit-ups), carrying heavy loads, and heavy gardening (such as digging or hoeing).

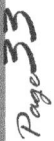

MUSCLE STRENGTHENING ACTIVITIES

- Muscle strengthening activities are exercises in which groups of muscles work or hold against a force or some weight. Muscle strengthening activities help build good muscle strength. When muscles do more work, It becomes stronger. Therefore, haing strong and healthy muscles enable us to perform everyday physical task.
- Ex. push-ups, sit-ups, squats, and lifting

Muscle-strengthening activities count if they involve a moderate to high level of intensity or effort and work the major muscle groups of the body: the legs, hips, back, chest, abdomen, shoulders, and arms. Muscle strengthening activities for all the major muscle groups should be done at least 2 days a week.

There is No specific or standard amount of time is recommended for muscle strengthening, but muscle-strengthening exercises should be performed to the point at which it would be difficult to do another repetition without help.

When resistance training is used to enhance muscle strength, one set of **8** to **12** repetitions of each exercise is effective, although two or three sets may be more effective for more dramatic results.

Development of muscle strength and endurance is progressive over time. Increases in the amount of weight or the days a week of exercising will result in stronger muscles.

Bone-Strengthening Activity

Bone Strengthening Activity

Weight-bearing
- Running, basketball, dancing

Resistance training
- Resistance bands, free weights, weight machines

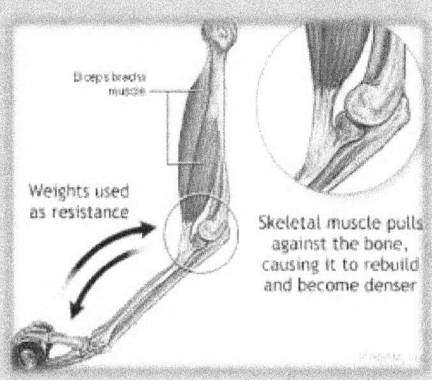

Weights used as resistance

Skeletal muscle pulls against the bone, causing it to rebuild and become denser

This kind of activity (sometimes called weight-bearing or weight-loading activity) produces a force on your bones that promotes bone growth and strength.

This force is commonly produced by impact with the ground.

Examples of bone-strengthening activity include jumping jacks, running, brisk walking, and weight-lifting exercises. As these examples illustrate, bone-strengthening activities can also be aerobic and muscle strengthening.

SUMMARY

AEROBIC ACTIVITIES	MUSCLE STRENGTHENING ACTIVITIES	BONE STRENGTHENING ACTIVITIES
During aerobic activity, oxygen is delivered to the muscles in our body allowing us to sustain the physical activity for few minutes.	Muscle contraction occurs during a muscle strengthening activity. The repetitive contractions during exercise cause damage to muscle fibers. However, these muscle fibers are ready to be repaired once they get damaged. There will be new muscle fibers produced to replace and repair those fibers taht were damaged. The muscles in the body then starts to grow	Bone growth is stimulated by the physical stress. As skeletal muscle contract, they pull their attachment on bones causing physical stress. This consequently stimulates bone tissue, making it stronger and thicker. Such bone strengthening activities can icrease bone density throughout our skeletal system.

Mechanism

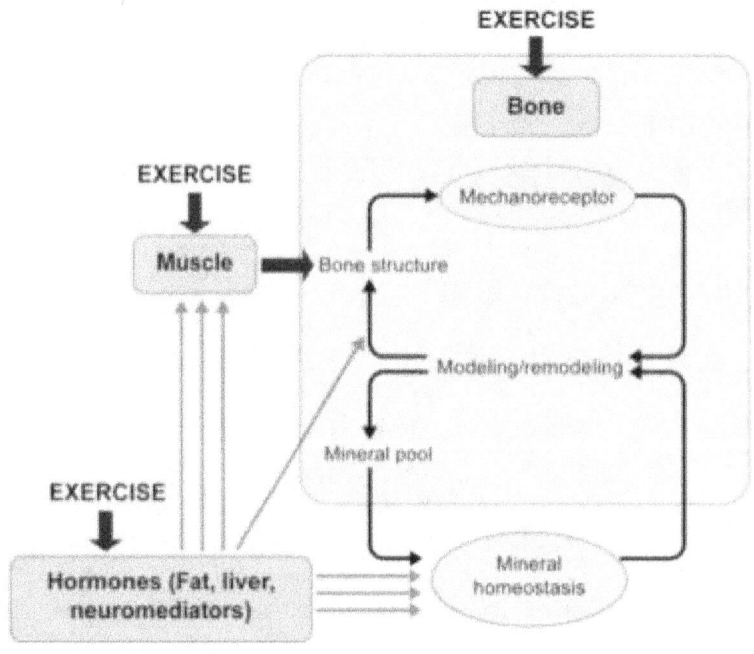

Vigorous-Intensity	<ul><li>Active games involving running and chasing, such as tag</li><li>Bicycle riding*</li><li>Jumping rope</li><li>Martial arts, such as karate</li><li>Running</li><li>Sports such as ice or field hockey, basketball, swimming, tennis or gymnastics</li><li>Cross-country skiing</li></ul>	<ul><li>Active games involving running and chasing, such as flag football</li><li>Bicycle riding*</li><li>Jumping rope</li><li>Martial arts such as karate</li><li>Running</li><li>Sports such as tennis, ice or field hockey, basketball, swimming, soccer</li><li>Vigorous dancing</li><li>Aerobics</li></ul>
Muscle-Strengthening	<ul><li>Games such as tug of war</li><li>Modified push-ups (with knees on the floor)</li><li>Resistance exercises using body weight or resistance bands</li><li>Rope or tree climbing</li><li>Sit-ups (curl-ups or crunches)</li><li>Swinging on playground equipment/bars</li></ul>	<ul><li>Cross-country skiing</li><li>Games such as tug of war</li><li>Push-ups</li><li>Resistance exercises with exercise bands, weight machines, hand-held weights</li><li>Climbing wall</li><li>Sit-ups (curl-ups or crunches)</li></ul>
Bone-Strengthening	<ul><li>Games such as hop-scotch</li><li>Hopping, skipping, jumping</li><li>Jumping rope</li><li>Running</li><li>Sports such as gymnastics, basketball, volleyball, tennis</li></ul>	<ul><li>Hopping, skipping, jumping</li><li>Jumping rope</li><li>Running</li><li>Sports such as gymnastics, basketball, volleyball, tennis</li></ul>

*Some activities, such as bicycling, can be moderate or vigorous intensity, depending upon level of effort.

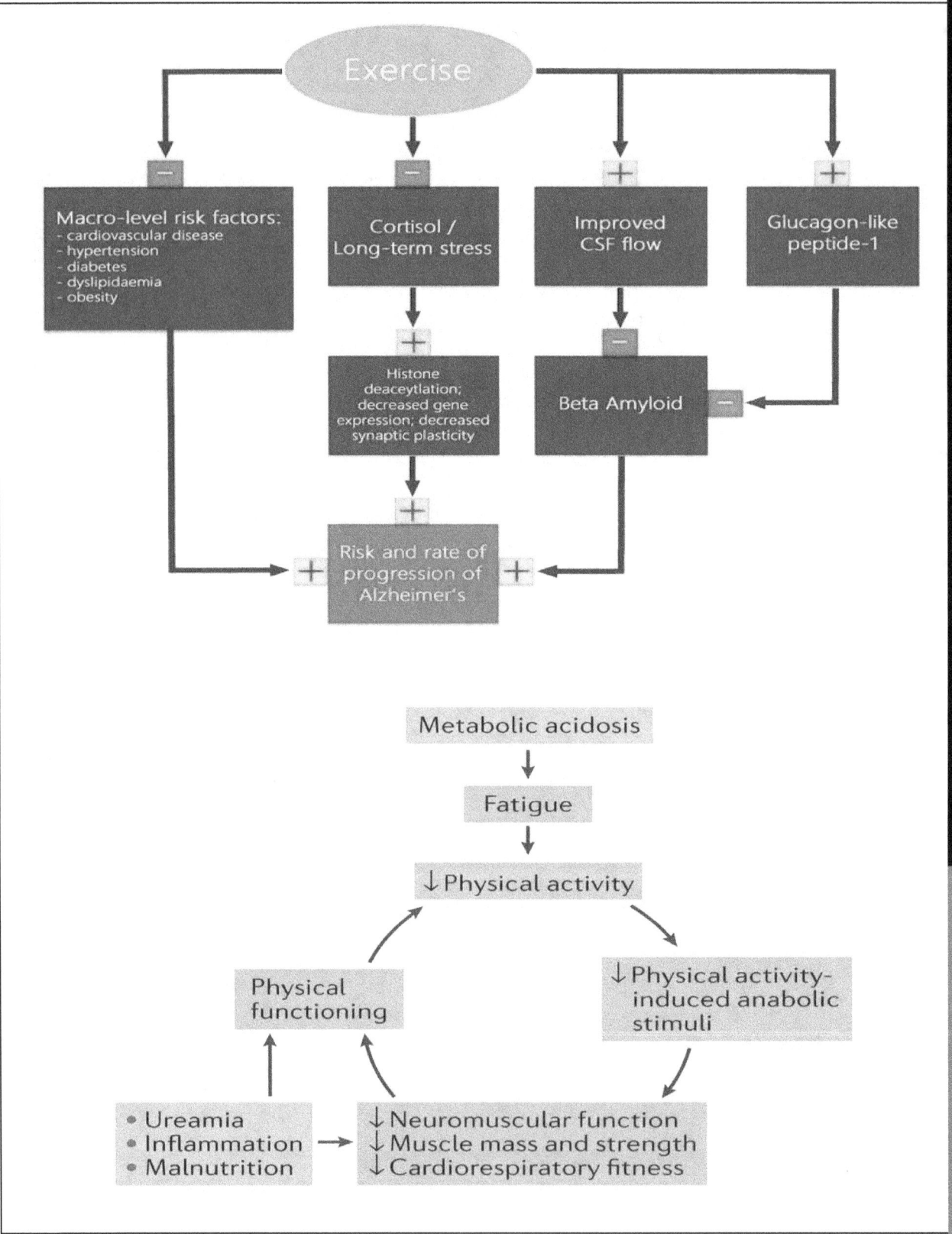

BENEFITS OF PHYSICAL FITNESS

The benefits of physical fitness are numerous and include better health, greater strength, more flexibility, increased energy, improved appearance, and a more positive attitude and mood. Regular exercise can lead to both immediate and long-term benefits. Regular physical activity has been shown to reduce the morbidity and mortality from many chronic diseases.

Physical Activity for Fitness

- Exercise: planned, structured, and repetitive bodily movement done to improve or maintain one or more components of physical fitness, such as endurance, flexibility, and strength.
- Physical Fitness is the ability to perform moderate to vigorous physical activity on a regular basis without excessive fatigue.
- Components of Physical Fitness
    - Cardiorespiratory fitness
    - Muscular strength
    - Muscular endurance
    - Flexibility
    - Body composition

Moderate Exercise	Vigorous Exercise
Hiking	Jogging, Running
Gardening or yard work	Heavy Yard Work
Dancing	Aerobics
Golfing (carrying clubs)	Basketball
Biking <10mph	Biking >10mph
Walking 3.5 mph	Walking 4.5 mph
	Swimming Laps
	Weightlifting (vigorous)

Move Something!

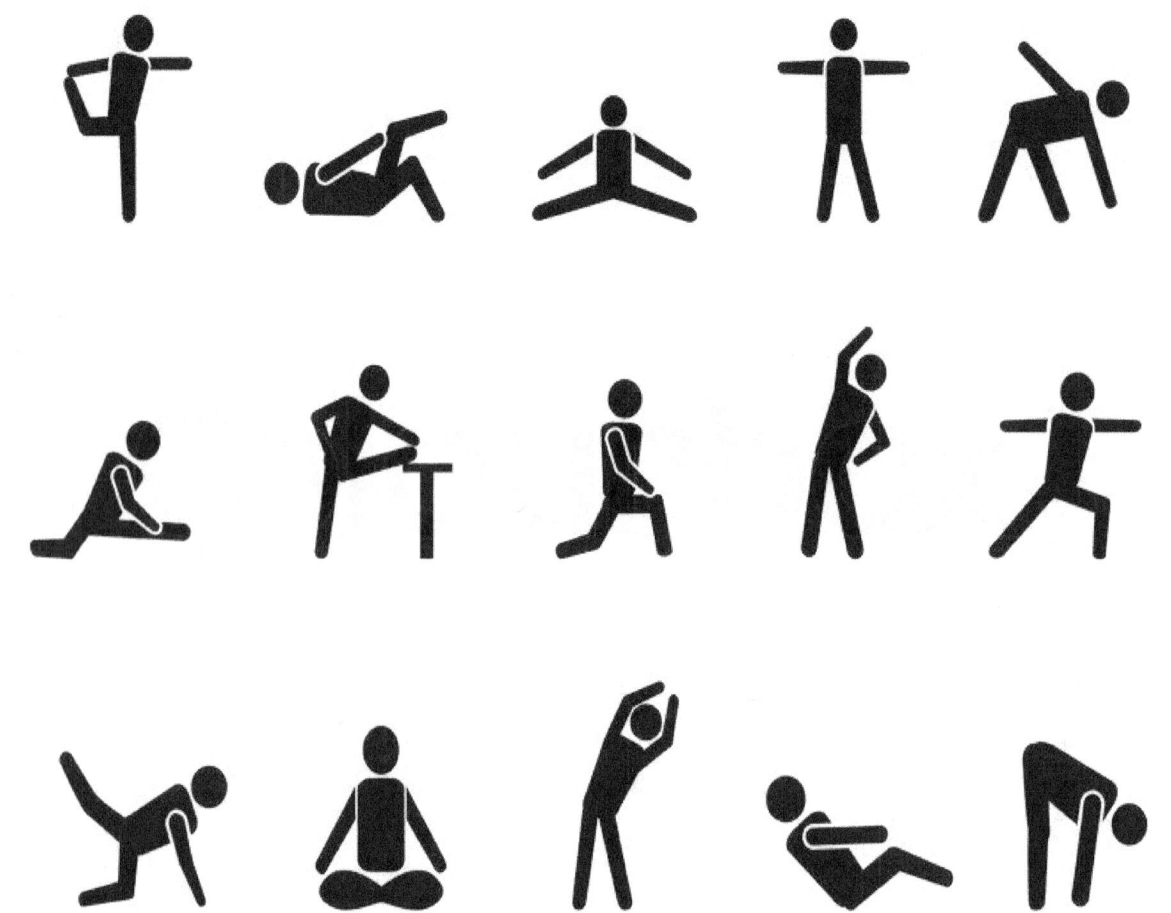

Chapter Two

Awesome Health Benefits of Moving!

*****

Studies clearly demonstrate that participating in regular physical activity provides many health benefits. There are many conditions affected by physical activity that occur with increasing age, with the serious conditions of heart disease and cancer leading.

Reducing risk of these conditions require that you devote time and participation in regular physical activity. There are also other benefits, such as increased cardiorespiratory fitness, increased muscular strength, and decreased depressive symptoms and blood pressure, require only a few weeks or months of participation in physical activity.

The health benefits of physical activity are seen in children and adolescents, young and middle-aged adults, older adults, women and men, people of different races and ethnicities, and people with disabilities and chronic conditions.

The health benefits of physical activity are also generally independent of body weight. Adults of all sizes and shapes gain health and fitness benefits by being habitually physically active.

The benefits of physical activity also outweigh the risk of injury and sudden heart attacks, two concerns that prevent many people from becoming physically active. In fact, the opposite is true – exercise helps prevent injuries and heart attacks!

The following chapters provide more detail on what is known from research studies about the specific health benefits of physical activity and how much physical activity is needed to get the health benefits.

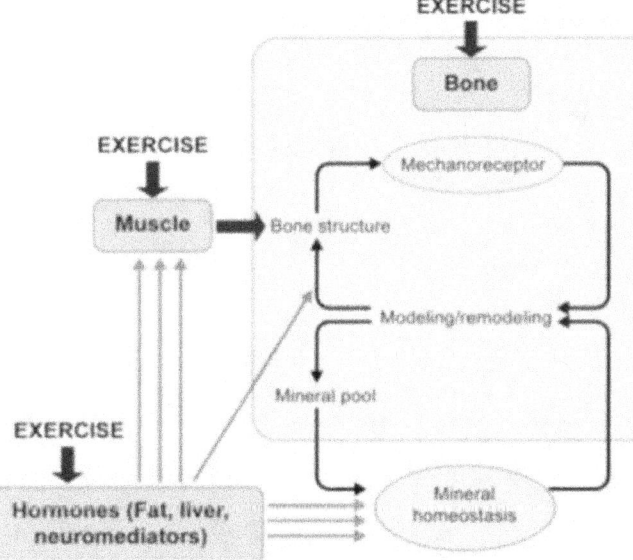

- Brief, vigorous exercise causes immediate structural and chemical changes in the DNA molecules within your muscles that benefit your health

- Endurance training also produces beneficial genetic changes that play a role in energy metabolism, insulin response, and muscle inflammation

- Increased blood flow from regular exercise adapts your brain to turn different genes on or off; many of these changes help protect against diseases such as Alzheimer's and Parkinson's

Virtually everyone would agree that exercise improves health, but the specific mechanisms by which it actually produces those benefits have been challenging to relay to people.

Fitness research has come a long way though, and modern science has made a number of interesting observations that help explain how exercise affects your body to cause it to strengthen, heal and to improve your health.

Part of the answer lies in the ability of exercise to affect your genetic expression; activating some genes, while deactivating others.

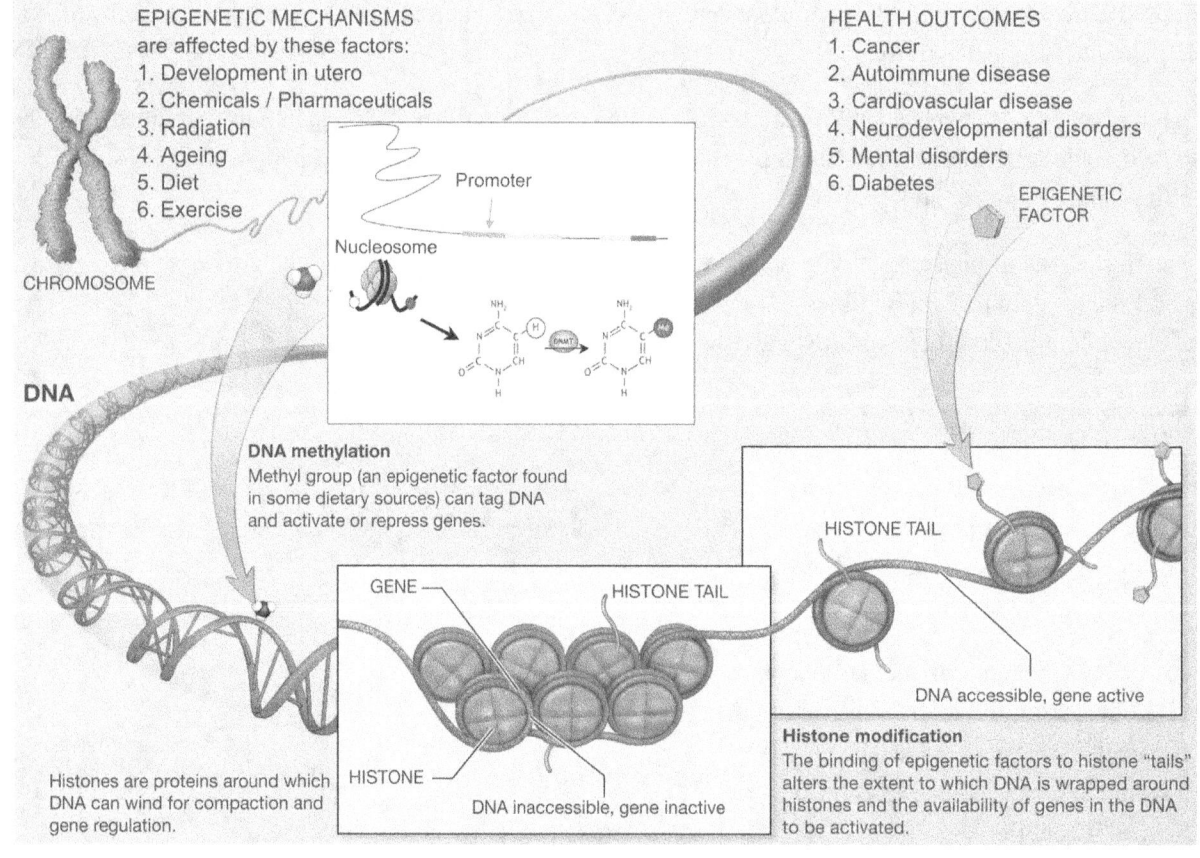

A previous *New York Times* (2016) article delved into the latest research on this front, noting that:

"The human genome is astonishingly complex and dynamic, with genes constantly turning on or off, depending on what biochemical signals they receive from the body. When genes are turned on, they express proteins that prompt physiological responses elsewhere in the body."

Epigenetics of Exercise

Far from being "written in stone," your genetic expression can be altered by influences coming from outside your gene. This influence alters the operation of your gene but does not affect the DNA blueprint itself. This process is known as "epigenetics," and occurs mainly through methylation.

Epigenetics is the science of studying the outside influences on your gene expression.

In **methylation** there are clusters of atoms, called **methyl** groups which attach to the outside of your gene like microscopic mollusks and makes your gene **more or less** able to receive and respond to biochemical signals from your body.

Methylation patterns can be altered by a variety of lifestyle changes, such as diet and exercise – together both Poor Diet and Lack of Exercise are the #2 Actual Cause of Death.

Toxic exposure also tends to affect your genetic expression, by altering the types of proteins a particular gene will express.

In this way, your environment, diet, and general lifestyle play a significant role in your state of health and development of disease.

By Moving YourSelf for at least 60 minutes a day with Cardio-Vascular Aerobics, you create the condition where your entire body is OPEN to receive and carry-out all the signals within your body.

Your body is created to Heal itself …. Being Sedentary alters and inhibits your bodies ability to communicate – so your body cannot send or receive the signals to heal.

When it comes to exercise, previous research has found that exercise can induce *immediate* changes in the methylation patterns of genes found in your muscle cells.

A study published in the journal *Cell Metabolism* in 2012 showed that while the underlying genetic code in the muscle remains unchanged, vigorous exercise — even if brief — causes positive structural and chemical changes in the DNA molecules within your muscles.

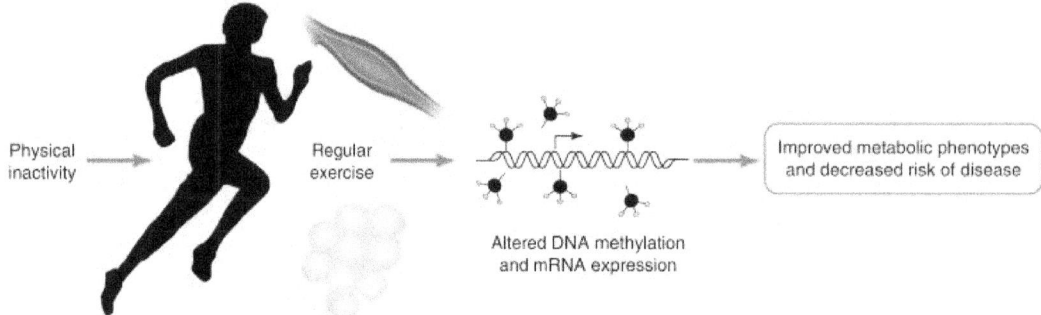

This gene activation is induced by **contraction of your muscle**, and this contraction-induced gene activation appears to be part of the chain of events that leads to the genetic reprogramming of your muscle for strength — as well as to many other structural and metabolic benefits of exercise.

You can Move YourSelf into Strength and Power!

Several of the genes affected by an acute bout of exercise are genes involved in your fat metabolism. Specifically, the study suggests that when you exercise, your body almost immediately experiences genetic activation that increases the production of these fat-busting proteins.

Previous studies have also identified and measured a wide variety of biochemical changes that occur during exercise. More than 20 different metabolites are affected, including compounds that help stabilize your blood sugar.

All of these biochemical changes create a positive feedback loop, resulting in improved health and physical performance.

You can Move YourSelf into your Healing, Health and into the Enjoyment of your Abundant Life!

How Endurance Training Affects Your Genes

The above kinds of findings led to another question: does endurance training (opposed to a brief intense bout of exercise) also affect methylation, and if so, how?

A Swedish study published in December 2014 sought to shed light on this question.

Scientists at the Karolinska Institute in Stockholm recruited 23 young and healthy men and women, brought them to the lab for a series of physical performance and medical tests, including a muscle biopsy, and then asked them to exercise half of their lower bodies for three months.

One of the obstacles in the past to precisely studying epigenetic changes has been that so many aspects of our lives affect our methylation patterns, making it difficult to isolate the effects of exercise from those of diet or other behaviors.

The Karolinska scientists overturned that obstacle by the simple expedient of having their volunteers bicycle using only one leg, leaving the other unexercised.

In effect, each person became his or her own control group. Both legs would undergo methylation patterns influenced by his or her entire life; but only the pedaling leg would show changes related to exercise."

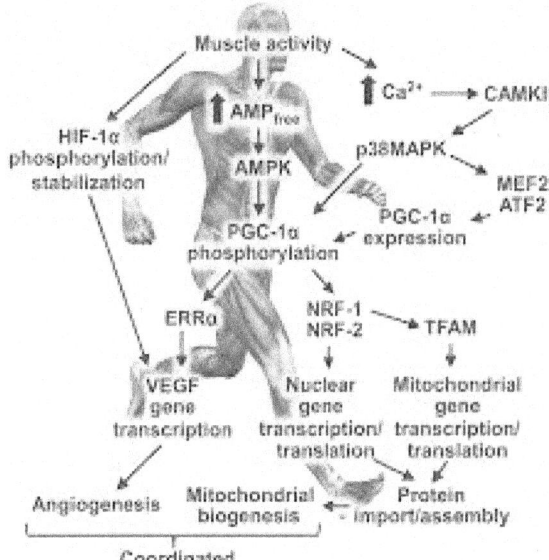

The volunteers performed their one-legged pedal exercise, at a moderate pace, for 45 minutes four times a week for three months. The result? The exercised leg was stronger than the unexercised leg, confirming that exercise led to physical improvement, as you would expect.

Genetic alterations within the cells of the muscles revealed there was more to the story however. More than 5,000 sites on the muscle cells' genome, biopsied from the exercised leg, had altered methylation patterns. These changes were not found in biopsied cells from the unexercised leg.

A majority of the methylation changes that occurred in the exercised leg play a role in:

- Energy metabolism
- Insulin response
- Muscle inflammation

These are all categories that are important in your Growth and Development and will allow you to Successfully Move YourSelf into the Enjoyment of Your Abundant Life!

Endurance Training versus High Intensity Exercise

By now you know that exercise — in all its forms, has a positive effect on your health and wellness. It has the power to affect your entire body, and your overall state of health.

Exercise is more than beneficial, it goes to the foundation of Life = MOTION!

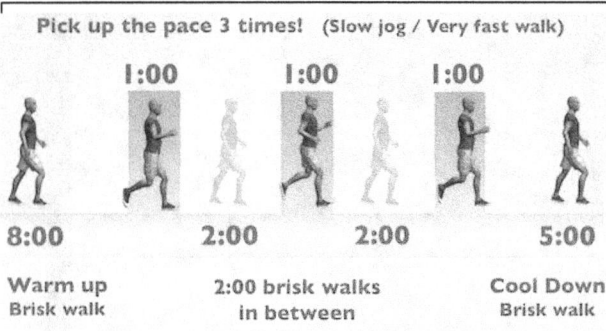

LIGHT INTERVAL TRAINING:
A 20 minute Walk-Jog Workout

Its beneficial impact on your insulin response (normalizing your glucose and insulin levels by optimizing insulin receptor sensitivity) is among the most important benefits of exercise, as insulin resistance is a factor that is found in most chronic disease.

Through endurance training, you can create a lifestyle change that is easily available and accomplished as well as having a solution that doesn't cost much money.

You can create the environment in Self that can induce changes that affect how your body manifests its or gene expression and get healthier and more functional muscles that ultimately improve our quality of life.

You can have the God-Body that will Successfully Move You into the Enjoyment of your Abundant Life!

High intensity interval training (HIIT) has been shown to be far more effective at producing positive results when in comparison to endurance training. While its concluded that endurance training does indeed induce your genetic alterations that promote good health, HIIT is known to do so, but in a far more efficient process.

There is mounting research which shows that by just focusing on endurance-type exercises, such as jogging on a treadmill, you could actually be excluding yourself from many of the most profound benefits of exercise that are derived from higher intensity levels.

Some of the latest research in high intensity exercise involves myokines – which are a class of cell-signaling proteins produced by your muscle fibers — and how they can combat diseases like metabolic syndrome and cancer.

These myokines — which are cytokines produced in your muscle — are very anti-inflammatory.

They also increase your insulin sensitivity and your glucose utilization inside the muscle.

The reason for this is because it induces a rapid and deep level of muscle fatigue. This triggers the synthesis of more contractile tissue, and all the metabolic components to support it — including more myokines.

The more you Move YourSelf, the more you create the cycle of your body creating Energy from using Energy!

This is HOW we create perpetual Motion and Abundant Life ….. By Moving SomeThing!

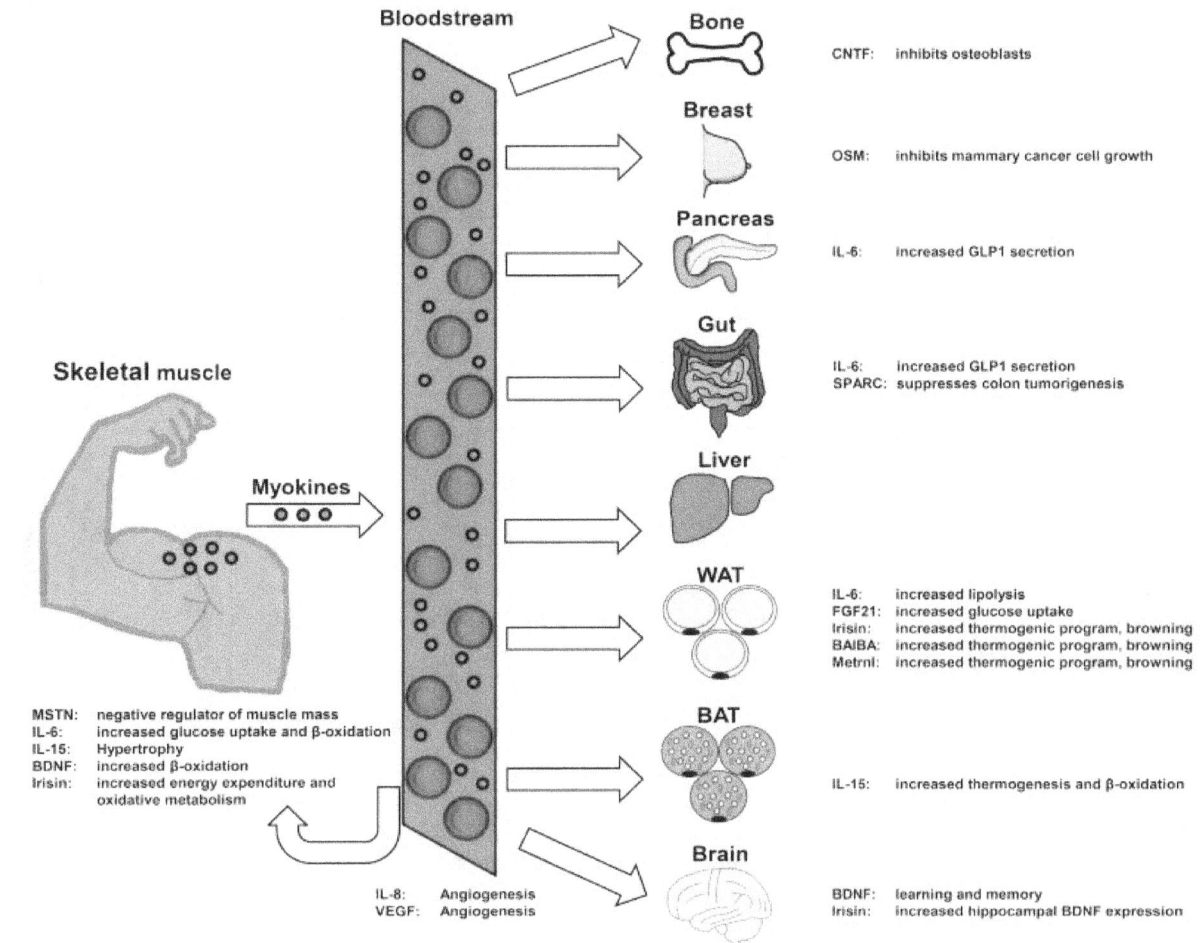

Many Biological Effects of Exercise

Getting back to the effects of exercise in general, a number of biological effects occur when you work out.

This includes changes in your:

- **Your Muscles** use glucose and ATP for contraction and movement. To create more ATP, your body needs extra oxygen, so breathing increases and your heart starts pumping more blood to your muscles. Without sufficient oxygen, lactic acid will form instead. Tiny tears in your muscles make them grow bigger and stronger as they heal.

- **Your Lungs**. As your muscles call for more oxygen (as much as 15 times more oxygen than when you're at rest), your breathing rate increases. Once the muscles surrounding your lungs cannot move any faster, you've reached what's called your VO2 max—your maximum capacity of oxygen use. The higher your VO2 max, the fitter you are.

- **Your Heart.** As mentioned, your heart rate increases with physical activity to supply more oxygenated blood to your muscles. The fitter you are, the more efficiently your heart can do this, allowing you to work out longer and harder. As a side effect, this increased efficiency will also reduce your *resting* heart rate. Your blood pressure will also decrease as a result of new blood vessels forming.

- **Your Joints and bones**, as exercise can place as much as five or six times more than your body weight on them. Peak bone mass is achieved in adulthood and then begins a slow decline, but exercise can help you to maintain healthy bone mass as you get older. Weight-bearing exercise is actually one of the most effective remedies against osteoporosis, as your bones are very porous and soft, and as you get older your bones can easily become less dense and hence, more brittle -- especially if you are inactive.

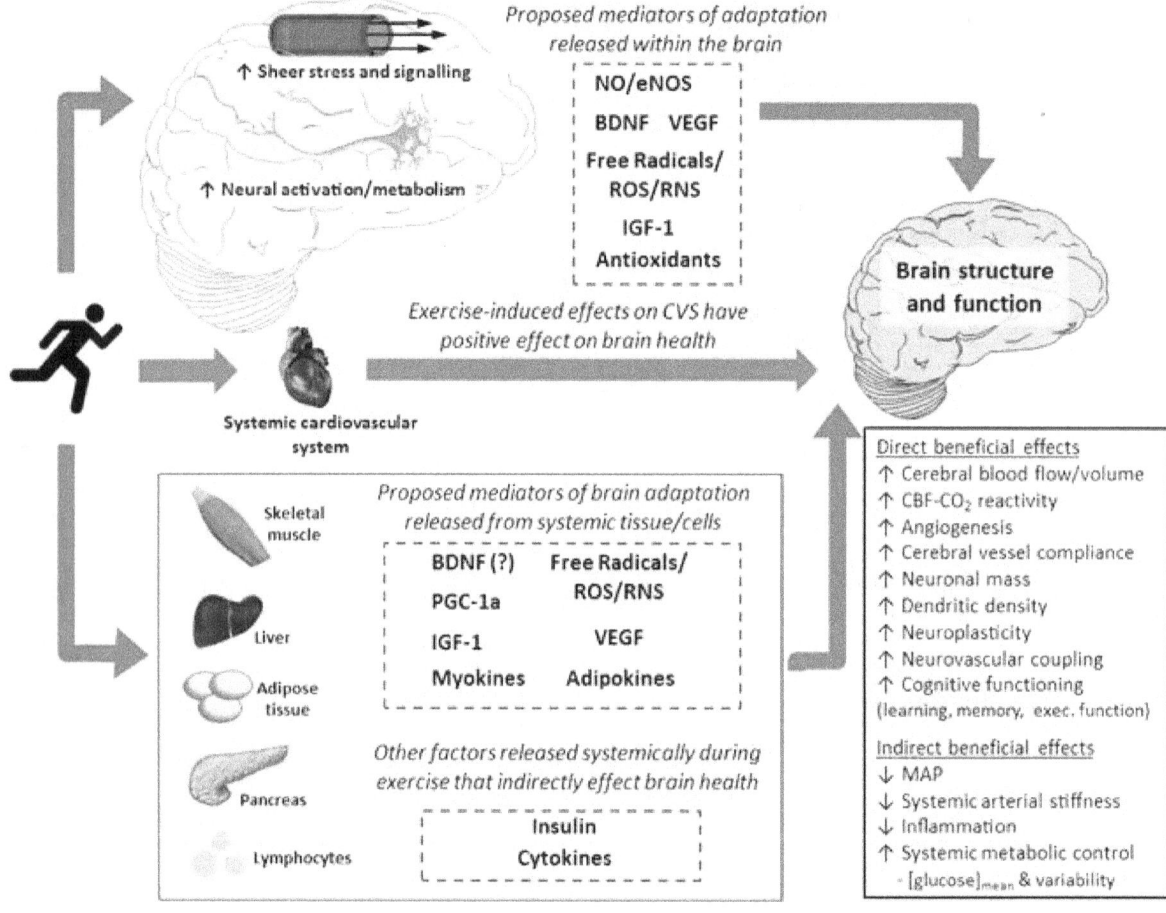

Exercise Is Important for Optimal Brain Health, Too

Mounting research also shows that exercise is as important for your brain function as it is for the rest of your body. In fact, it may be part and parcel of staying "sharp as a tack" well into old age.

For starters, the increased blood flow allows your brain to almost immediately function better. As a result, you tend to feel more focused after a workout.

More importantly though, exercising regularly will prompt the growth of new brain cells.

In your hippocampus, these new brain cells help boost memory and learning. It also helps *preserve* both gray and white matter in your brain, which prevents cognitive deterioration that can occur with age.

Genetic changes occur here, too. The increased blood flow adapts your brain to turn different genes on or off, and many of these changes help protect your brain against diseases such as Alzheimer's and Parkinson's.

A number of neurotransmitters are also triggered, such as endorphins, serotonin, dopamine, glutamate, and GABA. Some of these are well-known for their role in mood control. Not surprisingly, exercise is one of the most effective prevention and treatment strategies for depression.

Three of the mechanisms by which exercise produces these beneficial changes in your brain are:

- **Increasing Brain Derived Neurotrophic Factor (BDNF)**. Exercise stimulates the production of a protein called FNDC5, which in turn triggers the production of BDNF, which has remarkable rejuvenating abilities. In your brain, BDNF both preserves existing brain cells, and activates brain stem cells to convert into new neurons, effectively making your brain grow larger.

- **Decreasing BMP and boosting Noggin**: Bone-morphogenetic protein (BMP) slows down the creation of new neurons, thereby reducing neurogenesis. If you have high levels of BMP, your brain grows slower and less nimble. Exercise reduces the impact of BMP, so that your adult stem cells can continue performing their vital functions of keeping your brain agile.

In animal research, mice with access to running wheels reduced the BMP in their brains by half in just one week. In addition, they also had a notable increase in another brain protein called Noggin, which acts as a BMP antagonist. So, exercise not only reduces the detrimental effects of BMP, it simultaneously boosts the more beneficial Noggin as well.

This complex interplay between BMP and Noggin appears to be yet another powerful factor that helps ensure the proliferation and youthfulness of your neurons.

- **Reducing plaque formation**: By altering the way damaging proteins reside inside your brain, exercise may help slow the development of Alzheimer's disease.

Exercise Leverages Other Healthy Lifestyle Changes

While diet accounts for about 80 percent of the health benefits you get from a healthy lifestyle, exercise is the ultimate "leveraging agent" that kicks all those benefits up a notch. The earlier you begin and the more consistent you are, the greater your long-term rewards, but it's never too late to start. Even seniors can improve their physical and mental health—not to mention physical function—by starting up an appropriate exercise program. Strength training is particularly important for the elderly, and super-slow strength training tends to be both safer and more effective than many other alternatives.

I believe that, overall, high-intensity interval training really helps maximize the health benefits of exercise, while simultaneously being the most efficient and therefore requiring the least amount of time. That said, ideally, you should strive for a varied and well-rounded fitness program that incorporates a wide variety of exercises.

I also strongly recommend avoiding sitting as much as possible, and making it a point to walk more every day. A fitness tracker can be very helpful for this. I suggest aiming for 7,000 to 10,000 steps per day, *in addition to* your regular fitness regimen, not in lieu of it. The research is clearly showing that prolonged sitting is an independent risk factor for chronic disease and increases your mortality risk from *all* causes. So standing up more and engaging in non-exercise movement as much as possible is just as important for optimal health as having a regular fitness regimen.

Health Benefits Associated with Regular Physical Activity

Children and Adolescents
Strong evidence
• ■Improved cardiorespiratory and muscular fitness
• ■Improved bone health
• ■Improved cardiovascular and metabolic health biomarkers

- ■Favorable body composition

Moderate evidence

- ■Reduced symptoms of depression

Adults & Older Adults

Strong evidence

- ■Lower risk of early death
- ■Lower risk of coronary heart disease
- ■Lower risk of stroke
- ■Lower risk of high blood pressure
- ■Lower risk of adverse blood lipid profile
- ■Lower risk of type 2 diabetes
- ■Lower risk of metabolic syndrome
- ■Lower risk of colon cancer
- ■Lower risk of breast cancer
- ■Prevention of weight gain
- ■Weight loss, particularly when combined with reduced calorie intake
- ■Improved cardiorespiratory and muscular fitness
- ■Prevention of falls
- ■Reduced depression
- ■Better cognitive function (for older adults)

Moderate to strong evidence

- ■Better functional health (for older adults)
- ■Reduced abdominal obesity

Moderate evidence

- ■Lower risk of hip fracture
- ■Lower risk of lung cancer
- ■Lower risk of endometrial cancer
- ■Weight maintenance after weight loss
- ■Increased bone density
- ■Improved sleep quality

Reduced Risk of Your Premature Death

There is an abundance of Strong scientific evidence that shows that physical activity reduces the risk of your premature death (dying earlier than the average age-at-death for a specific population group) from the leading causes of death, such as heart disease and some cancers, as well as from other causes of death.

This effect is remarkable in two ways:

- ■First, only a few lifestyle choices have as large an effect on mortality as physical activity. It has been estimated that people who are physically active for approximately 7 hours a week have a 60% lower risk of dying early than those who are active for less than 30 minutes a week.
- ■Second, it is not necessary to do high amounts of physical activity or vigorous-intensity activity to reduce the risk of premature death. Studies show that there are substantially lower risks when people perform at least 150 minutes of at least moderate-intensity aerobic physical activity a week.

Can Exercise Make You Smarter?

There are many published physical benefits of regular exercise. But what effects does exercise have on our cognitive function?

Mental performance such as reaction time, perception and interpretation of visual images, and executive control processes has shown measurable improvements with moderately intense aerobic exercise.

After 15 minutes of exercise, your body begins to produce and secrete Endorphins (among other things).

Endorphins are chemicals or hormones for your Brain.

The electricity that is generated from exercise 'feeds' your Brain. Brain activity is measured through electricity or Electrical Energy.

The Electricity or Energy produced from exercise increases the electrical energy of your Brain.

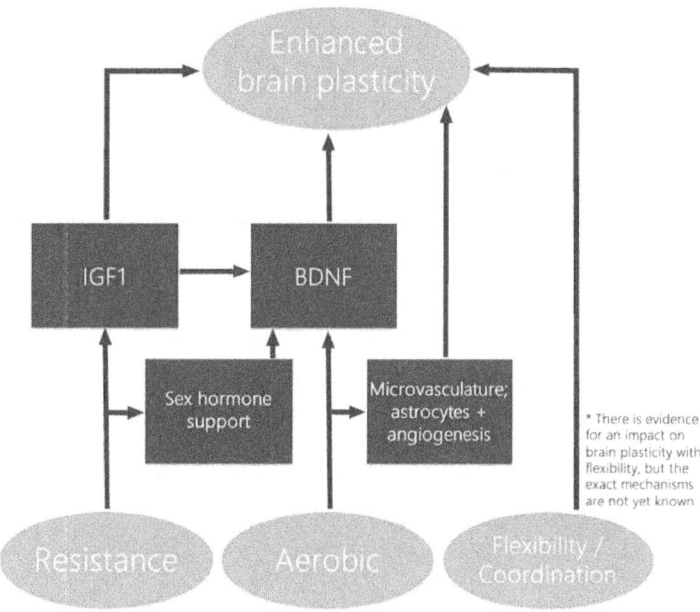

The most positive influences have been seen in executive control processes such as:

- •planning;
- •scheduling;
- •coordination of people, places, events, etc.;
- •working memory; and
- •inhibition.

These positive effects of exercising are related to increase in blood flow to your brain and stimulation of nerve cells.

Moderate exercise gives you a double benefit for your time spent. Not only will your fitness be improved, but your ability to concentrate and perform mental tasks will improve as well.

Research clearly demonstrates the importance of avoiding inactivity. Even low amounts of physical activity reduce the risk of dying prematurely.

The most dramatic difference in risk is seen between those who are inactive (30 minutes a week) and those with low levels of activity (90 minutes, or 1 hour and 30 minutes, a week).

The relative risk of dying prematurely continues to be lower with higher levels of reported moderate- or vigorous-intensity, leisure-time physical activity.

Exercise Fights Middle-Age Spread

A 20-year study of more than 3,500 men and women found that high activity levels led to less excess weight (5.7 fewer pounds gained each year in men and 13.4 fewer pounds gained each year in women) when compared to adults with low activity levels. The key is to start an exercise program before middle age. Sticking with the national guidelines of 30 minutes of moderate exercise each day had a significant effect over the two decades of the study.

All adults can gain this health benefit of physical activity. Age, race, and ethnicity do not matter. Men and women younger than 65 years as well as older adults have lower rates of early death when they are physically active than when they are inactive.

Physically active people of all body weights (normal weight, overweight, obese) also have lower rates of early death than do inactive people.

Cardiorespiratory Health

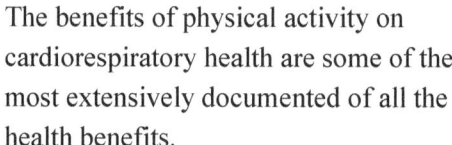

The effects of exercise on lung structures

In the long-term, regular exercise strengthens the respiratory system.
- The respiratory muscles (the diaphragm and intercostals) get stronger, so they can make the chest cavity larger.
 This larger chest cavity means more air can be inspired, therefore increasing your vital capacity.
- More capillaries form around the alveoli, so more gaseous exchange can take place.

Gas exchange can now take place more quickly meaning exercise can be maintained at a higher intensity for longer.

The benefits of physical activity on cardiorespiratory health are some of the most extensively documented of all the health benefits.

Cardiorespiratory health involves the health of the heart, lungs, and blood vessels.

Heart diseases and stroke are two of the leading causes of death in the United States.

Risk factors that increase the likelihood of cardiovascular diseases include smoking, high blood pressure (called hypertension), type 2 diabetes, and high levels of certain blood lipids (such as low-density lipoprotein, or LDL, cholesterol).

Low cardiorespiratory fitness is also a risk factor for heart disease.

People who do moderate- or vigorous-intensity aerobic physical activity have a significantly lower risk of cardiovascular disease than do inactive people.

Regularly active adults have lower rates of heart disease and stroke, lower blood pressure, better blood lipid profiles, and better fitness.

Significant reductions in risk of cardiovascular disease are observed at activity levels equivalent to 150 minutes a week of moderate-intensity physical activity.

Even greater benefits are seen with 420 minutes (7 hours) a week.

Long Term Effects of Exercise on the Respiratory System

Diaphragm and Intercostal Muscles:
They both get stronger due to the continued work they do during exercise.

Tidal Volume:
This will increase as the diaphragm and intercostal muscles contract stronger allowing the lungs to expand more.

Alveoli:
Due to the lungs expanding more, more alveoli can then be used. This allows gaseous exchange to increase allowing more oxygen in and more carbon dioxide out with each breath.

The evidence is strong that greater amounts of physical activity result in even further reductions in the risk of cardiovascular disease.

Metabolic Health

Regular physical activity strongly reduces the risk of developing type 2 diabetes as well as the metabolic syndrome.

The metabolic syndrome is a condition in which people have some combination of high blood pressure, a large waistline (abdominal obesity), an adverse blood lipid profile (low levels of high-density lipoprotein [HDL] cholesterol, raised triglycerides), and impaired glucose tolerance.

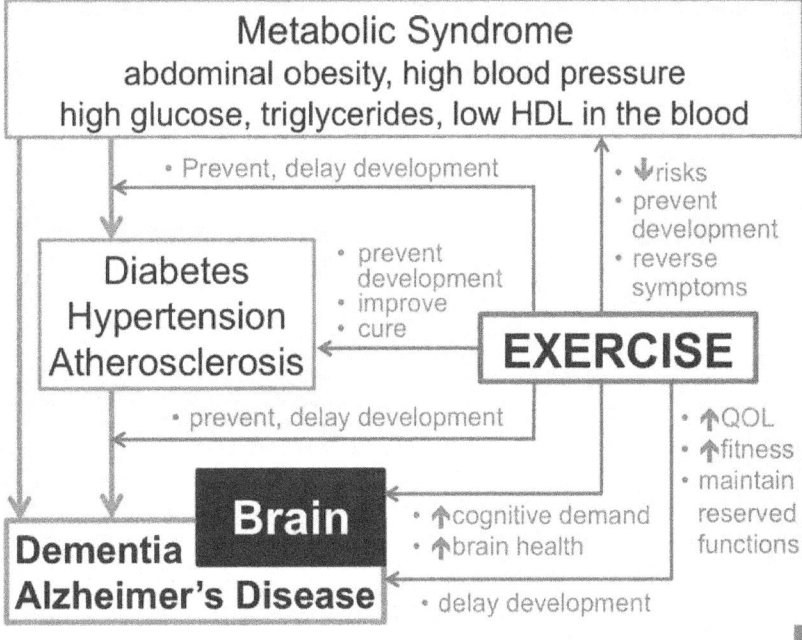

People who regularly engage in at least moderate-intensity aerobic activity have a significantly lower risk of developing type 2 diabetes than do inactive people.

Although some experts debate the usefulness of defining the metabolic syndrome, good evidence exists that physical activity reduces the risk of having this condition, as defined in various ways. Lower rates of these conditions are seen with 120 to 150 minutes (2 hours to 2 hours and 30 minutes) a week of at least moderate-intensity aerobic activity.

As you increase the time to 420 minutes a week – 1 hour a day, you increase the metabolic benefits!

As with cardiovascular health, additional levels of physical activity lower the risk even further. In addition, physical activity helps control blood glucose levels in persons who already have type 2 diabetes.

Exercise May Block Colds

It appears that being fit by exercising at least 5 days a week is associated with a reduction in upper respiratory tract infections. Those who exercised regularly had 43% fewer days with an upper respiratory tract infection compared to those who exercised no more than 1 day a week.

Recirculation of your immunoglobulins and neutrophils and your natural killer cells is increased with each aerobic exercise session.

Your natural killer cells are responsible for ridding your body of harmful bacteria and viruses!

Additionally, stress hormones that may suppress immunity are not elevated during moderate exercise. In addition to the reduced number of days with an upper respiratory tract infection, the severity of such infections was reduced as well.

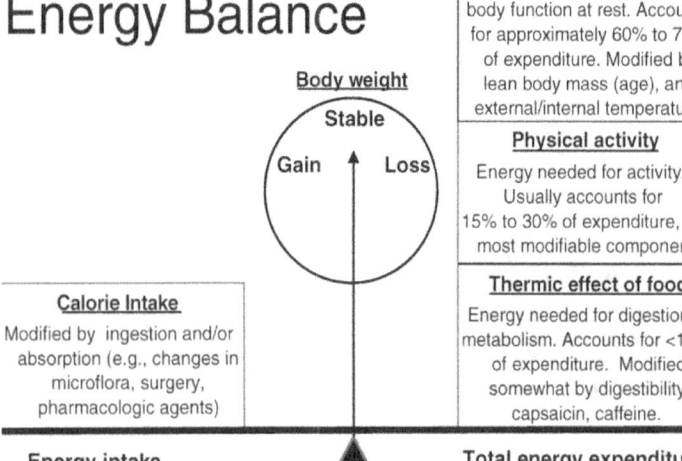

Weight and Energy Balance

Overweight and obesity occur when fewer calories are expended, including calories burned through physical activity, than are taken in through food and beverages.

Physical activity and caloric intake both must be considered when trying to control body weight.

Because of this role in energy balance, physical activity is a critical factor in determining whether a person can maintain a healthy body weight, lose excess body weight, or maintain successful weight loss.

People vary a great deal in how much physical activity they need to achieve and maintain a healthy weight. Some need more physical activity than others to maintain a healthy body weight, to lose weight, or to keep weight off once it has been lost.

Strong scientific evidence shows that physical activity helps people maintain a stable weight over time. However, the optimal amount of physical activity needed to maintain weight is unclear. People vary greatly in how much physical activity results in weight stability.

Many people need more than the equivalent of 150 minutes of moderate-intensity activity a week to maintain their weight.

Musculoskeletal Health

Bones, muscles, and joints support the body and help it move. Healthy bones, joints, and muscles are critical to the ability to do daily activities without physical limitations.

Preserving bone, joint, and muscle health is essential with increasing age. Studies show that the frequent decline in bone density that happens during aging can be slowed with regular physical activity. These effects are seen in people who participate in aerobic, muscle-strengthening, and bone-strengthening physical activity programs of moderate or vigorous intensity. The range of total physical activity for these benefits varies widely. Important changes seem to begin at 90 minutes a week and continue up to 300 minutes a week.

Hip fracture is a serious health condition that can have life-changing negative effects for many older people. Physically active people, especially women, have a lower risk of hip fracture than do inactive people.

Research studies on physical activity to prevent hip fracture show that participating in at least 120 to 300 minutes a week of physical activity that is of at least moderate intensity is associated with a reduced risk.

As we age...

- **Brain:** Decreased neural activity contributes to deterioration of musculoskeletal health
- **Muscle:** Loss of muscular mass, flexibility, and strength
- **Bones:** Density and strength of bones decreases
- **Joints:** Loss of cartilage and stiffening of ligaments and tendons reduces joint mobility

Imagine Turning It Up to 420 minutes a week …. We are talking Building your God-Body.

You need your body to carry you into your Abundant Life … So, by increasing your exercise to 1 hour a day …. 420 minutes a week …. You can keep your body Healthy and Strong!

Building strong, healthy bones is also important for children and adolescents. Along with having a healthy diet that includes adequate calcium and vitamin D, physical activity is critical for bone development in children and adolescents.

Bone-strengthening physical activity done 3 or more days a week increases bone-mineral content and bone density in youth.

Regular physical activity also helps people with arthritis or other rheumatic conditions affecting the joints. Participation in 300 to 420 minutes (5 to 7 hours) a week of moderate-intensity, low-impact physical activity improves pain management, function, and quality of life.

Very high levels of physical activity, however, may have extra risks. People who participate in very high levels of physical activity, such as elite or professional athletes, have a higher risk of hip and knee osteoarthritis, mostly due to the risk of injury involved in competing in some sports.

Progressive muscle-strengthening activities increase or preserve muscle mass, strength, and power. Higher amounts (through greater frequency or higher weights) improve muscle function to a greater degree. Improvements occur in younger and older adults.

Resistance exercises also improve muscular strength in persons with such conditions as stroke, multiple sclerosis, cerebral palsy, spinal cord injury, and cognitive disability. Though it does not increase muscle mass in the same way that muscle-strengthening activities do, aerobic activity also helps to slow the loss of muscle with aging.

Functional Ability and Fall Prevention

Functional ability is the capacity of a person to perform tasks or behaviors that enable him or her to carry out everyday activities, such as climbing stairs or walking on a sidewalk. Functional ability is key to a person's ability to fulfill basic life roles, such as personal care, grocery shopping, or playing with the grandchildren.

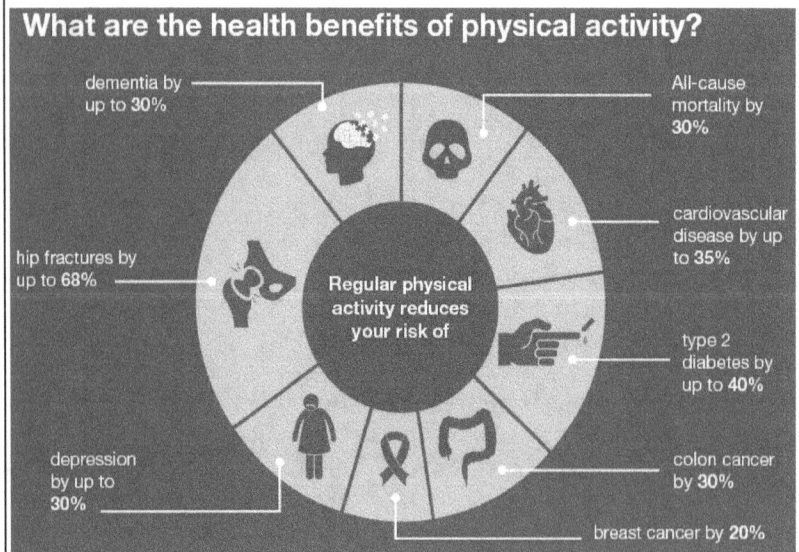

Loss of functional ability is referred to as functional limitation.

Middle-aged and older adults who are physically active have lower risk of functional limitations than do inactive adults. It appears that greater physical activity levels can further reduce risk of functional limitations.

Older adults who already have functional limitations also benefit from regular physical activity.

Typically, studies of physical activity in adults with functional limitations tested a combination of aerobic and muscle strengthening activities, making it difficult to assess the relative importance of each type of activity.

However, both types of activity appear to provide benefit.

Lower Cancer Risk

Physically active people have a significantly lower risk of colon cancer than do inactive people, and physically active women have a significantly lower risk of breast cancer.

Research shows that a range of moderate-intensity physical activity—between 210 and 420 minutes a week (3 hours and 30 minutes to 7 hours)—is needed to significantly reduce the risk of colon and breast cancer; **currently, the recommendation of 150 minutes a week does not provide a major benefit.**

It also appears that greater amounts of physical activity lower risks of these cancers even further, although exactly how much lower is not clear.

Although not definitive, some research suggests that the risk of endometrial cancer in women and lung cancers in men and women also may be lower among those who are regularly active compared to those who are inactive.

Finally, cancer survivors have a better quality of life and improved physical fitness if they are physically active, compared to survivors who are inactive.

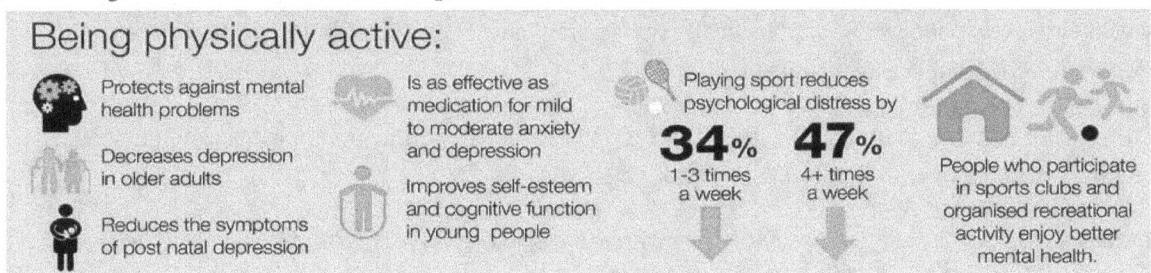

Mental Health

Physically active adults have lower risk of depression and cognitive decline (declines with aging in thinking, learning, and judgment skills). Physical activity also may improve your quality of sleep. Whether physical activity reduces distress or anxiety is currently unclear.

Mental health benefits have been found in people who do aerobic or a combination of aerobic and muscle-strengthening activities 5 to 7 days a week for 0 to 60 minutes at a time. Some research has shown that even lower levels of physical activity also may provide some benefits.

Regular physical activity appears to reduce symptoms of anxiety and depression for children and adolescents. Whether physical activity improves self-esteem is not clear – but if you Look Good You Feel Good and Exercise helps you to Look Good.

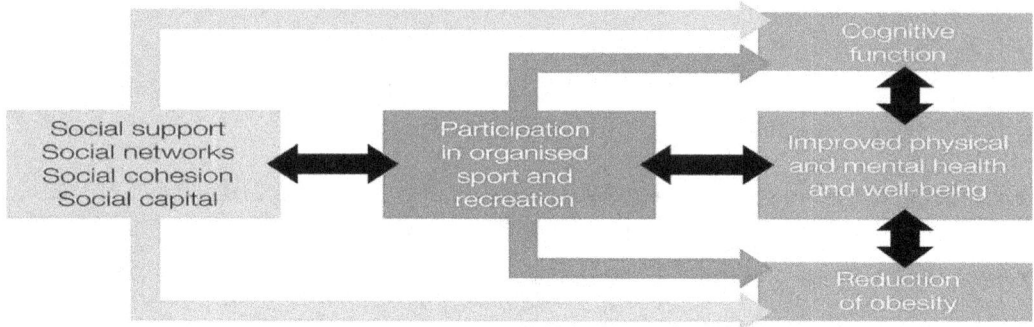

Lower Risk of Adverse Events

Some people hesitate to become active or to increase their level of physical activity because they fear getting injured or having a heart attack. Studies of generally healthy people clearly show that moderate-intensity physical activity, such as brisk walking, has a low risk of such adverse events.

The risk of musculoskeletal injury increases with the total amount of physical activity. As an example, a person who regularly runs 40 miles a week has a higher risk of injury than a person who runs 10 miles each week. However, people who are physically active may have fewer injuries from other causes, such as motor vehicle collisions or work-related injuries.

Depending on the type and amount of activity that physically active people do, their overall injury rate may be lower than the overall injury rate for inactive people.

The underlying factor is that you cannot have or create your Healing, Health and Wellness without Moving SomeThing – Moving YourSelf into the Enjoyment of Your Abundant Life!

WARNING: Bursts of Activity Can Trigger Heart Attacks

Researchers analyzed 14 studies of cardiac effects of episodic physical activity and found that it was associated with more than a three-fold increase in heart attack risk and a five-fold increase in sudden cardiac death risk in the short-term. Researchers concluded that there is a link between episodic physical activity (e.g., sexual activity) with the risk of heart attack and sudden cardiac death within one to two hours after the activity.

The risk was greatest for those who are not engaged in regular exercise. To reduce your risk of heart attack and sudden cardiac death, researchers suggest to make your physical activity more frequent and regular rather than episodic.

Overcoming Your Excuses for Not Exercising or Being Physically Active

Given the health benefits of regular physical activity, we might have to ask why two out of three (60%) Americans are not active at recommended levels.

Many technological advances and conveniences that have made our lives easier and less active, and many personal variables, including physiological, behavioral, and psychological factors, may affect our plans to become more physically active.

In fact, the 10 most common reasons adults cite for not adopting more physically active lifestyles are:

- ■do not have enough time to exercise;
- ■find it inconvenient to exercise;
- ■lack self-motivation;
- ■do not find exercise enjoyable;
- ■find exercise boring;
- ■lack confidence in their ability to be physically active (low self-efficacy);
- ■fear of being injured or have been injured recently;
- ■lack self-management skills, such as the ability to set personal goals or monitor progress
- ■lack encouragement, support, or companionship from family and friends; and
- ■do not have parks, sidewalks, bicycle trails, or safe and pleasant walking paths convenient to their homes or offices.

Understanding common barriers to physical activity and creating strategies to overcome them may help you make physical activity part of your daily life.

For Important Health Benefits

Adults should get a Minimum of:

- 5 hours and 30 minutes (330 minutes) of moderate-intensity aerobic activity (e.g., brisk walking) every week **and**

muscle-strengthening activities on 2 or more days a week that work all major muscle groups (legs, hips, back, abdomen, chest, shoulders, and arms).

OR

- 2 hour and 30 minutes (150 minutes) of vigorous-intensity aerobic activity (e.g., jogging or running) every week **and**

muscle-strengthening activities on 2 or more days a week that work all major muscle groups (legs, hips, back, abdomen, chest, shoulders, and arms).

OR

- An equivalent mix of moderate- and vigorous-intensity aerobic activity **and**

muscle-strengthening activities on 2 or more days a week that work all major muscle groups (legs, hips, back, abdomen, chest, shoulders, and arms).

For Even *Greater* Health Benefits

Adults should increase their activity to:

- 7 hours (420 minutes) each week of moderate-intensity aerobic activity **and**

muscle-strengthening activities on 2 or more days a week that work all major muscle groups (legs, hips, back, abdomen, chest, shoulders, and arms).

OR

- 3 hours and 30 minutes (210 minutes) each week of vigorous-intensity aerobic activity **and**

muscle-strengthening activities on 2 or more days a week that work all major muscle groups (legs, hips, back, abdomen, chest, shoulders, and arms).

OR

- An equivalent mix of moderate- and vigorous-intensity aerobic activity **and**

muscle-strengthening activities on 2 or more days a week that work all major muscle groups (legs, hips, back, abdomen, chest, shoulders, and arms).

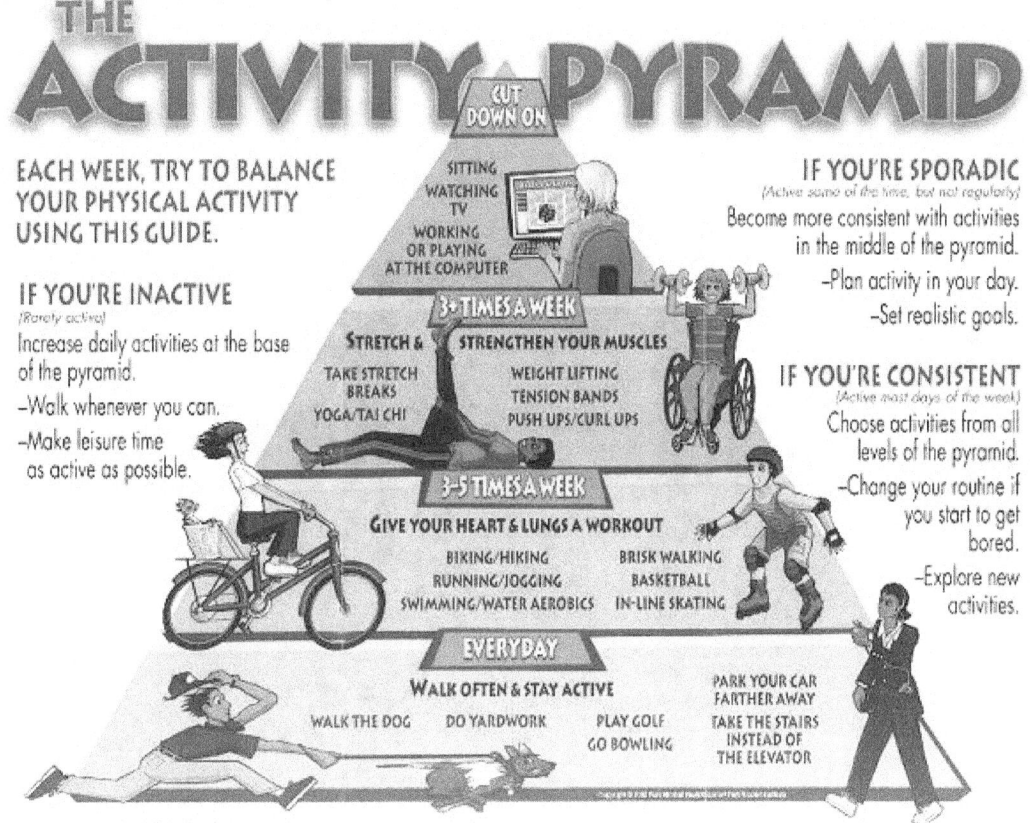

Epigenetics

This is a new branch of genetics that is shedding light on the "nature vs. nurture" debate.
"Epi" means "above" or "on top of" so epigenetics refers to modifications that occur on top of your genes. Environmental factors actually cause your cells and genetic code to change over your lifetime. Your genetic code itself is always the same, but genes can be "turned on" or "turned off."

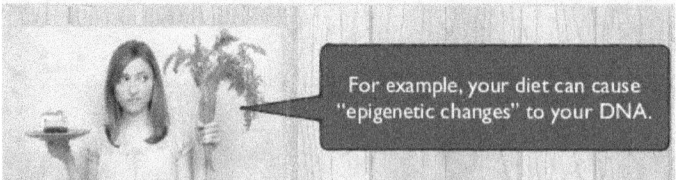

For example, your diet can cause "epigenetic changes" to your DNA.

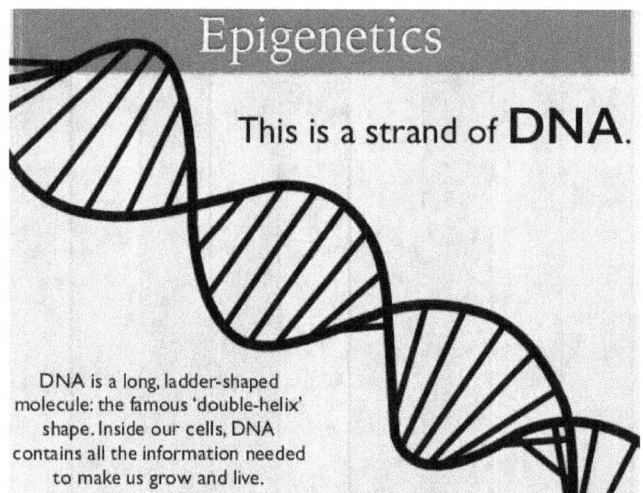

Epigenetics

This is a strand of **DNA**.

DNA is a long, ladder-shaped molecule: the famous 'double-helix' shape. Inside our cells, DNA contains all the information needed to make us grow and live.

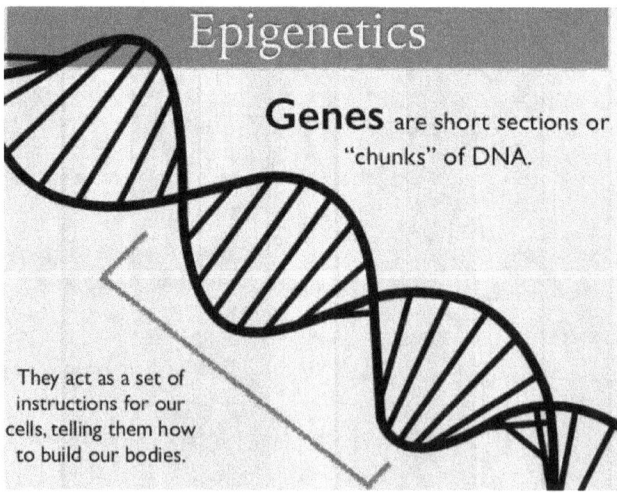

Epigenetics

Genes are short sections or "chunks" of DNA.

They act as a set of instructions for our cells, telling them how to build our bodies.

Epigenetics

Throughout your life, and depending on specific conditions, a chemical called methyl attaches to genes. This chemical "switches" on or off only a selection of your genes.

This process is known as **gene regulation**.

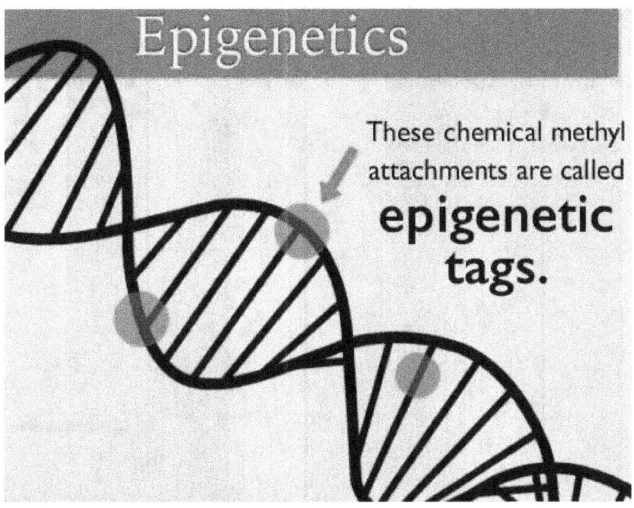

Epigenetics

These chemical methyl attachments are called **epigenetic tags.**

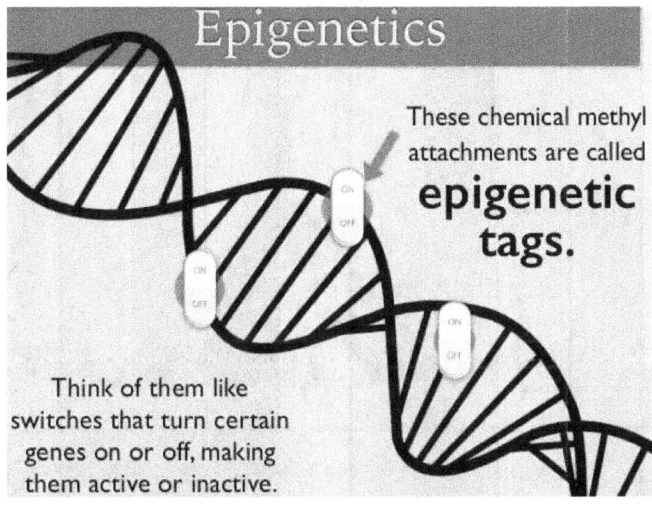

Epigenetics

These chemical methyl attachments are called **epigenetic tags.**

Think of them like switches that turn certain genes on or off, making them active or inactive.

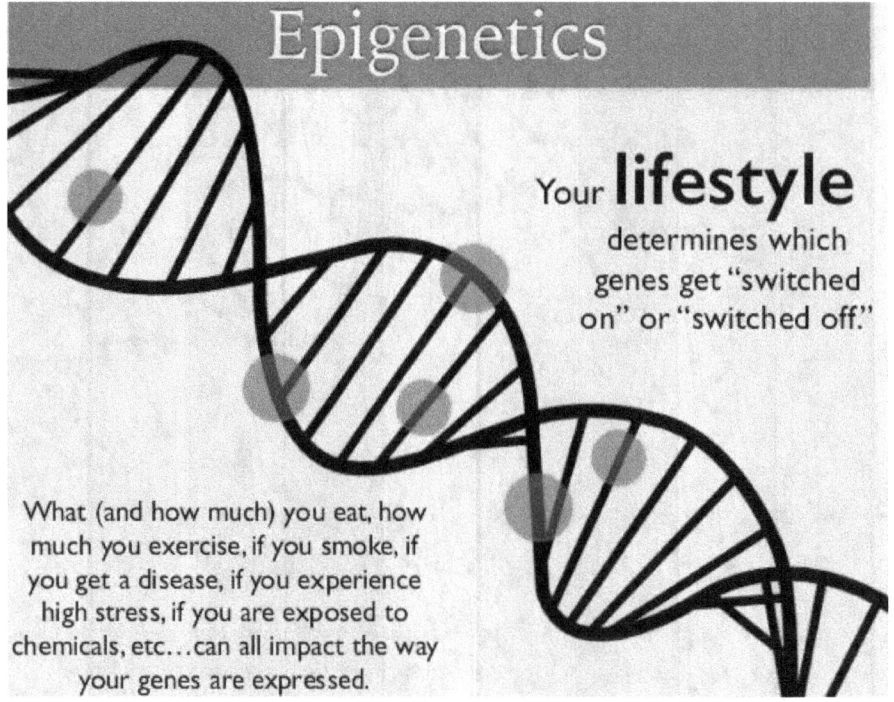
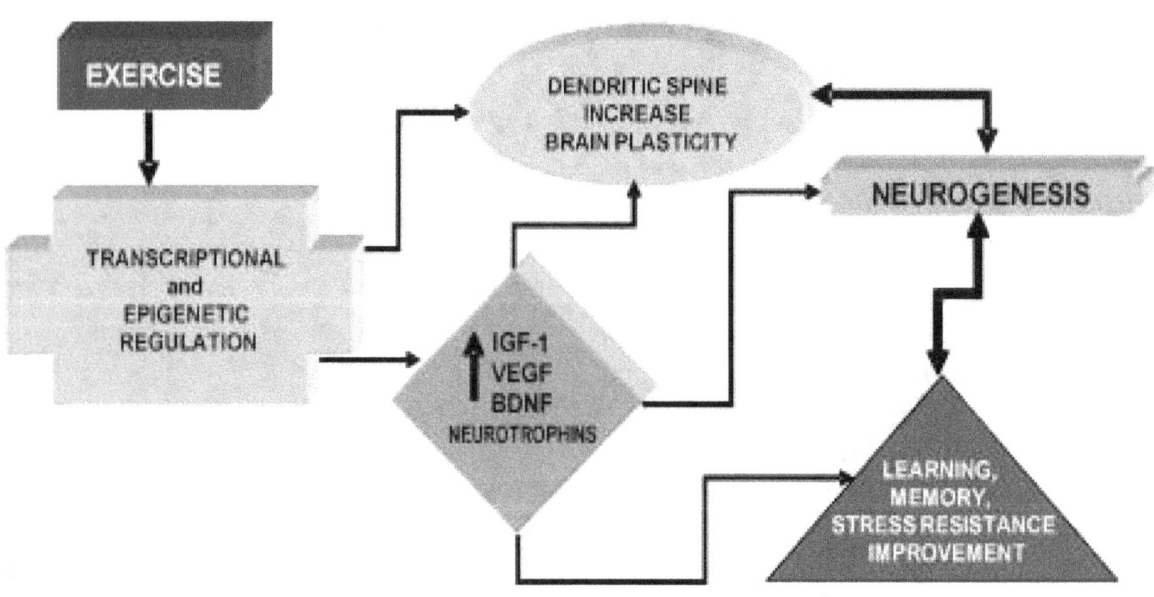

The 2010 American Cancer Society study published in the American Journal of Epidemiology followed 123,216 individuals (69,776 women and 53,440 men) from 1993-2006. See the alarming results:

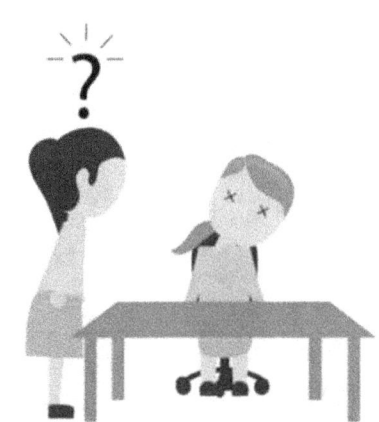

Women who sit more than 6 hours a day were

94%

more likely to die during the time period studied than those who were physically active and sat less than 3 hours a day.

Men who sit more than 6 hours a day were

48%

more likely to die during the time period studied than those who were physically active and sat less than 3 hours a day.

Findings were independent of physical activity levels (the negative effects of sitting were just as strong in people who exercised regularly).

SITTING SO MUCH SHOULD SCARE YOU

People across the U.S. are sitting almost all day, living an excessively sedentary lifestyle. They don't like it, they know it's bad for them, but they are doing it anyway.

How Sedentary is the Typical American Each Day?

Sedentary *21 Hours*
Active *3 Hours*

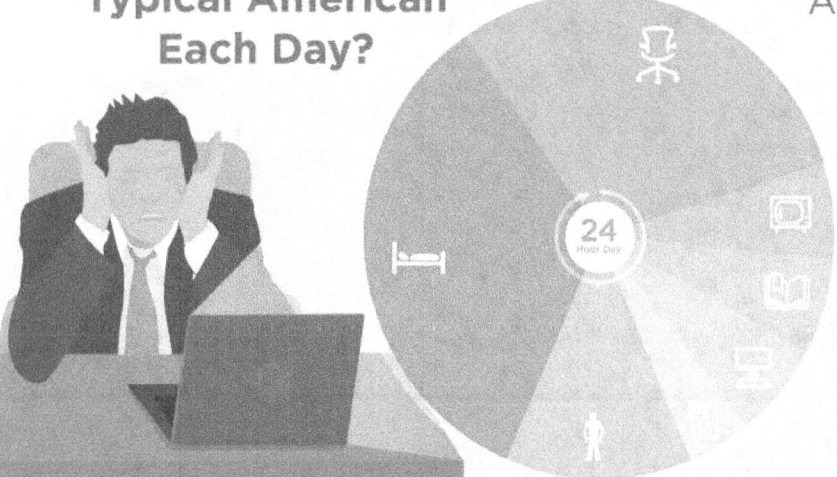

- **Sleeping** — 8 Hours
- **Sitting at Work** — 7.5 Hours
- **Watching TV** — 1.5 Hours
- **Leisure Time** — 1.5 Hours
- **On Home Computer** — 1.5 Hours
- **Eating** — 1 Hour
- **Active/Standing** — 3 Hours

Supreme Health & Fitness! *Health & Wellness Series ... Vol 3!*

THE DANGERS OF SITTING DISEASE

Sitting disease is a concept created by the scientific community to address the problems associated with sitting all day and living a sedentary lifestyle. However, it is not a disease recognized by the medical community. Is your workforce in danger?

HOW MANY U.S. EMPLOYEES ARE AFFECTED?

86% of U.S. workers sit for the entire workday

Upon starting a new, desk-bound job, people gain, on average **16 LBS. WITHIN 8 MONTHS**

When home & leisure activities are included, many people are sitting between **8 TO 13 HOURS PER DAY**

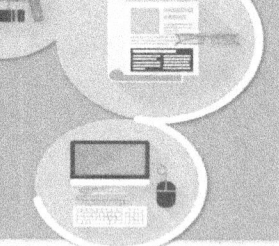

WHY IS THIS A PROBLEM?

Sitting all day increases the risks of multiple major health concerns:

- CANCER
- OBESITY
- MUSCULOSKELETAL PROBLEMS
- CARDIOVASCULAR DISEASE
- DIABETES
- EARLY DEATH

WOMEN WHO SPENT 6+ HRS. PER DAY SITTING WERE 94% MORE LIKELY TO DIE from increased risk factors compared to physically active women who only sat 3 hours per day.

Inactive men were **48% MORE LIKELY** to die than those who were physically active.

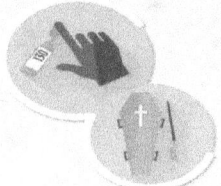 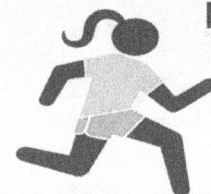

workers who remain sedentary for **10 YEARS** double their risk of developing **COLON CANCER**

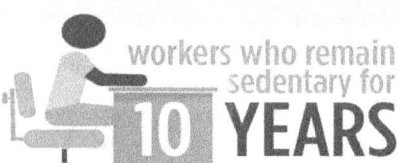 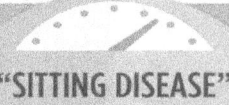

"SITTING DISEASE" affects everyone who sits — regardless of whether that person is a healthy weight or whether or not they smoke.

Even with regular exercise, people who sit for the majority of their day **SHORTEN THEIR LIFE SPAN**

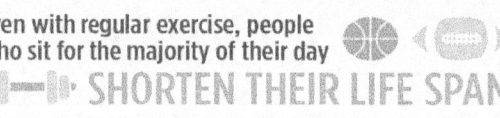

Employees who sit for more than **11** hours every day increase their **RISK OF DEATH** in the next 3 years by **40%**

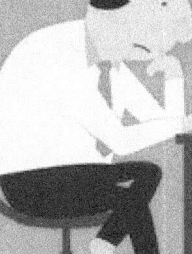

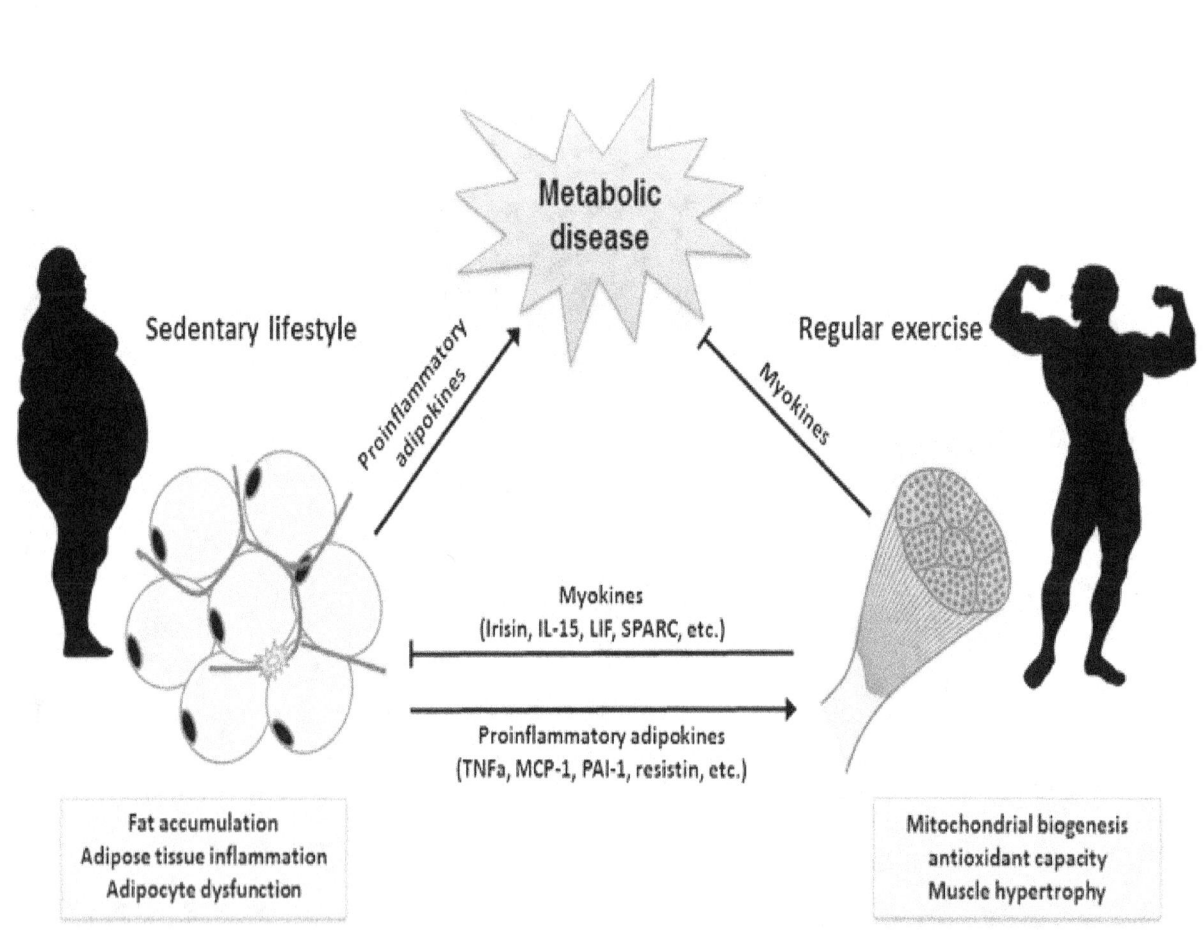

Chapter Three

Sitting Disease – Death By Sedentary

*****

- Sitting for more than eight hours a day is associated with a 90 percent increased risk of type 2 diabetes

- Those who sit the most have a 147 percent increased relative risk of cardiovascular events compared to those who sit the least; all-cause mortality is increased by 50 percent

- Sitting also increases lung cancer 54 percent; uterine cancer by 66 percent, and colon cancer by 30 percent

If you're like most people, unfortunately you spend a vast majority of your day sitting down, whether its in your office, commuting to and from work, watching TV in the evening… Research shows that the average American spends at least nine to 10 hours of their day sitting.

There are certain occupations, such as telecommunications employees spend an average of 12 hours sitting each day. And, the more sedentary you are at work, the more sedentary you will tend to be at home as well.

Even on weekends, the average person sits for eight hours. This behavior can be more problematic than you might think, as the human body was designed to be in more or less constant movement throughout the day.

I have personally suffered from lower -back issues for several years. I found that merely getting up for a few minutes even six times an hour would not help eliminate my back pain but stopping sitting altogether did.

The science and evidence shows that prolonged sitting actively promotes dozens of chronic diseases, including overweight and type 2 diabetes, even if you're very fit. This is really a conundrum as one would assume that physically fit people could get away with sitting.

However, research shows that maintaining a regular fitness regimen *cannot* counteract the accumulated ill effects of sitting eight to 12 hours a day in between bouts of exercise.

This is very strong evidence to seriously consider eliminating as much sitting as you can.

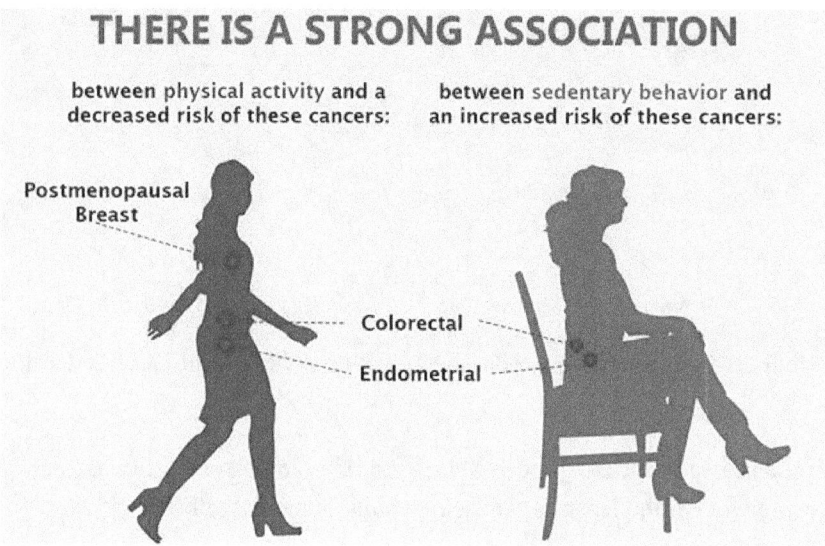

Sitting really is the new smoking and it increases your rate of lung cancer by over 50 percent.

Who would have known that sitting is far more dangerous than second hand smoke?

Analysis Concludes: Sitting Kills, Even if You Exercise

There's really compelling evidence showing that when you sit for lengths of time, disease processes set in that independently raise your mortality risk, even if you eat right, exercise regularly and are very fit; even a professional or Olympic level athlete.

The most recent systematic review looked at 47 studies of sedentary behavior and discovered that the time a person spends sitting each day produces detrimental effects that outweigh the benefits reaped from exercise.

Sitting was found to increase your risk of death from virtually all health problems, from type 2 diabetes and cardiovascular disease to cancer and all-cause mortality. For example, sitting for more than eight hours a day was associated with a 90 percent increased risk of type 2 diabetes.

Other research has found that those who sit the most have a **112%** increased Relative Risk of diabetes, and a **147%** increased relative risk of cardiovascular events compared to those who sit the least.

All-cause mortality is also increased by **50%**.

In fact, chronic sitting has a mortality rate similar to smoking. And, the less you exercise, the more pronounced the detrimental effects of sitting.

To counteract the ill effects of prolonged sitting, the authors of the featured review suggest that you:

- Keep track of how much you're sitting each day, and make an effort to reduce it, little by little, each week

- Use a standing desk at work. Although standing up frequently is better than constant sitting I am now strongly convinced that avoiding sitting completely is far preferable and has better metabolic effects.

- When watching TV, stand up and/or walk around during commercial breaks.

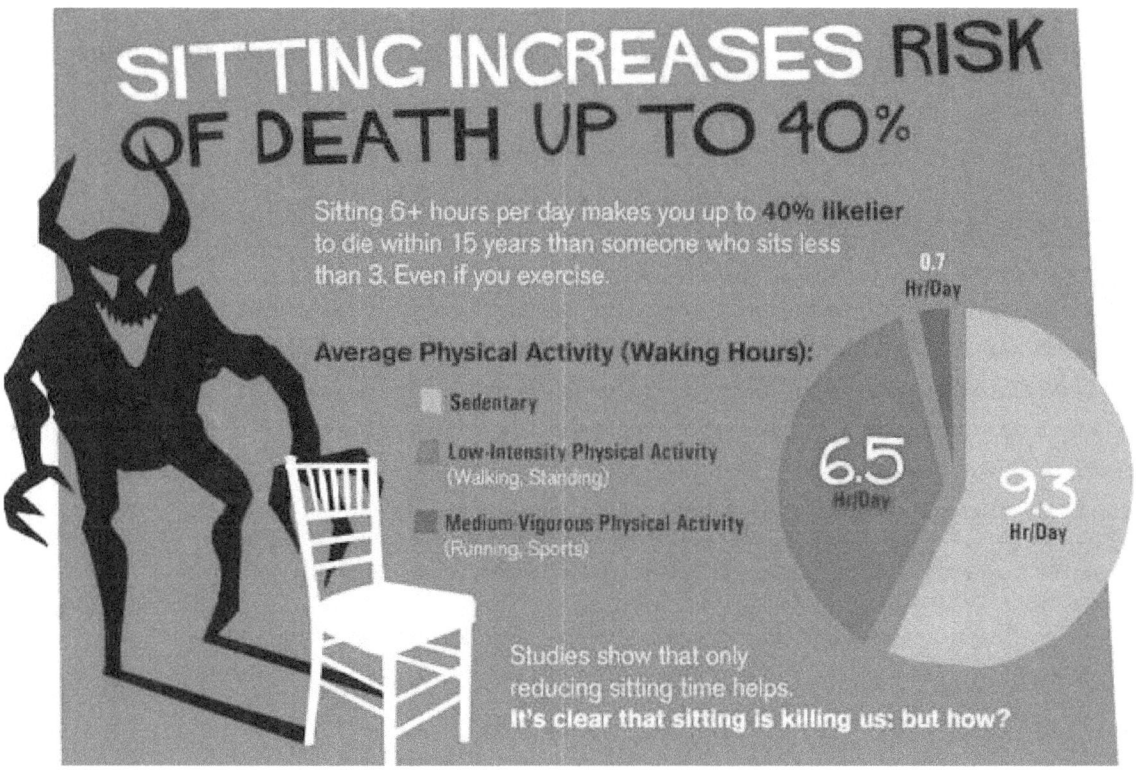

More Studies Highlighting Debilitating Effects of Sitting

Part one in a two-part series of articles published in the *British Medical Journal* (BMJ) at the beginning of January 2016, also highlights the hazards of our modern sedentary lifestyle, suggesting that public policy needs to be reassessed and updated to focus on increasing movement during work hours.

The article summarizes the findings from the 2015 Inaugural Active Working Summit, where a number of health effects of sitting were reviewed, including cancer and mental health.

There is one study presented at the summit found that sitting increases:

- Lung cancer by 54%
- Uterine cancer by 66%
- Colon cancer by 30%

The reason for this increased cancer risk is thought to be linked to weight gain and associated biochemical changes, such as alterations in hormones, metabolic dysfunction, leptin dysfunction, and inflammation — all of which promote cancer.

Research also shows that your risk for anxiety and depression rises right along with hours spent in your chair.

Why Sitting Causes So Much Harm

Dr. James Levine, co-director of the Mayo Clinic and the Arizona State University Obesity Initiative, and author of the book **Get Up! Why Your Chair Is Killing You and What You Can Do About It**, has dedicated a good part of his career to investigating the health effects of sitting. His investigations show that when you've been sitting for a long period of time and then get up, a number of molecular cascades occur. For example, within 90 seconds of standing up, the muscular and cellular systems that process blood sugar, triglycerides, and cholesterol—which are mediated by insulin—are activated.

All of these molecular effects are activated simply by carrying your own bodyweight.

These cellular mechanisms are also responsible for pushing fuel into your cells and, if done regularly, will radically decrease your risk of diabetes and obesity. In short, at the molecular level, your body was designed to be active and on the move all day long.

When you stop moving for extended periods of time, it's like telling your body it's time to shut down and prepare for death …. The longer you are inactive, the more your body inadvertently prepares for its own death.

You are literally teaching or programming your body to DIE!

Inactivity—sitting—is not supposed to be a way of life.

As a consequence of sitting, your blood sugar levels, blood pressure, cholesterol, and toxic buildup all rise.

As noted by Dr. Levine, while we clearly need to rest from time to time, that rest is supposed to break up activity—not the other way around!

"[T]his very unnatural [sitting] posture is not only bad for your back, your wrists, your arms, and your metabolism, but it actually switches off the fundamental fueling systems that integrate what's going on in the bloodstream with what goes on in the muscles and in the tissues," he says.

The solution to these adverse events do not involve a prescription — all you need to do is *Move Something .... Move YourSelf into Your Abundant Life!* and avoid sitting down as much as possible.

If you've been sitting down for a full hour, you've sat too long, and the cellular mechanisms involved in the maintenance of your body and health are shutting down.

If you have a sit-down job I would strongly encourage you to present this information to your employer and get a stand-up desk.

What We Learned Amazed Us

After Aleternating Between Sitting and Standing for 30 Days:

 **71%** Reported Feeling More Energized

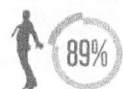 **89%** Almost All Reported Feeling Better

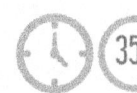 **35%** Increased Standing Time To More Than 60 Minutes Per Day

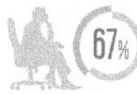 **67%** Reported an Improvement In Comfort

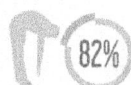 **82%** Felt Less Fatigue and More Allert

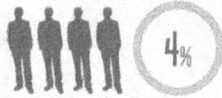 **4%** 4 people said they lost some extra pounds

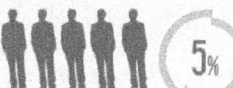 **5%** 5 people said they had improved indurance at the gym

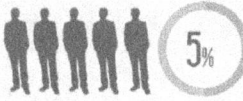 **5%** 5 people said they tripled personal standing time to stand 90 minutes a day.

 **x38** 38 people claim that Zero Gravity relieves previous levels of discomfort

Avoiding Sitting is the First Step Toward a Healthier Lifestyle

The World Health Organization (WHO) recommends getting at least 150 minutes of physical activity per week, but I say this may be too **underachieving** of a goal for many people — particularly the young trying to grow and develop and the elderly who are trying to start to regenerate their cells and improve their overall health and wellness.

When all else fails, you simply avoid sitting still as much as possible.

In a paper titled, "Recommendations for Physical Activity in Older Adults", Professor Phillip Sparling and colleagues write:

"There is now a clear need to reduce prolonged sitting. Secondly, evidence on the potential of high intensity interval training in managing the same chronic diseases, as well as reducing indices of cardiometabolic risk in healthy adults, has emerged. This vigorous training typically comprises multiple 3-4 minute bouts of high intensity exercise interspersed with several minutes of low intensity recovery, three times a week.

We argue that when advising patients on exercise doctors should encourage people to increase their level of activity by small amounts rather than focus on the recommended levels. These include finding ways to do more lower intensity lifestyle activity..."

It is Killing us

94% MORE LIKELY TO DIE

The 2010 American Cancer Society Study published in the American Journal of Epidemiology following 123,216 individuals

from 1993-2006. The alarming results:

53,440 & 69,776

Women who were inactive and sat over 6 hours a day — 94% more likely to die during the time period studied then those who were physically active and sat less than 3 hours a day.

Men who were inactive and sat over 6 hours a day — 48% more likely to die than their standing counterparts.

Findings were independent of physical activity levels (the negative effects of sitting were just as strong in people who exercised regularly).

Medical experts have started referring to long periods of physical inactivity and its negative consequences as "sitting disease."

A Fitness Tracker Can Be a Helpful Tool

Part of the solution may also be to reassess your use of technology to create your Health and Wellness instead of having it contribute to a sedentary lifestyle. Your TV, for example, can increase your sedentary time by hours each day, so consider trading some of that sedentary time for something more active. That doesn't mean that all technology is detrimental though.

I'm very excited about the amount of technology being devoted to health, like the wearable fitness trackers for example, which can measure your activity levels and track how long and how well you sleep. It's hard to change a habit if you're not tracking it, and devices like these can help you modify your behavior over time, such as motivating you to walk more, and get in bed earlier to get your eight hours of sleep.

I recommend aiming for 7,000 to 10,000 steps per day, over and above any exercise regimen you may have, and to shoot for at least 6 – 8 hours of sleep each night.

With a fitness tracker, you can track all of this and more.

When Sitting Is Unavoidable - Keep Your Posture in Mind

While it's certainly possible to limit sitting, it's still an unavoidable part of most people's lives.

The question then becomes, how can you limit the risks associated with sitting?

Paying attention to your posture is one way. A recent CNN article suggests "sitting smarter" by incorporating yoga postures and being aware of your breathing and presents a five-point yoga-based posture check that can make for healthier sitting.

Also familiarize yourself with your body's signals to shift or move. Following the recommendations by "posture guru" Esther Gokhale may also go a long way toward improving posture-related pain associated with prolonged sitting, and will likely help ameliorate the worst risks of sitting.

The basics of healthy sitting include the following points:

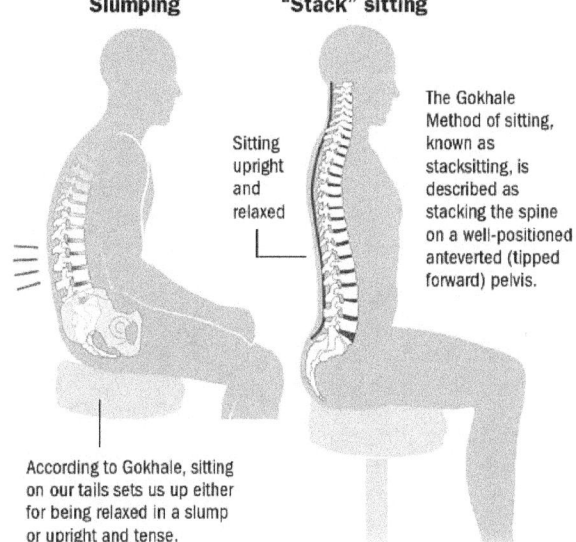

Sit up straight!
The basis of the Gokhale Method is sitting, standing, sleeping and walking the way our ancestors did. While medical professionals have expressed skepticism about Esther Gokhale's research and claims, her book has been highly praised by Amazon customers.

Slumping — Sitting upright and relaxed

"Stack" sitting — The Gokhale Method of sitting, known as stacksitting, is described as stacking the spine on a well-positioned anteverted (tipped forward) pelvis.

According to Gokhale, sitting on our tails sets us up either for being relaxed in a slump or upright and tense.

- **Stack sitting**: In order to allow the bones in your spine to stack well and permit the muscles alongside them to relax, sit with your behind sticking out behind you, but not exaggeratedly so.

  Now, when you breathe, each in-and-out breath will automatically lengthen and settle your spine. This gentle movement stimulates circulation and allows natural healing to go on even while you sit.

While conventional advice tells you to tuck in your pelvis to maintain an S-shaped spine, Esther has found that a J-spine is far more natural. A J-spine refers to a posture where your back is straight, your lumbar relatively flat, and your buttocks are protruding slightly.

By tucking your pelvis, you lose about a third of the volume in your pelvic cavity, which squishes your internal organs. This can compromise any number of them in a variety of ways. This is further compounded if you're both "tucked" and "hunched" while sitting.

- **Stretch sitting**. Another way to elongate your spine is by using your back rest as a traction device. You will need either a towel or a specially designed traction cushion for this purpose. This simple maneuver brings your back away from the back rest, lengthens your spine, and then roots you higher up against the back rest.

This position helps you maintain an elongated spine, and by getting traction on your discs, you allow them to rehydrate and prevent the nerves from being impinged between your vertebrae. It will also help flatten out your lumbar area, and this alone can sometimes provide immediate pain relief if you have sciatic nerve root pain.

I want you to please remember that sitting should be your last resort when you have no alternative.

It is far better for you to stand than sit. It might take a bit to adjust but once you do it will be every bit as comfortable as sitting.

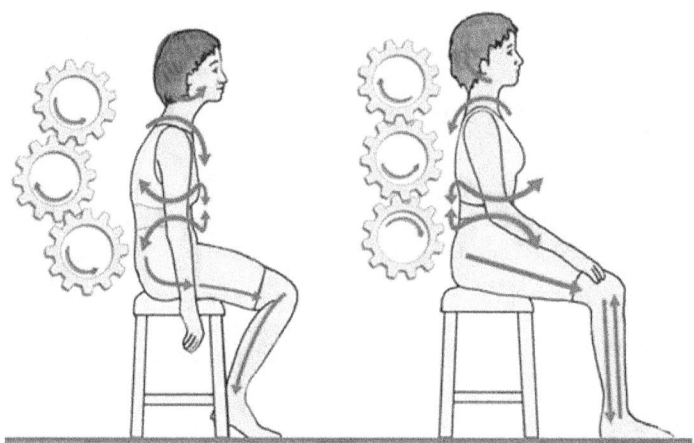

Make Walking a Part of Your Daily Routine

The evidence is overwhelming at this point—10,000 studies and growing—that prolonged sitting will reduce your lifespan by promoting dozens of chronic diseases, even if you exercise regularly.

Stand Up Every 20 Minutes

Science has previously recommended standing up and doing exercises at your desk every 10-15 minutes to counteract the ill effects of sitting, but after reading Dr. Levine's book, I'm convinced even that may be insufficient if you're seeking optimal health.

< 20 minutes	> 20 minutes
No harm done	Physiological changes

I really think or I should say that I know that the answer is to stand up as much as possible.

We should not sit longer than 20 minutes at one given time!

With that being said, I must say that I realize some people may be limited by work policies and/or other factors and eliminating sitting altogether is too lofty a goal.

I'm simply suggesting you take a closer look at how you spend your day and find ways to stand up or move more often. Especially for your Health and Wellness!

Remember, as a general rule, if you've been sitting for one hour, you've sat too long. At bare minimum, avoid sitting for more than 50 minutes out of every hour.

I believe high intensity training, non-exercise activities like walking 7,000 to 10,000 steps a day and avoiding sitting whenever possible is an ideal combination for optimizing your health. Walking is our BEST Exercise and I recommend walking in addition *to* your regular fitness regimen.

If you're currently doing *nothing* in terms of regimented exercise, walking is certainly a great place to start. For many, simply getting and staying out of your chair is a first step that can bring you closer to a healthier lifestyle. As you become more used to low level, non-exercise activity, you're more likely to get motivated enough to start exercising more vigorously.

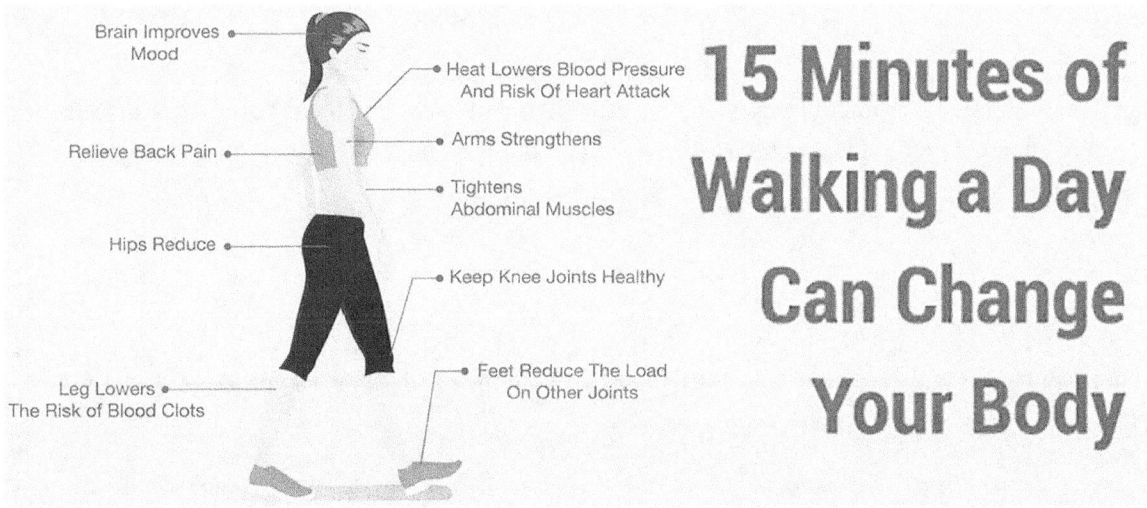

3 Quick Exercises To Combat Dangers Of Sitting Too Much

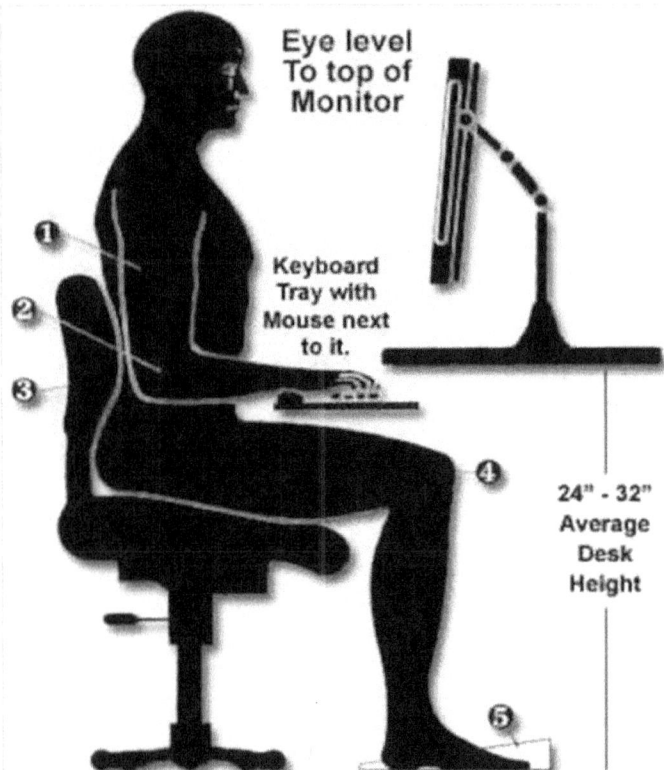

As we have discussed, Sitting too much each day has a negative impact on your health and shortens your life span. While you may not initially feel the pain, soreness, or other effects early on, there will come a point you start to feel it and wonder what happened. It's better to get in the habit of doing stretching exercises to help keep a healthy spine.

Note that these are stretching exercises not workouts. Both types of exercises are necessary for good health.

Studies have shown that even people who regularly work out can suffer from the negative impacts of sitting too many hours each day.

Common health problems that are associated with sitting too much are an increased risk of heart disease, cancer, and diabetes.

What can you do if you have to sit for hours each day?

Start doing the following basic exercises on a daily basis and you can literally Save YourSelf:

#1 Stretch Your Thoracic Spine

To stretch your thoracic spine (middle back), get on your hands and knees and then move one arm under you until your shoulder touches the ground. Hold the stretch for 30 seconds. Repeat on the other side.

#2 Stretch Your Hip Flexors

Sitting for long periods each day tightens the hip flexors. A simple way to stretch your hip flexors is to stand and lift your foot up toward your butt. Grab your foot with the hand on the same side of the body and hold for 30 seconds. Repeat with the opposite side.

#3 Stretch Your Glutes

Lastly, you need to stretch the glutes because they weaken from sitting so much as well. One way to relax the glute muscles is to sit on a foam roller and rest your ankle on your other leg above the knee. Lean back putting your weight on the same-side glute and roll around on the foam roller massaging any sore spots. Switch legs and target the other side massaging out the sore areas.

Most people are sitting too long in the day, so it's important to start doing these exercises, especially if you have a desk job. Working out regularly is not enough to protect your body from the negative impacts of sitting because physical activity does not stretch and massage those key areas: thoracic spine, hip flexors, and glutes.

The Important thing is for you to BE ACTIVE and constantly Move SomeThing ….. Move YourSelf into the Enjoyment of Your Abundant Life!

A Body IN Motion Stays IN MOTION …. Create the Motion of Your Abundant Life!

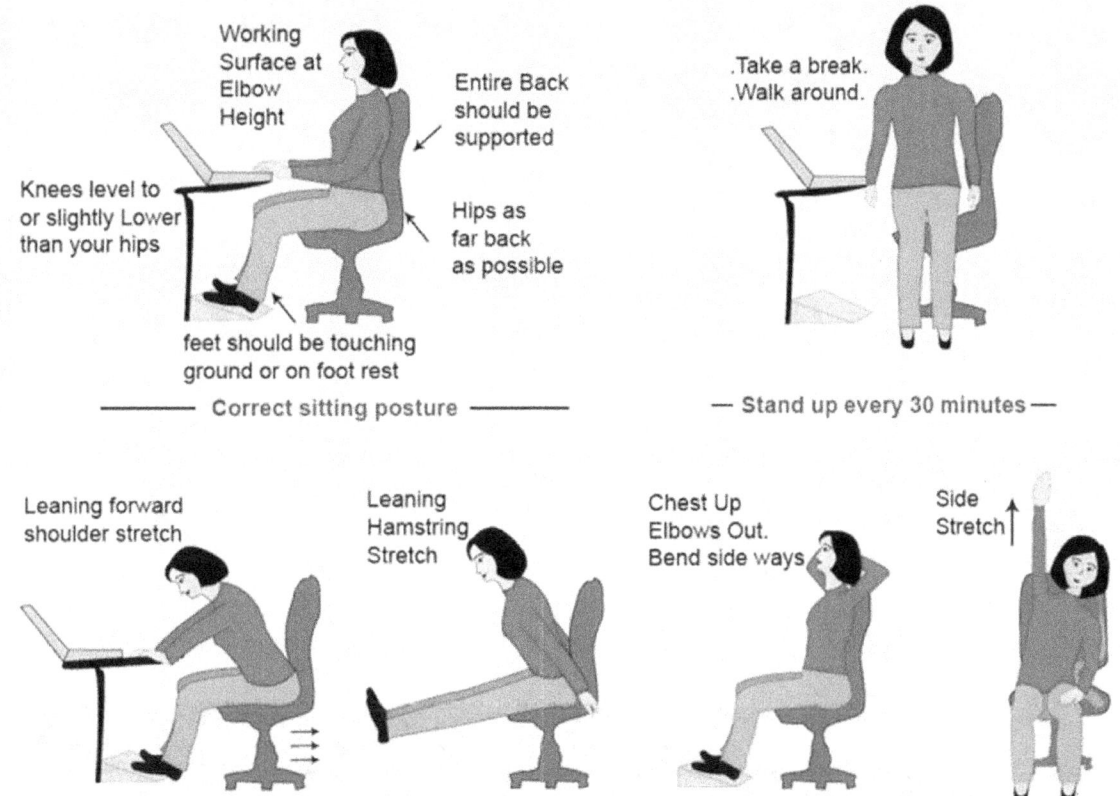

"Sitting Disease" by the numbers

Our modern sedentary lifestyles, both at home and in the workplace, are costly for us and for our employers.

WE ARE SITTING TOO MUCH

Average hours of seated commute + average hours of seated homelife = too much sitting!

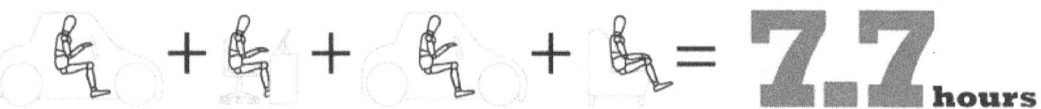

= **7.7 hours**

A 2008 Vanderbilt University study of 6,300 people published in the *American Journal of Epidemiology* estimated that the average American spends 55% of waking time (7.7 hours per day) in sedentary behaviors such as sitting.

94% more likely to die

IT IS KILLING US

MEDICAL EXPERTS HAVE STARTED REFERRING TO LONG PERIODS OF PHYSICAL INACTIVITY AND ITS NEGATIVE CONSEQUENCES AS "SITTING DISEASE."

The 2010 American Cancer Society study published in the *American Journal of Epidemiology* followed 123,216 individuals (69,776 women and 53,440 men) from 1993–2006. The alarming results:

Women who were inactive and sat over 6 hours a day were **94% more likely to die** during the time period studied than those who were physically active and sat less than 3 hours a day.

Men who were inactive and sat over 6 hours daily were **48%** more likely to die than their standing counterparts.

Findings were independent of physical activity levels (the negative effects of sitting were just as strong in people who exercised regularly).

A January 2010 *British Journal of Sports Medicine* article suggests that people who sit for long periods of time have an increased risk of disease.

In 2010 the University of Queensland, Australia, School of Population Health reported, "Even when adults meet physical activity guidelines, sitting for prolonged periods can compromise metabolic health."

3 out of 4

Full-Time Employees of Large Companies Wish They Didn't Spend Most of Their Working Hours Sitting (Ipsos study)

67% of U.S. office workers wish their employers offered them desks that could be adjusted so they could work either seated or standing. (Ipsos study)

WE WANT CHANGE

OVER HALF (~**60%**) OF EMPLOYEES SURVEYED WERE CONVINCED THEY WOULD BE MORE PRODUCTIVE IF THEY HAD THE OPTION TO WORK ON THEIR FEET. (Ipsos study)

Standing a little more each day tones muscles, improves posture, increases blood flow, ramps up metabolism and burns extra calories. Join the Uprising at www.juststand.org

Move Something!

We know sitting too much is bad, and most of us intuitively feel a little guilty after a long TV binge. But what exactly goes wrong in our bodies when we park ourselves for nearly eight hours per day, the average for a U.S. adult? Many things, say four experts, who detailed a chain of problems from head to toe.

REPORTING BY BONNIE BERKOWITZ; GRAPHIC BY PATTERSON CLARK

ORGAN DAMAGE

Heart disease
Muscles burn less fat and blood flows more sluggishly during a long sit, allowing fatty acids to more easily clog the heart. Prolonged sitting has been linked to high blood pressure and elevated cholesterol, and people with the most sedentary time are more than twice as likely to have cardiovascular disease than those with the least.

Overproductive pancreas
The pancreas produces insulin, a hormone that carries glucose to cells for energy. But cells in idle muscles don't respond as readily to insulin, so the pancreas produces more and more, which can lead to diabetes and other diseases. A 2011 study found a decline in insulin response after just one day of prolonged sitting.

Colon cancer
Studies have linked sitting to a greater risk for colon, breast and endometrial cancers. The reason is unclear, but one theory is that excess insulin encourages cell growth. Another is that regular movement boosts natural antioxidants that kill cell-damaging — and potentially cancer-causing — free radicals.

MUSCLE DEGENERATION

Mushy abs
When you stand, move or even sit up straight, abdominal muscles keep you upright. But when you slump in a chair, they go unused. Tight back muscles and weak abs form a posture-wrecking alliance that can exaggerate the spine's natural arch, a condition called hyperlordosis, or swayback.

Tight hips
Flexible hips help keep you balanced, but chronic sitters so rarely extend the hip flexor muscles in front that they become short and tight, limiting range of motion and stride length. Studies have found that decreased hip mobility is a main reason elderly people tend to fall.

Limp glutes
Sitting requires your glutes to do absolutely nothing, and they get used to it. Soft glutes hurt your stability, your ability to push off and your ability to maintain a powerful stride.

LEG DISORDERS

Poor circulation in legs
Sitting for long periods of time slows blood circulation, which causes fluid to pool in the legs. Problems range from swollen ankles and varicose veins to dangerous blood clots called deep vein thrombosis (DVT).

Soft bones
Weight-bearing activities such as walking and running stimulate hip and lower-body bones to grow thicker, denser and stronger. Scientists partially attribute the recent surge in cases of osteoporosis to lack of activity.

Mortality of sitting
People who watched the most TV in an 8.5-year study had a 61 percent greater risk of dying than those who watched less than one hour per day.
- 61%
- 33%
- 14%
- 4%

Hours of TV per day: 1-2, 3-4, 5-6, 7+

TROUBLE AT THE TOP

Foggy brain
Moving muscles pump fresh blood and oxygen through the brain and trigger the release of all sorts of brain- and mood-enhancing chemicals. When we are sedentary for a long time, everything slows, including brain function.

Strained neck
If most of your sitting occurs at a desk at work, craning your neck forward toward a keyboard or tilting your head to cradle a phone while typing can strain the cervical vertebrae and lead to permanent imbalances.

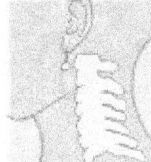
Proper alignment of cervical vertebrae

Sore shoulders and back
The neck doesn't slouch alone. Slumping forward overextends the shoulder and back muscles as well, particularly the trapezius, which connects the neck and shoulders.

BAD BACK

Inflexible spine
Spines that don't move become inflexible and susceptible to damage in mundane activities, such as when you reach for a coffee cup or bend to tie a shoe. When we move around, soft disks between vertebrae expand and contract like sponges, soaking up fresh blood and nutrients. When we sit for a long time, disks are squashed unevenly and lose sponginess. Collagen hardens around supporting tendons and ligaments.

Disk damage
People who sit more are at greater risk for herniated lumbar disks. A muscle called the psoas travels through the abdominal cavity and, when it tightens, pulls the upper lumbar spine forward. Upper-body weight rests entirely on the ischial tuberosity (sitting bones) instead of being distributed along the arch of the spine.

Lumbar region bowed by shortened psoas

THE RIGHT WAY TO SIT
If you have to sit often, try to do it correctly. As Mom always said: "Sit up straight."
- Not leaning forward
- Shoulders relaxed
- Elbows bent 90 degrees
- Arms close to sides
- Lower back may be supported
- Feet flat on floor

So what can we do? The experts recommend...

Sitting on something wobbly such as an exercise ball or even a backless stool to force core muscles to work. Sit up straight and keep your feet flat on the floor in front of you so they support about a quarter of your weight.

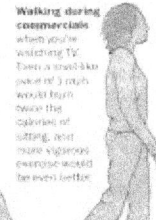
Stretching the hip flexors for three minutes per side once a day, like this.

Walking during commercials when you're watching TV. Even a snail-like pace of 1 mph would burn twice the calories of sitting, and more vigorous exercise would be even better.

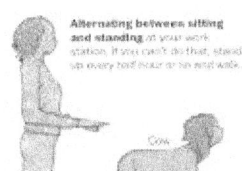
Alternating between sitting and standing at your work station. If you can't do that, stand up every half hour or so and walk.

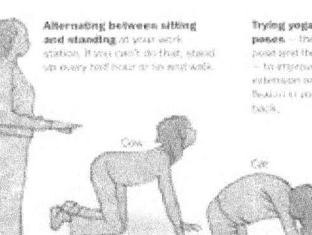
Trying yoga poses — the cow pose and the cat — to improve extension and flexion of your back.

Cow / Cat

The experts
Scientists interviewed for this report:

James A. Levine, inventor of the treadmill desk and director of Obesity Solutions at Mayo Clinic and Arizona State University

Charles E. Matthews, National Cancer Institute investigator and author of several studies on sedentary behavior

Jay Dicharry, director of the REP Biomechanics Lab in Bend, Ore., and author of Anatomy for Runners

Tal Amasay, biomechanist at Barry University's Department of Sport and Exercise Sciences

---

Supreme Health & Fitness!   Health & Wellness Series ... Vol 3!

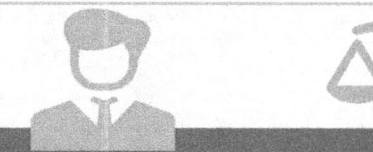  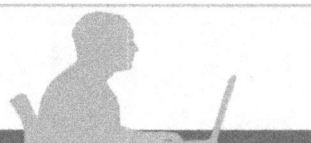

STANDING vs. SITTING

✓ Burns more calories and improves circulation.

✓ Conventional comfort preventing achy legs.

✗ Standing solutions are often expensive.

✗ Puts pressure on your spine and promotes obesity.

In a 24 hour period, we typically spend:

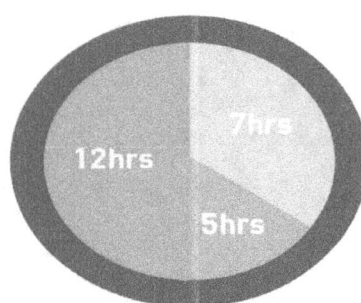

- Sitting — 7hrs
- Sleeping — 12hrs
- Active — 5hrs

Studies Have Shown...

That we have a better ability to concentrate whilst being seated. However, this ability is reduced for every hour of continual sitting. Therefore a mixture of sitting and standing throughout the day achieves optimal cognitive function.

Studies conducted by M.C. Schraefel and Kenneth J. Andersen at the University of Southampton, UK (2012)

An 8-hour working day...

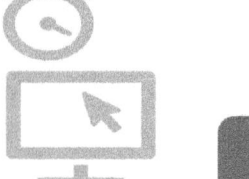

1530 Cals

Risk of cardiovascular disease drops by **50%**

354 Calories

1176 Cals

Over the course of a year, a person standing up burns over 92,000 calories more than one sitting down. That's the equivalent of doing 38 marathons a year!

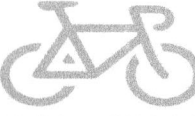 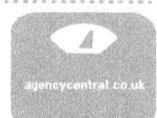 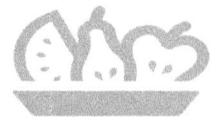

Stay Active | Stay Aware | Stay Healthy

Move Something!

Is Sitting Down Getting You Down?

1 in 2 Americans sits 6+ hours per day

9.3 HOURS — The amount an average person spends sitting each day

2 in 3 Americans watch 2+ hours of TV per day

increase in sitting **8%** From Year 1980 To Year 2000

80% of jobs require no physical activity

Stand Up to Health Concerns
Common conditions associated with sitting too much

- Neck and back pain
- Heart disease
- Degenerative disc disease
- Stroke
- Diabetes
- Cancer
- Hip pain
- Muscle stiffness
- Poor balance and mobility

1 in 10 premature deaths worldwide is caused by lack of exercise

That's as many deaths as smoking cigarettes causes!

Fight Back on Your Feet

Decrease daily sitting
Sitting under 3 hours per day increases lifespan **by 2 years**

54% Sitting most of the day increases risk of dying from a heart attack by 54%

Break up sedentary periods with walks
- Stand up every 15 minutes
- Walk 10 minutes for every hour of sitting

Replace your office chair
- Adjust desk to work while standing
  - You burn 10–60 calories more per hour of standing than sitting!
- Sit on an exercise ball
  - Forces good posture for back health
  - Promotes movement

Turn off the TV
Men who watch 3+ hours of TV per day have a 64% higher chance of dying from heart attack

Risk increases 11% with each additional hour of TV

Supreme Health & Fitness! — *Health & Wellness Series ... Vol 3!*

Chapter Four

Pre-Mature Death Risk Factors - Lack of Exercise & Obesity

*****

- New data suggests at least twice as many deaths occur due to a lack of exercise than due to obesity
- A brisk 20-minute walk each day may reduce your risk of premature death by up to 30 percent

Would you take a brisk 20-minute walk each day if you knew it could reduce your risk of premature death by up to 30 percent? Well… lace up your walking shoes, because that's what scientists from the University of Cambridge revealed.

Everyone in the study benefited from the modest increase in physical activity, regardless of whether they were normal weight, overweight, or obese.

In fact, the researchers believe that increasing exercise is even more important than reducing obesity in terms of public health.

Their data suggests that at least twice as many deaths occur due to a lack of exercise than due to obesity.

This is really astounding, considering one in five US deaths are associated with obesity.

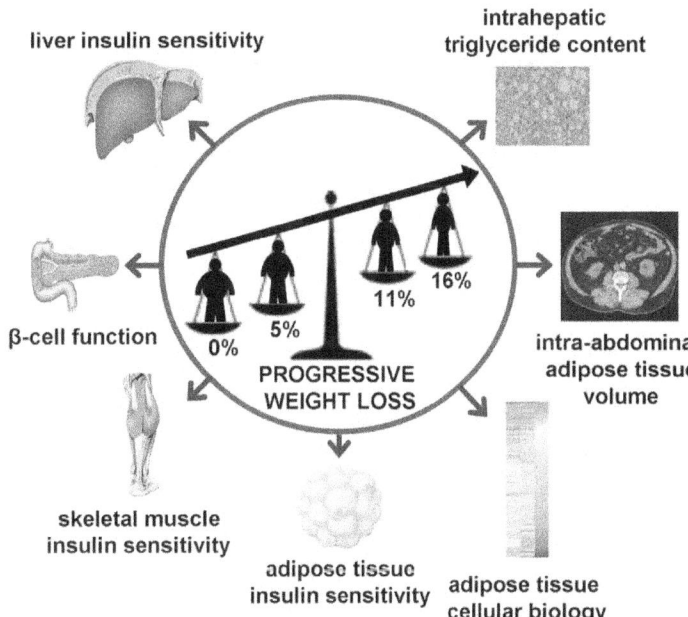

The studies author, Ulf Ekelund, from the Medical Research Council Epidemiology Unit at the University of Cambridge told *TIME*.

"This is a simple message: just a small amount of physical activity each day could have substantial health benefits for people who are physically inactive."

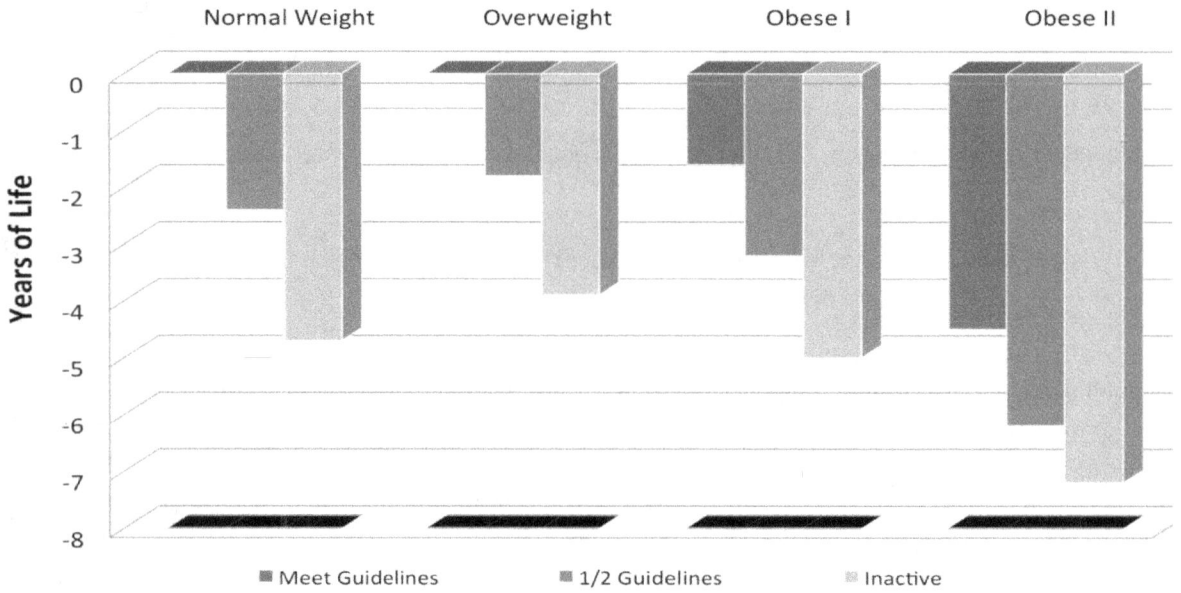

Obese class I = BMI 30-34.9 Obese class II = BMI 35+

If You Want to Live Longer... Move SomeThing!

If you are currently living a sedentary lifestyle, the mere act of incorporating some moderate activity most days of the week can **significantly** reduce your mortality rate…. That means extending your LIFE!

Past research showed that just meeting the LOW minimum requirement of 30 minutes of moderate physical activity a day, five days a week, can reduce your risk of death *from any cause* by 19 percent.

Those who engaged in moderate intensity activity even more -- a full seven days a week -- further reduced their risk of death, from 19 to 24 percent. A separate study also found that, compared to those who exercised daily and often vigorously, sedentary people had a six times greater risk of dying from heart disease over the course of 15 years.

Increasing to a minimum of completing at least 60 minutes (just 420 minutes a week) a day of Cardiovascular Aerobics as your base, will allow you to create the environment in yourself that will give your body the Motion and energy it needs to make your Life-Span LIMITLESS!

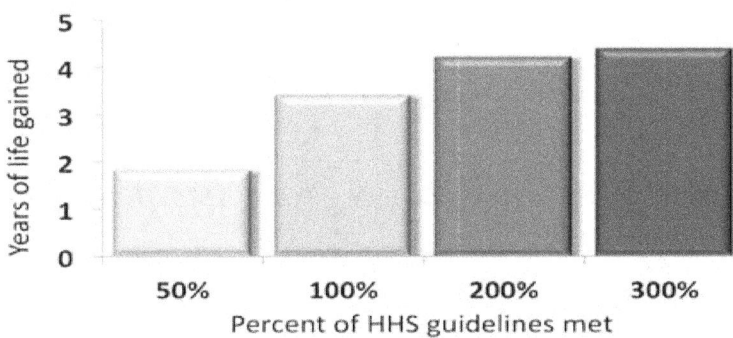

The greatest gains are often seen among people who go from being sedentary to physically activity, although benefits also increase with exercise frequency and intensity (to a point, of course, as overdoing it will backfire).

As Samantha Heller, an exercise physiologist at New York University Medical Center, told CBS News:

"If you look at the human body, you will notice the odd, irregular shapes of the bones and muscles. Just the musculoskeletal architecture of the human body shows that it is designed to move. The adaptations the body makes to regular exercise are nothing short of 'astounding," she said.

Aerobic exercise ignites the body's immune system, improves mental function, boosts energy, strengthens muscles and bones, and reduces the risk for chronic diseases such as heart disease, cancer and diabetes, she said.

'If we do not move, we will not be able to move,' Heller said. 'Gee, I am so sorry I exercised today' is something no one has ever said."

Exercise Improves the Quality of Your Life, Not Just the Quantity

Part of what makes exercise so useful is that it not only extends your life but also adds quality of life to those extra years. All of those movements that you might now take for granted – walking up and down stairs, carrying in groceries, climbing a ladder to change a light bulb – can start to become more difficult by the time you're in your 70s.

This is when sarcopenia (age-related muscle loss) tends to accelerate.

You might start to feel weaker and find you can't do things, physically, that you used to do. But exercise can *change* that by helping you to maintain your muscle mass and strength (and even *increase* your muscle size).

At the same time, exercise lowers your risk of chronic diseases so much that researchers described it as "the best preventive drug" for many common ailments, from psychiatric disorders to heart disease, diabetes, and cancer.

A body IN Motion STAYS IN MOTION ….. A Body At-Rest STAYS AT-REST ….. WHICH ONE ARE YOU?

YOU CAN PUT YOURSELF IN MOTION TO STAY IN MOTION = YOUR ABUNDANT LIFE!

Psychological Benefits of Physical Activity

- Improves health-related quality of life.
- Improves one's mood.
- Alleviates symptoms associated with mild depression.
- Reduces anxiety.
- Aids in managing stress.
- Enhances self-concept, self-esteem, self-efficacy, and self-confidence.
- Offers opportunities for affiliation with others.

Your Entire Body Benefits from Exercise

Numerous beneficial biochemical changes occur during exercise, including alterations in more than 20 different metabolites involved in fat burning and metabolism, among other things, like optimizing insulin/leptin receptor sensitivity. As stated by Dr. Timothy Church, director of preventive medicine research at the Pennington Biomedical Research Center in Baton Rouge, exercise indeed affects *your entire body*—from head to toe—in beneficial ways.

This includes changes in your:

- **Muscles**, which use glucose and ATP for contraction and movement. Tiny tears in your muscles make them grow bigger and stronger as they heal. Gaining more muscle through resistance exercises has many benefits, from losing excess fat to maintaining healthy bone mass and preventing age-related muscle loss as you age. The *intensity* of your resistance training can achieve a number of beneficial changes on the molecular, enzymatic, hormonal, and chemical level in your body.

- **Lungs**. As your muscles call for more oxygen, your breathing rate increases. The higher your VO2 max—your maximum capacity of oxygen use—the fitter you are.

- **Heart.** Your heart rate increases with physical activity to supply more oxygenated blood to your muscles. The fitter you are, the more efficiently your heart can do this, allowing you to work out longer and harder.

    Your blood pressure will also decrease as a result of new blood vessels forming.

- **Brain.** The increased blood flow also benefits your brain, allowing it to almost immediately function better. Exercising regularly also promotes the growth of new brain cells, boosting your capacity for memory and learning. A number of neurotransmitters are also triggered, such as endorphins, serotonin, dopamine, glutamate, and GABA. Some of these are well-known for their role in mood control. Exercise, in fact, is one of the most effective prevention and treatment strategies for depression.

- **Joints and Bones.** Exercise can place as much as five or six times more than your body weight on them which builds them to become Stronger! Weight-bearing exercise is one of the most effective remedies against osteoporosis, as your bones are very porous and soft. If you **don't** apply the science of Eating To Live, then as you get older your bones can easily become less dense and more brittle -- especially if you are also inactive.

Are You Sedentary? Try This to Get More Movement

Unfortunately, OVER more than half of American men, and 60 percent of American women, *never* engage in *any* vigorous physical activity lasting more than 10 minutes per week.

I believe high-intensity exercises are an important part of a healthy lifestyle, however perhaps equally important is simply *moving* more while sitting less.

PHYSICAL
- Better health
- Improved quality of life
- Improved fitness
- Better posture
- Better balance
- Stronger heart
- Fight off illnesses better
- Weight control
- Stronger muscles
- Stronger bones

MENTAL
- Reduce depression
- Reduce anxiety
- Reduce and prevent stress
- Sleep better
- Increase cognitive functioning
- Increase mental alertness
- Feeling more energetic
- Relaxation

SOCIAL
- Social integration
- Meet new people
- Build social skills
- Strengthen relationships
- Enjoy others' company
- Increase family time
- Build new friendships

EMOTIONAL
- Increase feelings of happiness
- Positive mood & affect
- Increase feeling of self-worth
- Better self-esteem
- Better self-confidence
- Increase feelings of success
- Lower sadness
- Lower tension
- Lower anger

Let's Test YourSelf!

I recommend using a pedometer, or something similar to keep track of your daily movement. At first, you may be surprised to realize just how little you move each day. This way you can successfully correct your exercise imbalance!

Sitting really is the new smoking, as sitting more than 8 hours a day will actually increase your risk of lung cancer by over 50%, far worse than exposure to second-hand smoke.

Setting a small goal of 7,000 to 10,000 steps a day (which is just over three to five miles, or 6-9 kilometers) can go a long way toward getting more movement into your life.

If you fit in your 7,000 to 10,000 steps a day, you'll enjoy a significant health boost. One study found that walking for two miles a day or more can cut your chances of hospitalization from a severe episode of chronic obstructive pulmonary disease (COPD) by about half.

Another study found that daily walking reduced the risk of stroke in men over the age of 60. Walking for at least an hour or two could cut a man's stroke risk by as much as one-third, and it didn't matter how brisk the pace was. Taking a three-hour long walk each day slashed the risk by two-thirds. As you become accustomed to this regular movement, you can then add in high-intensity interval training (HIIT), which will allow you to reap all the rewards that exercise has to offer. Personally, I seek to walk between 13,000 and 16,000 steps, or 7 to 9 miles a day. I use this uninterrupted quiet time to read about one new book a week.

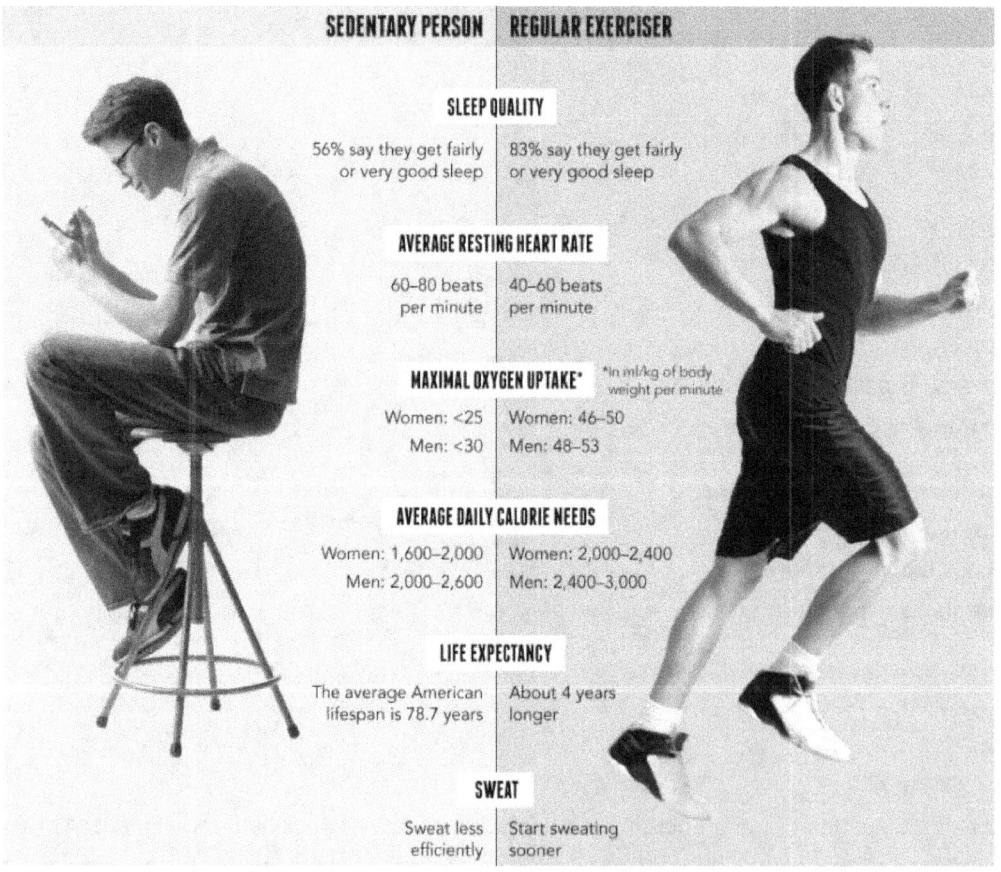

Optimize Your Exercise Benefits with High-Intensity Movements

Walking 7,000-10,000 steps is, ideally, *in addition to*, not in place of, your normal exercise program. This might sound like a lot, but when you incorporate HIIT into your workouts, you get the benefits in a fraction of the time. HIIT such as Peak Fitness mimics the movements of our hunter-gatherer ancestors, which included short bursts of high-intensity activities, but *not* long-distance running. This, researchers say, is what your body is hard-wired for. Basically, by exercising in short bursts, followed by periods of recovery, you recreate exactly what your body needs for optimum health.

Twice-weekly sessions, which require no more than 20 minutes from start to finish, can help you:

- Lower your body fat
- Improve your muscle tone
- Boost your energy and libido
- Improve athletic speed and performance
- Naturally increase your body's production of human growth hormone (HGH)—a synergistic, foundational biochemical underpinning that promotes health and longevity

Can you find 20 minutes twice a week to lower your risk of chronic disease, feel better, and live longer?

I thought so ….. OF COURSE YOU CAN!

All you have to DO is Move something!

What Are You Moving?

YourSelf!

Where Are You Going?

Your Abundant Life!

LET'S GO!!!!

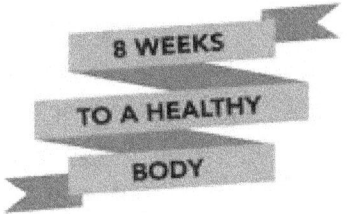

8 WEEKS TO A HEALTHY BODY

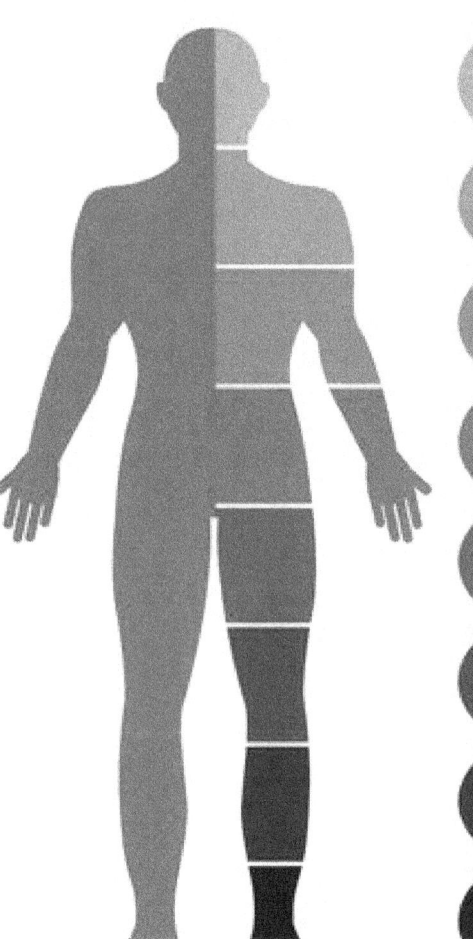

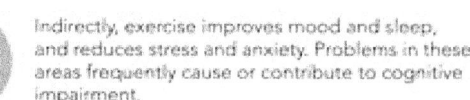
Indirectly, exercise improves mood and sleep, and reduces stress and anxiety. Problems in these areas frequently cause or contribute to cognitive impairment.

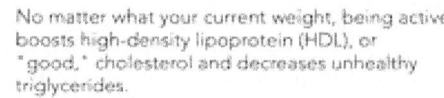
No matter what your current weight, being active boosts high-density lipoprotein (HDL), or "good," cholesterol and decreases unhealthy triglycerides.

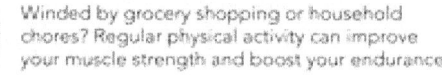
Winded by grocery shopping or household chores? Regular physical activity can improve your muscle strength and boost your endurance.

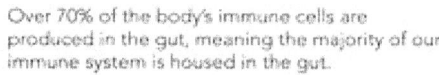
Over 70% of the body's immune cells are produced in the gut, meaning the majority of our immune system is housed in the gut.

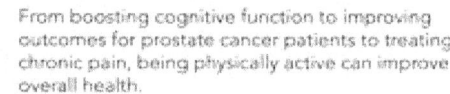
From boosting cognitive function to improving outcomes for prostate cancer patients to treating chronic pain, being physically active can improve overall health.

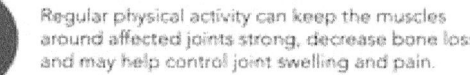
Regular physical activity can keep the muscles around affected joints strong, decrease bone loss and may help control joint swelling and pain.

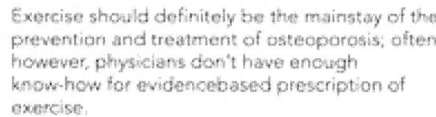
Exercise should definitely be the mainstay of the prevention and treatment of osteoporosis; often however, physicians don't have enough know-how for evidencebased prescription of exercise.

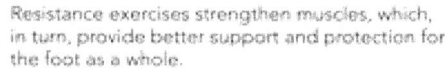
Resistance exercises strengthen muscles, which, in turn, provide better support and protection for the foot as a whole.

Move Some(Thing)!

THE BRAIN BENEFITS OF EXERCISE

- INCREASES PRODUCTION OF NEUROCHEMICALS THAT PROMOTE BRAIN CELL REPAIR
- IMPROVES MEMORY
- LENGTHENS ATTENTION SPAN
- BOOSTS DECISION-MAKING SKILLS
- PROMPTS GROWTH OF NEW NERVE CELLS AND BLOOD VESSELS
- IMPROVES MULTI-TASKING AND PLANNING

Move Something!

WHAT CAN EXERCISE DO TO YOUR BRAIN?

Only 20 minutes of exercise can provide many benefits.

LEARNING
A 2012 study found that even one exercise session can help you retain physical skills by enhancing what's commonly known as "muscle memory" or "motor memory".

LONG TERM MEMORY
Weightlifting for as little as 20 minutes can boost your long-term memory by 10%. Exercise releases the stress hormone norepinephrine, a chemical messenger in the brain that plays a strong role in memory.

REDUCE DEPRESSION RISK
Exercise boosts the body's production of PGC-1alpha, which breaks down depression-causing kynurenine. Researchers have concluded that you reduce the risk of getting depression when you exercise.

BETTER, FASTER, STRONGER
Recent research from the University of Illinois shows that the brain's white matter becomes more fibrous and compact with physical exercise. The more streamlined and compact your white matter is, the faster and more efficiently your brain functions.

HEAD AND HEART
Exercise is good for cardiovascular health, which benefits brain functioning- a healthy heart is better at pumping blood and oxygen to the brain. A recent study found that older adults who exercised more and whose aortas were in better condition performed better on cognitive tests.

BOOST CREATIVITY
Researchers at Stanford University found that walking can increase creativity up to 60%.

Supreme Health & Fitness! *Health & Wellness Series ... Vol 3!*

Breathing during exercise

Muscle cell respiration increases – more oxygen is used up and levels of CO_2 rise.

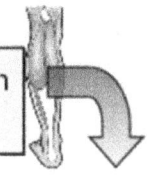

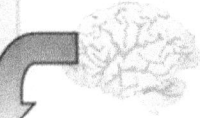

The brain detects increasing levels of CO_2 – a signal is sent to the lungs to increase breathing.

Breathing rate and the volume of air in each breath increase. This means that more gaseous exchange takes place.

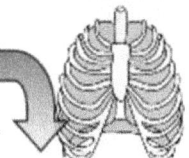

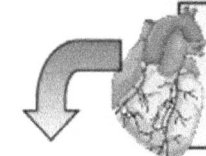

The brain also tells the heart to beat faster so that more blood is pumped to the lungs for gaseous exchange.

More oxygenated blood gets to the muscles and more CO_2 is removed.

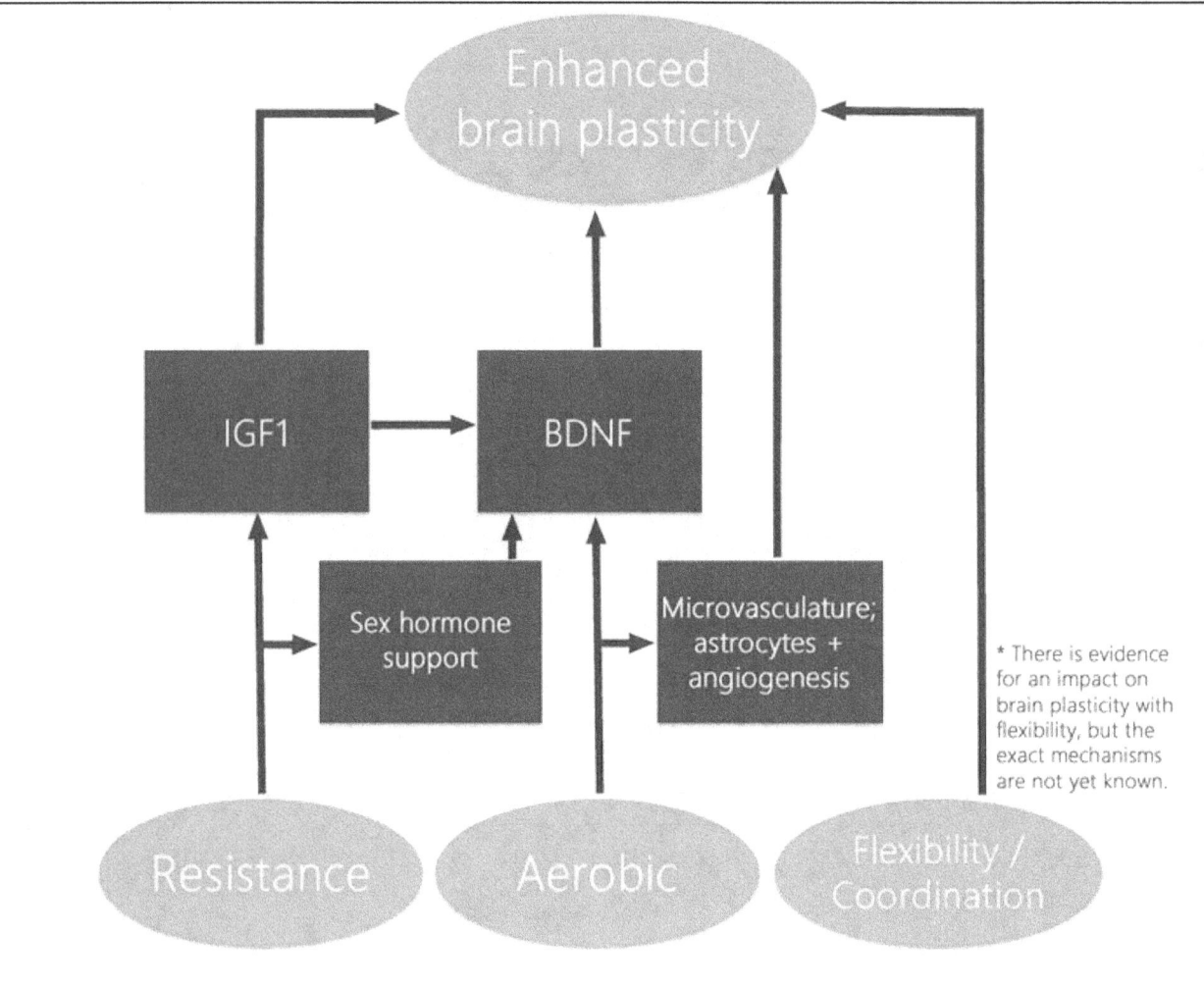

Chapter Five

Exercise and Your Brain Health & Power

*****

Scientists have been linking physical exercise to brain health for many years. In fact, compelling evidence shows that physical exercise helps build a brain that not only resists shrinkage but increases cognitive abilities.

For example, we now know that exercise promotes a process known as neurogenesis, i.e. your brain's ability to adapt and grow new brain cells, regardless of your age.

This means you can Move YourSelf to Build your Brain!

The featured article in *Real Simple*, magazine highlights a number of brain-boosting benefits of exercise, including the following.

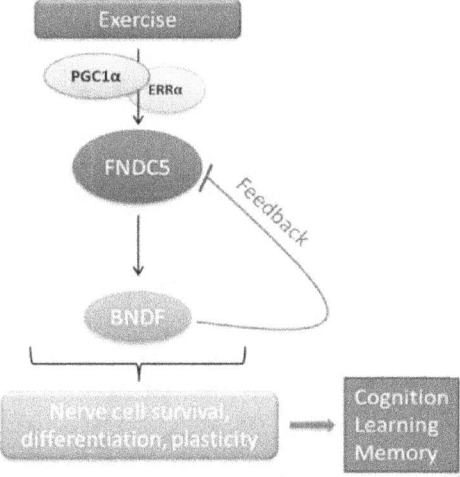

Exercise Shields You from Stress and Depression

Exercise is one of the "secret weapons" to overcoming depression, and studies have shown its efficiency typically surpasses that of antidepressant drugs. In fact, research has shown that in most cases these drugs *work no better than a placebo* – and can also have serious side effects.

One of the ways exercise promotes mental health is by normalizing insulin resistance and boosting natural "feel good" hormones and neurotransmitters associated with mood control, including endorphins, serotonin, dopamine, glutamate and GABA.

Swedish researchers have also teased out the mechanism by which exercise helps reduce stress and related depression. As it turns out, mice with well-trained muscles have higher levels of an enzyme that helps metabolize a stress chemical called **kynurenine**.

Their finding suggests that exercising your muscles actually helps rid your body of stress chemicals that can lead to depression. According to the authors:

"Our initial research hypothesis was that trained muscle would produce a substance with beneficial effects on the brain. We actually found the opposite: well-trained muscle produces an enzyme that purges the body of harmful substances. So, in this context the muscle's function is reminiscent of that of the kidney or the liver."

Recent research has also shown the clear links between inactivity and depression. Women who sat for more than seven hours a day were found to have a 47 percent higher risk of depression than women who sat for four hours or less per day. Those who didn't participate in any physical activity at all had a **99 percent** higher risk of developing depression than women who exercised.

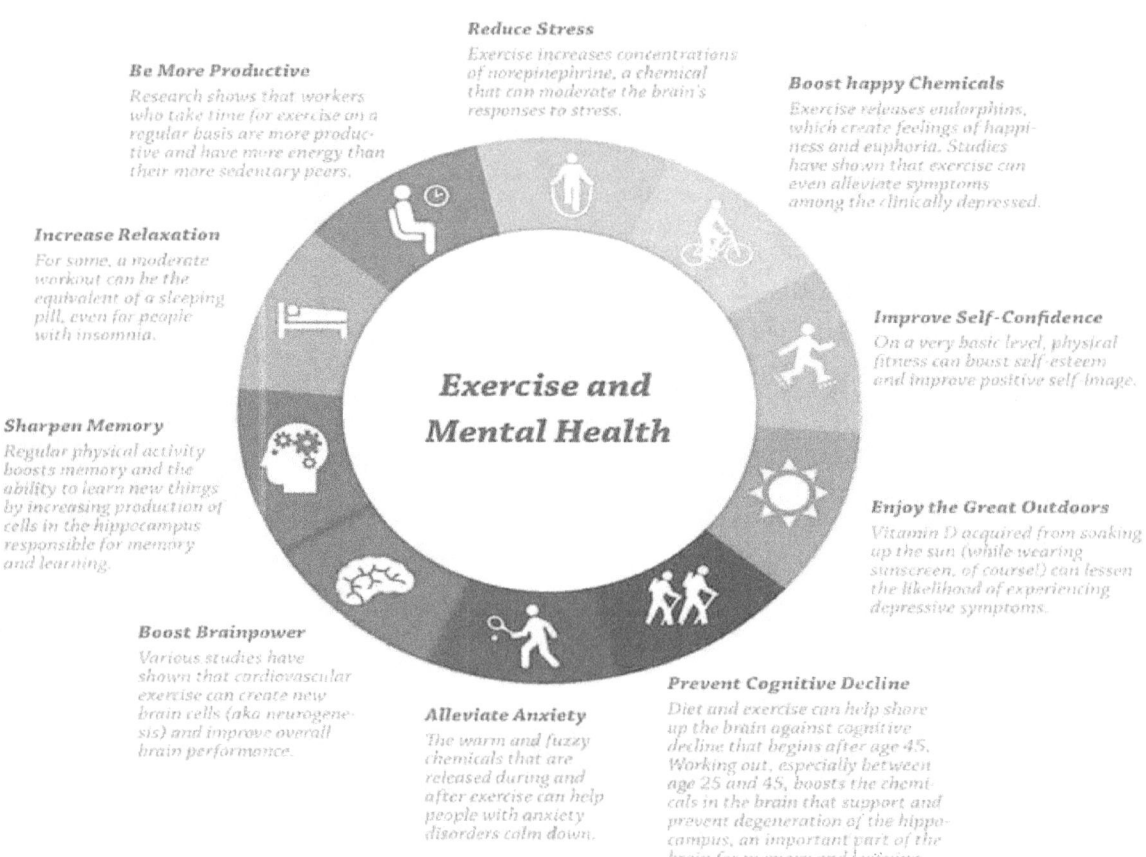

To Boost Creativity, Get Moving!

As noted in the featured article, exercise can also boost your creativity, and help you come up with new solutions to problems. For example, researchers at Stanford University found that walking can increase creativity up to 60 percent. Even a casual stroll around your office can be helpful.

According to the authors:

"Four experiments demonstrate that walking boosts creative ideation in real time and shortly after... Walking opens up the free flow of ideas, and it is a simple and robust solution to the goals of increasing creativity and increasing physical activity."

Exercise Boosts Brain Growth and Regeneration

As mentioned earlier, fascinating research shows that your brain is capable of rejuvenating and regenerating itself throughout your life. This information is completely contrary to what I was taught in medical school. At that time, it was believed that once neurons die, there's nothing you can do about it. Hence deterioration and progressive memory decline was considered a more or less inevitable part of aging. **Fortunately, that's simply not true.**

According to John J. Ratey, a psychiatrist who wrote the book *Spark: The Revolutionary New Science of Exercise and the Brain*, there's overwhelming evidence that exercise produces large cognitive gains and helps fight dementia. The featured article cites research showing that those who exercise have a greater volume of gray matter in the hippocampal region of their brains, which is important for memory.

According to the authors:

"After controlling for age, gender, and total brain volume, total minutes of weekly exercise correlated significantly with volume of the right hippocampus. Findings highlight the relationship between regular physical exercise and brain structure during early to middle adulthood."

Exercise also prevents age-related shrinkage of your brain, preserving both gray and white matter in your frontal, temporal, and parietal cortexes, thereby preventing cognitive deterioration.

The authors stated that:

"These results suggest that cardiovascular fitness is associated with the sparing of brain tissue in aging humans. Furthermore, these results suggest a strong biological basis for the role of aerobic fitness in maintaining and enhancing central nervous system health and cognitive functioning in older adults."

Similar findings have been found by other scientists.

For example, one observational study that followed more than 600 seniors, starting at age 70, found that those who engaged in the most physical exercise showed the least amount of brain shrinkage over a follow-up period of three years.

Exercise and Your Capillary Density

In general, exercise improves the heart's ability to pump blood and increases the natural ability of blood to carry oxygen to cells throughout the body. With exercise, blood circulation to the brain is thus increased and the brain receives more oxygen and glucose, both of which are crucial to brain function. The brain is the body's most active organ and it requires the most energy. Although it accounts for only 2% of our body weight, it uses between 20% and 30% of the body's energy.

Despite this need for a large amount of energy, the brain can not store any oxygen or glucose. It is therefore necessary for the blood stream to deliver a constant supply of these essential substances, and it does this by circulating continuously through the brain.

A person can feel a lack of oxygen after only a few seconds. When you stand up too quickly and become dizzy, this is an example of loss of blood flow to the brain that can be sensed.

Diabetics who give themselves too much insulin can drop their blood sugar level and faint, and can die unless they quickly increase the level of glucose in the brain. Adequate blood circulation and the vast network of blood vessels that serve the brain and allow for blood flow are thus critical. The 400 miles of blood vessels in the human brain have a surface area of approximately 100 square feet.

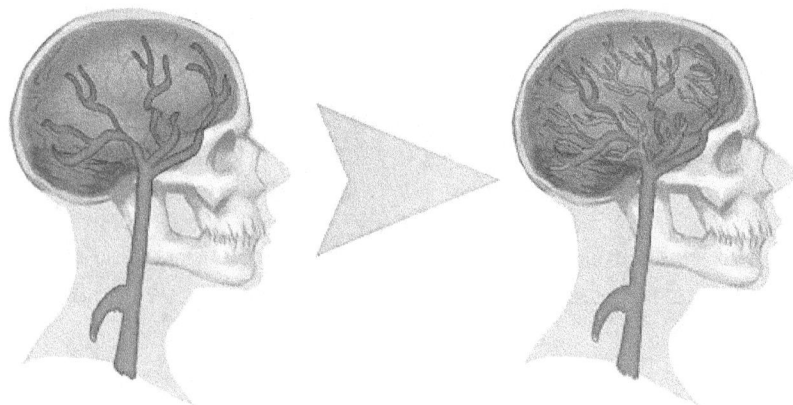

Angiogenesis - the formation of new blood vessels - can occur even in adulthood and is correlated with neurogenesis.

The health of these vessel walls is very important for proper brain function. In addition to delivering a constant supply of oxygen, glucose, and other important nutrients to the brain, blood flow to and from the brain also removes harmful toxins. So overall, having a proper functioning vascular(blood vessel) system is absolutely necessary for optimal brain health and functioning.

When blood flow to the brain is increased, the body responds by forming new blood vessels to bring the extra blood to nerve cells. This process, known as **angiogenesis**, is directly connected to neurogenesis, the process of making new nerve cells.

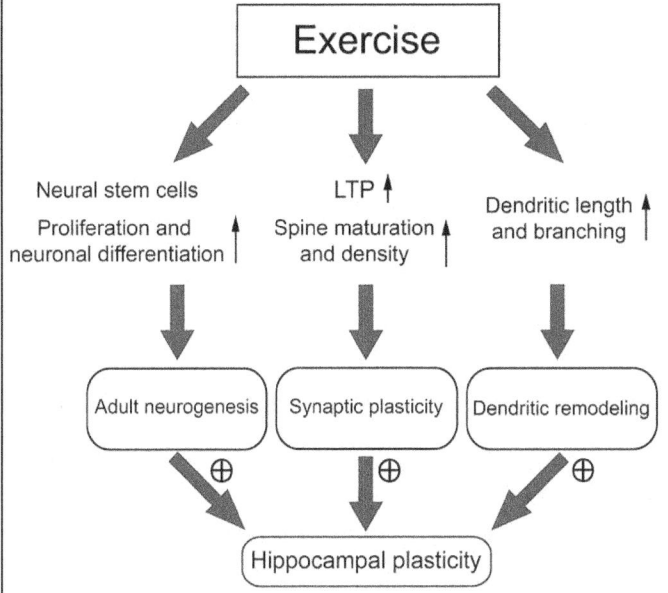

It was initially believed that angiogenesis, much like neurogenesis, was limited to certain periods of development or in response to pathological insults. It has since been discovered that angiogenesis naturally occurs when physical activity is increased, and can be induced by exposure to a complex environment or exercise.

Therefore, the formation of new blood vessels is not restricted to developmental periods but extends into mature adulthood and beyond.

For example, in the dentate gyrus, a brain structure that experiences a great amount of neurodegeneration on account of HD, new nerve cells are clustered close to blood vessels.

These nerve cells can only grow and be healthy when there is enough blood flow to the brain.

This means you DON'T have to grow old!

This means you CAN STAY YOUNG!

This means you Can Successfully Enjoy Your Abundant Life!

Researchers believe that decreased blood flow to the brain as a result of fewer blood vessels contributes to the decline in new cell production among older individuals. Moreover, exercise has been shown to increase angiogenesis and nerve cell proliferation throughout the brain in various animal models like mice and fruit flies.

It turns out that there is a good reason why exercise seems to "clear your head." Your heart rate increases as you exercise, increasing blood flow to the brain, which enhances waste removal and provides much-needed oxygen and glucose.

You can literally Move YourSelf into Mental Health, Clarity and Wellness!

All you have to Do is Move YourSelf!

In a test, students had a one-minute blast of oxygen given to them immediately before being given a list of words to remember. On average, the students who took the oxygen remembered two to three more words from a list of 15 than those who did not. Students who took oxygen while playing the Tetris computer game on its most demanding level were also shown to play significantly better.

Composite of 20 student brains taking the same test

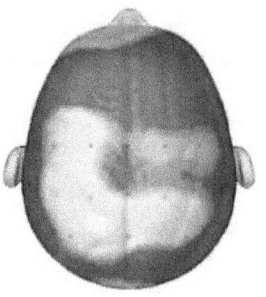 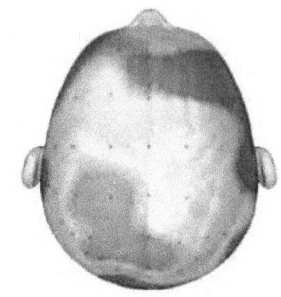

After sitting quietly After 20 minute walk

Exercise can act very similarly to having a one minute blast of oxygen. If performed on a consistent basis, exercise has the effect of providing a dose of continuous oxygen to the brain, such that the cognitive boosts can be continually maintained as well.

The increase in blood circulation because of exercise can induce the formation of new blood vessels that can, in turn, facilitate the creation of new nerve cells.

You Can Grow Your Brain!

Exercise and Your Cognitive Maintenance

Even people who do not have HD experience a moderate amount of neurodegeneration as part of the normal aging process. Here, the signals that nerve cells use to communicate with one another become less powerful and less efficient. This decreased ability for nerve cells to communicate makes it harder for the brain to adapt to outside influences and generate new nerve cells.

The inability to create new nerve cells leads to losses in brain tissue and impaired functioning. Indeed, imaging studies in elderly humans have shown some noticeable atrophy in the brain.

One of the consequences of atrophy is that older adults typically perform more poorly than younger adults on a broad range of cognitive measures.

Despite such declines in cognitive and motor processes during the course of aging in people, recent findings suggest that physical exercise can minimize some, but not all, kinds of cognitive decline.

A recent study showed that older adults who exercised throughout life had less brain tissue loss and performed significantly better on cognitive tests than adults who exercised infrequently.

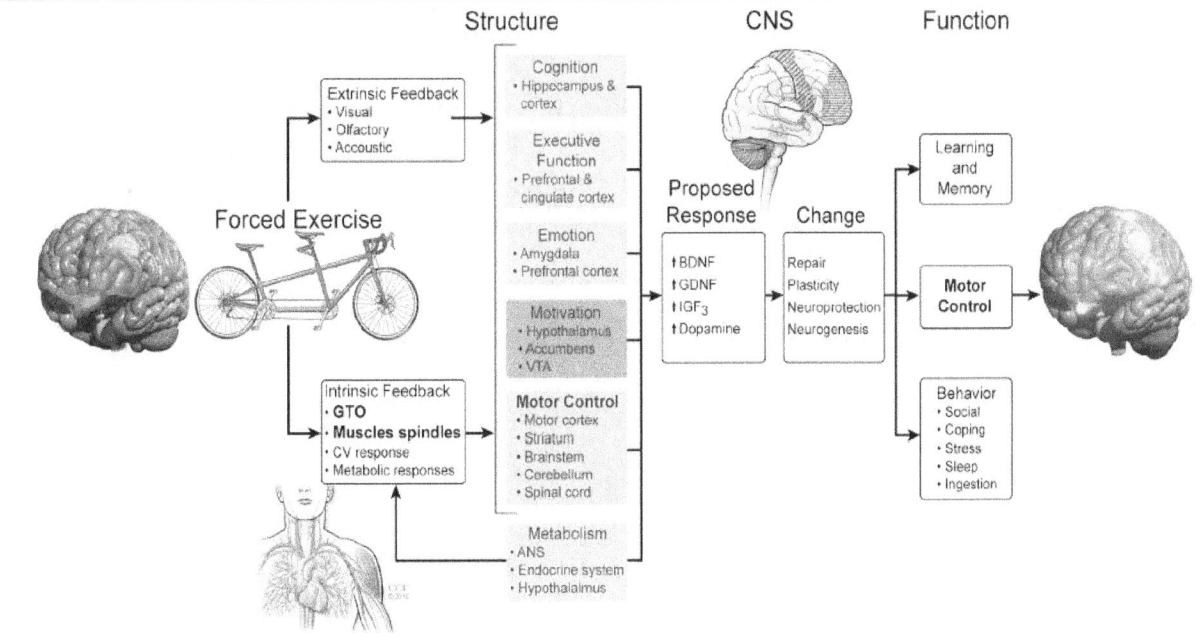

It turns out that the areas in your brain that are associated with mental decline due to aging are the same areas that are the most responsive to exercise.

Researchers have found that people who exercise a lot have more gray matter and white matter in the brain, particularly in the frontal lobe, temporal lobe, and parietal lobe. The lobes of your brain are composed of both gray matter and white matter.

Gray matter is where all your nerve centers are located.

White matter connects your gray matter together.

The amount of gray matter and white matter declines naturally, affecting the functioning of the lobes and contributing to a decline in cognitive functioning and processing ability.

Your frontal lobes of the brain have a lot to do with what people call higher-level cognition, where we synthesize information, and store data we've just acquired. If the frontal lobes are not functioning properly, then you can easily forget a phone number you just looked up or the name of a person you just met.

Your temporal lobes consolidate short-term memories and build them into long-term memories. Damage to temporal lobes can also result in altered personality and affective behavior.

Your parietal lobes allow us to construct a spatial coordinate system to represent the world around us. Damage to the parietal lobes can result in neglecting part of the body or space, which can impair many self-care skills such as dressing and washing.

Deterioration of each of these lobes is associated with some sort of mental decline.

Exercise appears to exert its effects partially by protecting against a loss of gray matter and white matter, thereby preserving the structure and function of the lobes in your brain.

With your lobes able to function better, the onset and progression of various cognitive deficits are likely to be delayed.

Rule #1: Exercise boosts brain power.

- Best business meeting: walking at about 1.8 miles per hour.
- Aerobic exercise improves executive functions. No need to run triathlons.
- Exercise improves cognition for two reasons:
  - Increases oxygen flow into the brain
  - Acts directly on the molecular machinery of the brain itself

Studies on exercise reveal that it DOES indeed play an influential role in slowing down your cognitive decline.

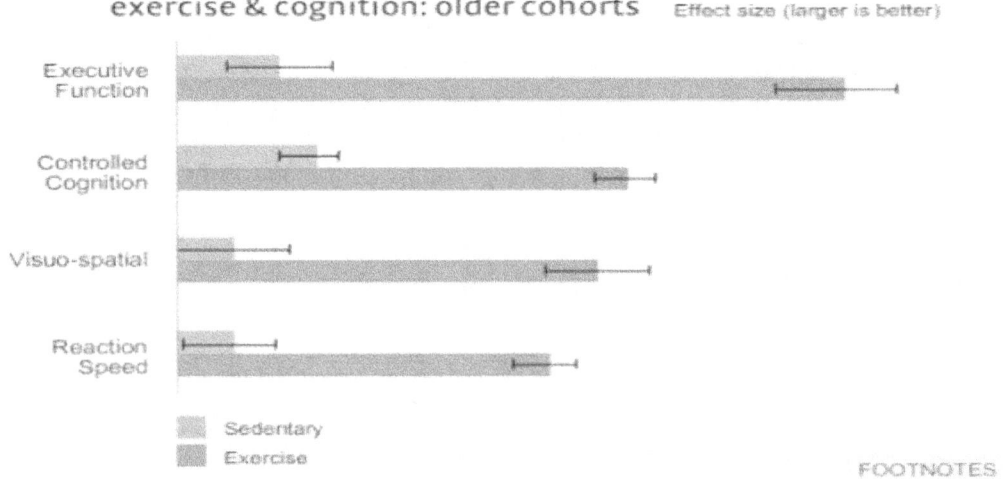

Physical exercise has long been recognized as an effective and economic strategy to promote brain health in humans.

The cellular and structural changes in the brains of exercised animals, including enhancements of neurogenesis and synaptogenesis, dendritic remodeling, and synaptic plasticity, have been considered as the key biological alterations accounting for exercise-elicited benefits to brain health.

However, what transduces body movements into the above-mentioned changes remains largely unknown. Emerging theories indicate that physical activity triggers the release of various factors into the circulation from skeletal muscle (neurotrophins, myokines, and cytokines) and/or adipose tissue (adipokines).

Now let's take a brief review of several of these molecules that are potentially implicated in this process, including neurotrophic factors (BDNF, IGF-1, and VEGF), adipokines (adiponectin and irisin), and myokines/cytokines (IL-15).

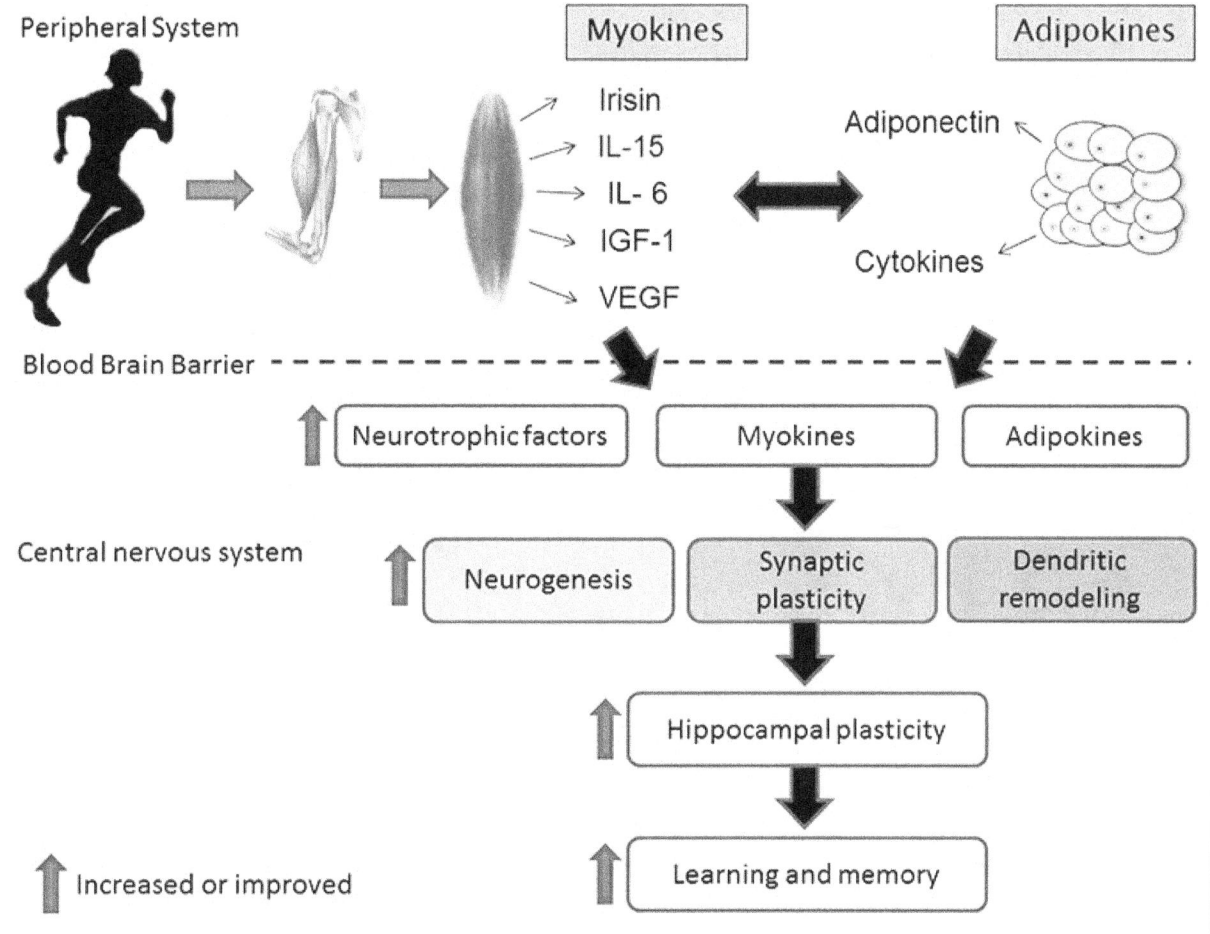

The relationship, whether its causal or concomitant, between the levels of these molecules (particularly in your blood) and brain function after exercise may help to identify biomarkers that can serve as objective indicators to evaluate exercise therapy on diseased or ageing brain.

In addition, unmasking biomarkers may be instrumental in elucidating the mechanisms mediating exercise-induced brain health, thereby contributing to novel drug discovery for treatments to maintain brain health.

How Exercise Affects Your Brain Power

One of the mechanisms by which your brain benefits from physical exercise is via a protein called **Brain Derived Neurotrophic Factor** (BDNF). Exercise initially stimulates the production of a protein called **FNDC5**, which in turn triggers the production of BDNF.

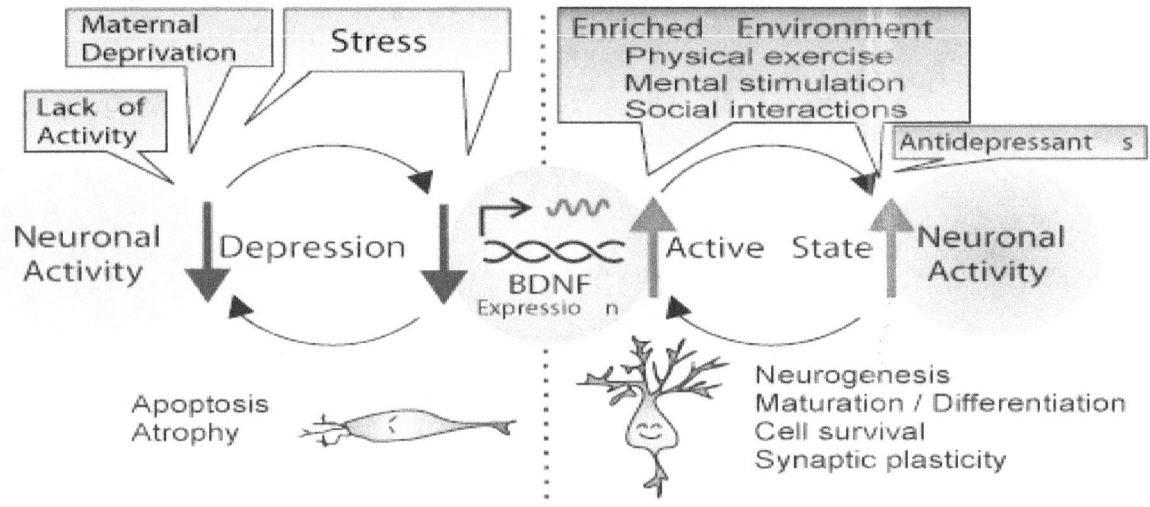

BDNF is a remarkable rejuvenator in several respects. In your brain, BDNF not only preserves existing brain cells, it also activates brain stem cells to convert into new neurons, and effectively makes your brain grow larger.

Research confirming this includes a study by Kirk Erickson, PhD, in which seniors aged 60 to 80 who walked 30 to 45 minutes, three days per week for one year, increased the volume of their hippocampus by two percent. The hippocampus is a region of your brain important for memory. Erickson told WebMD:

"Generally in this age range, people are losing one to three percent per year of hippocampal volume. The changes in the size of the hippocampus were correlated with changes in the blood levels of the brain-derived neurotrophic factor (BDNF)."

Erickson also found that higher fitness levels were associated with a larger prefrontal cortex. He called exercise *"one of the most promising non-pharmaceutical treatments to improve brain health."*

Two additional mechanisms by which exercise protects and boosts your brain health include the following:

- **Reducing plaque formation**: By altering the way damaging proteins reside inside your brain, exercise may help slow the development of Alzheimer's disease.

In one animal study, significantly fewer damaging plaques and fewer bits of beta-amyloid peptides, associated with Alzheimer's, were found in mice that exercised.

- **Decreasing BMP and boosting Noggin**: Bone-morphogenetic protein (BMP) slows down the creation of new neurons, thereby reducing neurogenesis. If you have high levels of BMP, your brain grows slower and less nimble. Exercise reduces the impact of BMP, so that your adult stem cells can continue performing their vital functions of keeping your brain agile.

In animal research, mice with access to running wheels reduced the BMP in their brains by half in just one week. In addition, they also had a notable increase in another brain protein called Noggin, which acts as a BMP antagonist. So, exercise not only reduces the detrimental effects of BMP, it simultaneously boosts the more beneficial Noggin as well.

This complex interplay between BMP and Noggin appears to be yet another powerful factor that helps ensure the proliferation and youthfulness of your neurons – *Your Fountain Of Youth!*

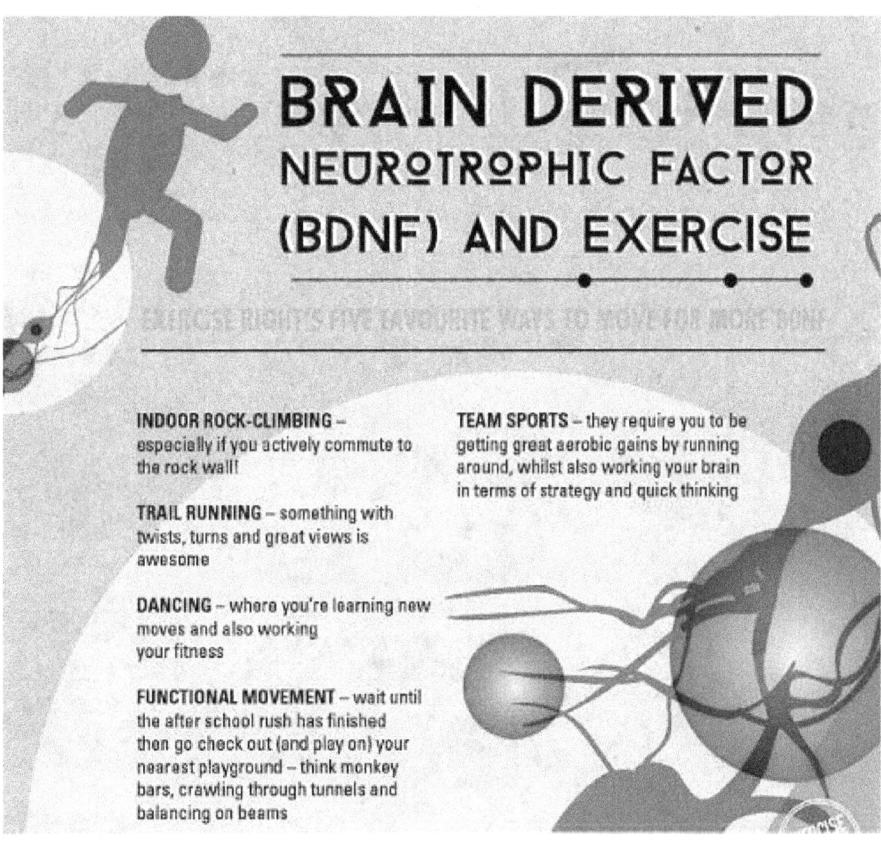

Brain Derived Neurotrophic Factor (BDNF) has been referred to as a fertilizer for your brain. It is a substance that is found in your brain and helps to maintain the life of your brain cells, as well as grow new ones. You've probably heard all about 'neuroplasticity' and how we used to think our brains, once adult, were like a lump of concrete – unable to change and grow.

Scientists now believe our brains are more like plastic – able to adapt, grow and change depending on what we do with them. BDNF is widely accepted as being a key player in this 'plastic' ability of the brain – its presence has been shown to make brain cells in petri dishes sprout new branches (necessary activity for a cell to make new connections!).

Low levels of BDNF have been associated with depression, anxiety, poor memory and brain degeneration as seen in conditions such as Alzheimer's and dementia.

Top 5 reasons you should want more BDNF

- **Improved learning and memory**
- May trigger the **production of more serotonin** (hello happy feelings!)
- Helps with **new skill acquisition**
- **Improved mood** (exercise increases BDNF as much or even more than taking antidepressants does)
- **Lower rates of Alzheimer's disease and dementia in older age** may be related to higher levels of BDNF.

Are you getting the picture? Better mood, better mental performance, healthier brain as you age…

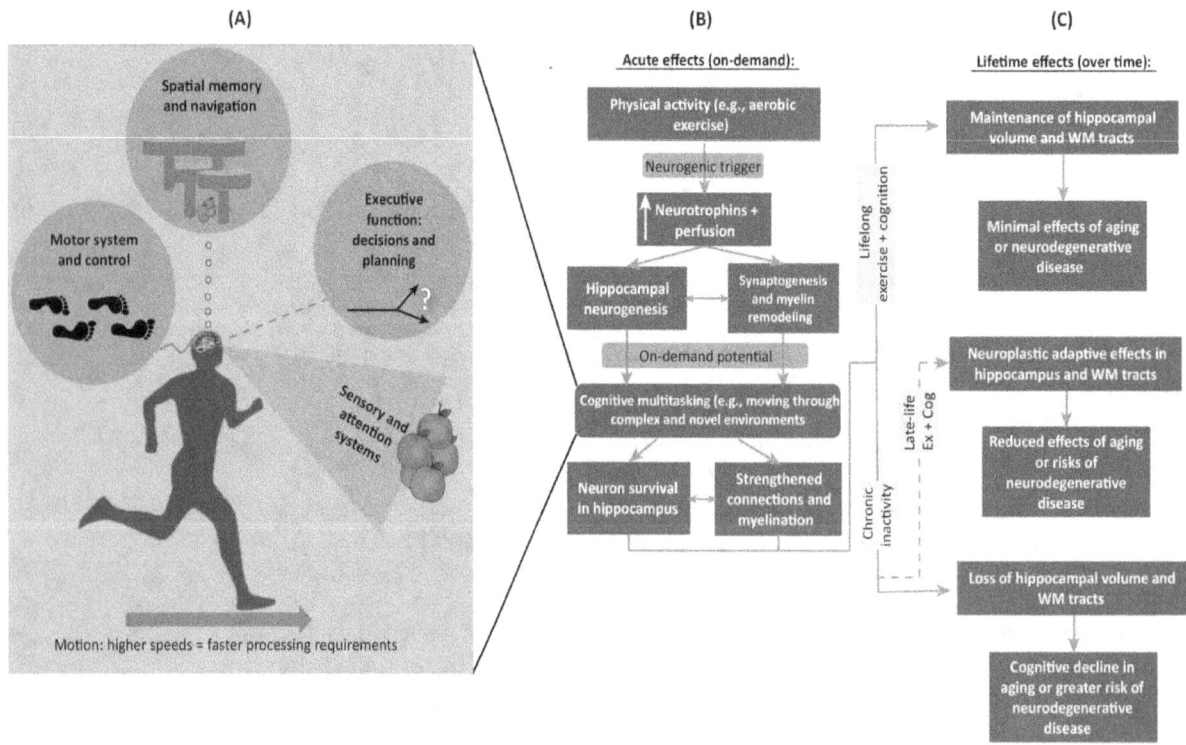

Exercise Prevents Both Your Brain and Muscle Decay

Showing the interconnectedness between muscle and brain health, BDNF also expresses itself in your **neuro-muscular** system where it protects your neuro-motors from degradation. Your neuromotor is the most critical element in your muscle. Without your neuromotor, your muscle is like an engine without ignition.

Neuro-motor degradation is part of the process that explains age-related muscle atrophy.

So BDNF is actively involved in both your muscles *and* your brain, and this cross-connection appears to be a major part of the explanation for why a physical workout can have such a beneficial impact on your brain tissue. It, quite literally, helps prevent, and even reverse, your brain decay as much as it prevents and reverses your age-related muscle decay.

The most important message from studies like these is that mental decline is by no means inevitable, and that exercise is as good for your brain as it is for the rest of your body.

And All you have to DO is Move SomeThing ….. Move Your Self into the Successful Enjoyment of Your Abundant Life ….. Youth and Mentally SHARP!

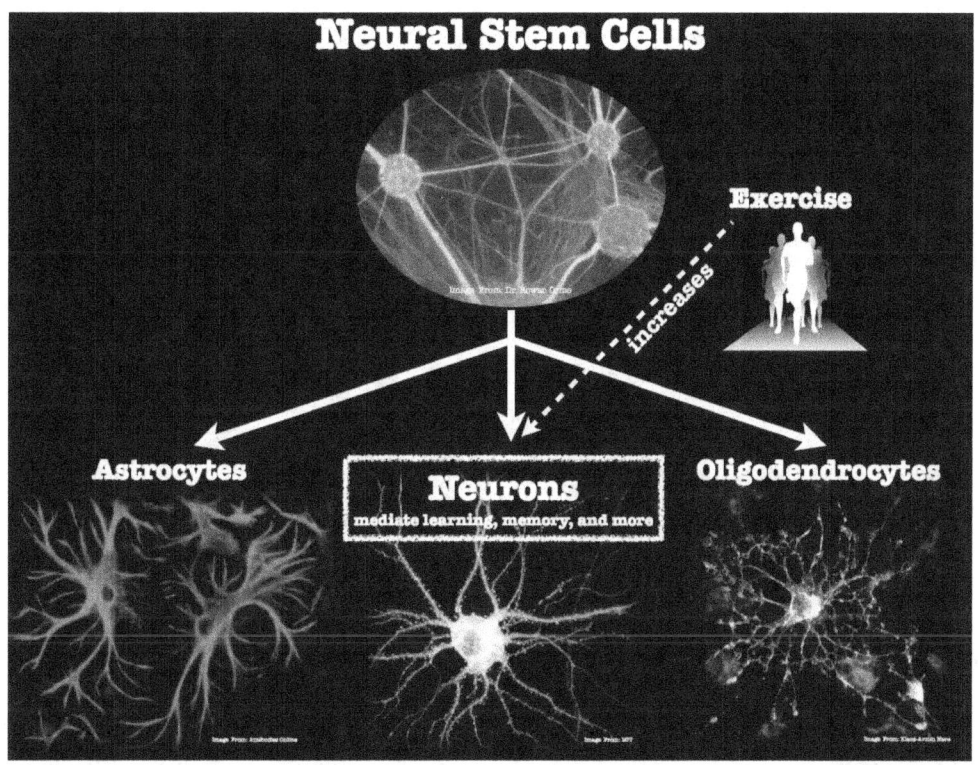

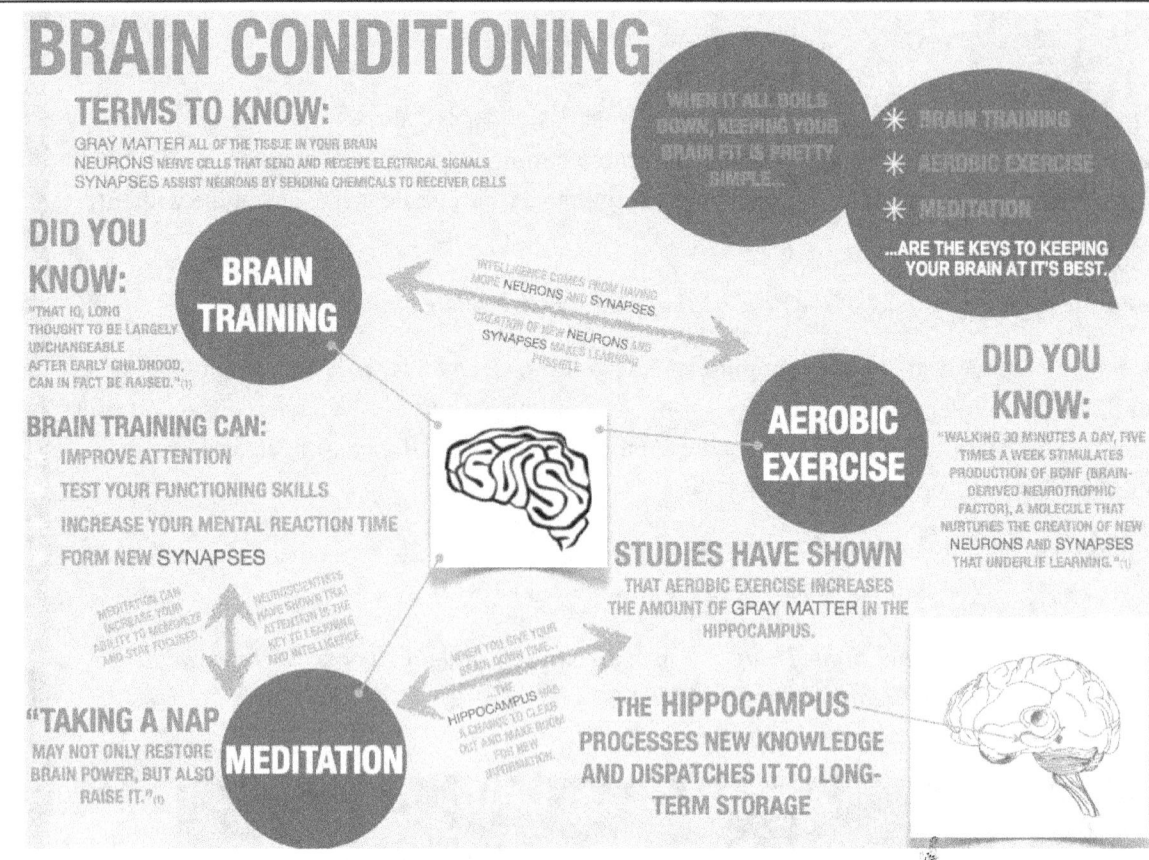

Diet & Fasting Also Plays a Role

Fasting IS the CURE for over 90% of any ills or disease.

Its also very Interesting that both fasting and exercise trigger very similar genes and growth factors that recycle and rejuvenate both your brain and muscle tissues.

These growth factors include BDNF and muscle regulatory factors (MRFs). These growth factors signal brain stem cells and muscle satellite cells to convert into new neurons and new muscle cells respectively.

This also helps explain why exercise while fasting can help keep your brain, neuro-motors, and muscle fibers biologically young.

For more information on how to incorporate intermittent fasting into your exercise routine for maximum benefits, please see my previous article, "High-Intensity Interval Training and Intermittent Fasting - A Winning Combo."

Besides the issue of when you eat, what you eat is of great importance.

Manufactured and processed Sugar suppresses your BDNF, which helps explain why a low-sugar diet in combination with regular exercise is so effective for protecting memory and staving off depression.

Sugar, and fructose in particular, will also obliterate your body's production of human growth hormone (HGH) when consumed within two hours after a workout, and HGH production is a *major* benefit of high intensity interval training (HIIT).

Exercise Can Help Keep You Sharp Well Into Old Age

While it's never too late to start exercising, the earlier you begin and the more consistent you are, the greater your long-term rewards.

Having an active lifestyle is really an investment in your future well-being, both physically and mentally.

I believe that, overall, high-intensity interval training really helps maximize the health benefits of exercise, while simultaneously being the most efficient and therefore requiring the least amount of time. That being said, ideally, you'll want to strive for a varied and well-rounded fitness program that incorporates a wide variety of exercises.

Actions of BDNF

- Sustains the viability of neurons (neuroprotection)
- Increases dendritic arborization and the number of synapses.
- BDNF gene is suppressed by stress (via cortisol).
- Decreased BDNF levels lead to neuronal atrophy and neuronal death.
- BDNF levels are low in depression, but increase with antidepressant treatment.
- Exercise increases BDNF levels.

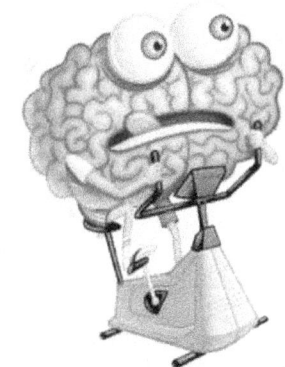

I also strongly recommend avoiding sitting as much as possible, and making it a point to walk more every day. The science is really clear on this point: ***you do not have to lose your mind with advancing age.***

Move Something!

Your brain has the capacity to regenerate and grow throughout the entire human lifespan, and exercise is perhaps the most potent way to ensure your brain's continued growth and rejuvenation.

- •Energetic challenges (e.g., exercise and energy restriction) induce BDNF signaling.
- •BDNF enhances neuronal bioenergetics and promotes optimal brain health.
- •BDNF signaling improves peripheral energy metabolism and cardiovascular function.
- •Deficits in BDNF may contribute to metabolic morbidity and associated diseases.

Emerging findings suggest that brain-derived neurotrophic factor (BDNF) serves widespread roles in regulating energy homeostasis by controlling patterns of feeding and physical activity, and by modulating glucose metabolism in peripheral tissues.

BDNF mediates the beneficial effects of energetic challenges such as vigorous exercise and fasting on cognition, mood, cardiovascular function, and on peripheral metabolism. By stimulating glucose transport and mitochondrial biogenesis BDNF bolsters cellular bioenergetics and protects neurons against injury and disease.

By acting in the brain and periphery, BDNF increases insulin sensitivity and parasympathetic tone.

Genetic factors, a 'couch potato' lifestyle, and chronic stress impair BDNF signaling, and this may contribute to the pathogenesis of metabolic syndrome. Novel BDNF-focused interventions are being developed for obesity, diabetes and neurological disorders.

All you have to DO is Move something!

What Are You Moving?

YourSelf!

Where Are You Going?

Your Abundant Life!

LET'S GO!!!!

Brain Facts that Need to be Respected Every Day!

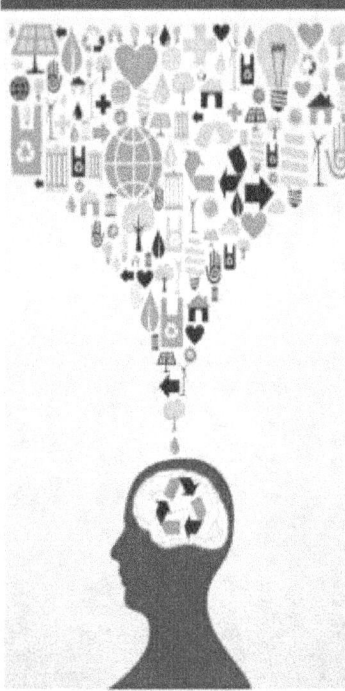

Fact # 1:
Although the human brain is only 2% of the body weight, it receives about:

- 15% of the cardiac output
- 20% of total body oxygen consumption
- 25% of total body glucose utilization

The brain is the most metabolically active organ and therefore prone to oxidative and inflammatory stress damage, which may deteriorate cognitive function.

Fact # 2:
The human brain is in a constant state of change such that:

- During the lifespan new neurons may be formed while others will die and new synapses are created while others are eliminated.

- Brain cerebral systems are not purely hard-wired and can be significantly influenced by many non-genetic factors such as physical activity, cognitive activity, sleep and nutrition.

Proposed Benefits of Aerobic Fitness on Cognitive Function Based on Current Research

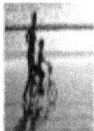 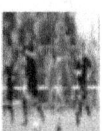 =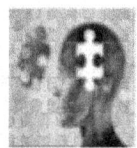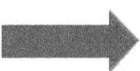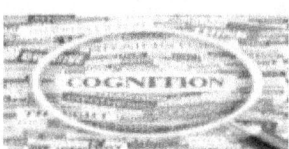

Proposed Biological Mechanisms Affected by Exercise | Examples of Potential Benefits of Exercise for Children and Teens

Proposed Biological Mechanisms Affected by Exercise		Examples of Potential Benefits of Exercise for Children and Teens
Cerebral blood flow increases to deliver more oxygen and nutrients and remove waste products from brain regions responsible for learning and memory.	**Neurogenesis** spurs the growth of new nerve cells in an important brain memory center called the hippocampus.	Helps to enhances scholastic performance, and brain development and improve brain activation, especially in low-academic performers, compared to low-fit children
Angiogenesis creates new brain blood vessels to help maintain and expand volume in key regions such as the hippocampus that are associated with cognitive function.	**Neuroplasticity** develops new brain connections by promoting changes in neural pathways and synapses for healthy development, learning, memory, and recovery from brain damage.	Helps to develop frontal cortex and medial temporal lobe (hippocampus) brain function for better memory forming, organizing and storing, cognitive control, and improved attention, accuracy and focus.
Neuroprotection associated with increases in the body's natural antioxidant defense system and other functions to defend brain health.	**Healthy brain signals** increase levels of (1) brain-derived neurotrophic factor (BDNF), a chemical that improves brain synapses and (2) endorphins that promote a feeling of well-being.	Helps to improve executive function mental processes that helps connect past experience with present action. It helps to support functions such as planning, organizing, strategizing, paying attention to and remembering details, and managing time and space.

Recent Aerobic Fitness and Cognition Research Highlights: Children & Teens

Research provides evidence supporting the beneficial effects of regular exercise in improving memory and accuracy in teens. The beneficial effects were region-specific and associated with the serum levels of some neurotrophic factors. (Lee, et al. Psychoneuroendocrinology. 2014; 39:214-224).

Research suggests that aerobic fitness can enhance brain connectivity and microstructure during neurodevelopment in fit children compared to their low fit peers (Herting et al. Develop Cog Neurosci. 2014; 7:65-75).

Study found that aerobic fitness facilitated cognitive performance in lower-performers who demonstrated the most improvements in response accuracy and focus measures following the end of exercise. (Drollette et al. Develop Cognitive Neuroscience. 2014; 7:53-64).

Study shows that compared to less fit children, highly fit children have larger sub-cortical brain structures, more efficient brain activation and neuro-processing during cognitive tasks, better working memory, attention and improved academic performance. (Haapala. J Human Kinetics.2013; 36:55-68).

Research finds that aerobic fitness during childhood enhances specific fMRI activation of brain frontal cortex function involved in cognitive control related to improved attention and focus. (Chaddock-Heyman et al. Frontiers in Human Neuroscience. 2013; 7(72):1-13).

Study found no differences in performance at initial learning between higher fit and lower fit participants. However, during the retention session higher fit children outperformed lower fit children. (Raine et al. PLOS ONE. 2013; 8(9): e72666).

Research reveals that exercise appears to improve the activation of brain neural circuitry supporting improved cognitive function in overweight children. (Krafft et al. Obesity. 2013; doi:10.1002/oby.20518).

Findings show that a single bout of aerobic physical activity in the form of *exergaming* (active video games) enhances children's executive decision making function across a wide age range compared to sedentary gaming. (Best. Developmental Psychology. 2012; 48(5):1501-1510).

Study suggests that daily moderate intensity walking is helpful for maintaining cognitive performance, with implication in scholastic performance. (Drollette et al. Med & Sci Sports & Exercise. 2012;44(10):2017-2024).

Study shows that students in a moderately physical activity program improved overall performance on standard academic tests by 6% compared to a decrease of 1% for sedentary controls. (Donnelly and Lambourne et al. Preventive Medicine. 2011; 52:536-542).

Research and a literature review suggest that aerobic fitness may influence brain health and cognition leading to enhanced scholastic performance and more effective cognitive function, which is important for adaptive behavior and cognitive development. (Hillman et al. Prev Med. 2011; 52S:S21-S28; Davis et al. Health Psychol. 2011; 30(10):91-98)

Findings show that higher-fit children have greater brain hippocampal volumes, efficiency of neural networks and enhanced relational memory performance compared to lower-fit children. (Chaddock et al. Brain Research. 2010;1358:172-183; Voss et al. Neuroscience.2011; 199:166-176)

Recent Aerobic Fitness and Cognition Research Highlights: Young and Middle Aged Healthy Adults

Research with 20 year old males showed that a single bout of moderate aerobic exercise for about 30 minutes improved post exercise cognition, most prominently for memory, reasoning and planning by between 20-35% and decreased the time taken to perform the tests (Nanda et al. J Clin Diagnostic Res. 2013;7(9):1883-1885).

Study findings suggest that simultaneous light to moderate-intensity physical activity during vocabulary learning facilitated memorization of new material in young adults (19-33 years) (Schmidt-Kassow et al. PLOS ONE.2013; 8(5): e64172; Schmidt-Kassow et al. Neuro-science Letters.2010; 482:40-44).

In young to middle age adults (18-45 years), research findings provided compelling data to suggest that greater levels of physical exercise are associated with larger volume of the brain hippocampus (Killgore et al. Scientific Reports. 2013; 3:3457).

Cerebrovascular blood flow velocity was significantly improved irrespective of age after 12 weeks of a cycling exercise program for all adult regardless of ages but the response was greater for younger adults (18-28 years of age) compared to older adults (58-68 years of age). (Murrell, et al. Age. 2013; 35(3):905-910).

In healthy young to middle age adults, research indicates that physical exercise is associated with higher intelligence (IQ) in women, whereas exercise was only slightly associated with higher IQ in men (Killgore and Schwab. Percept Mot Skills. 2012; 115(2):605-617).

Research findings suggest that regardless of age (young (19-29 years and older 59-65 years) adults' cognitive (executive function) was improved with exercise and higher cerebrovascular blood flow was strongly associated with improved cognition (Lucas et al. Exp Gerontol. 2012; 47(8):541-551).

Aerobic fitness improved cognitive attention processing only in younger adults (18-22 years) when compared to older adults (61-73 years) (Pontifex et al. Psycho-physiology. 2009; 46(2):379-387).

Students (averaging 20 years) with mild to moderate intellectual disabilities who participated in 8-weeks of moderate aerobic training performance showed significantly improved in processing speed by over 100%. (Pastula et al. J Strength Conditioning Research. 2012; 26(12):3441-3448).

Cognitive Function Benefits Associated with Exercise for Seniors: Overview

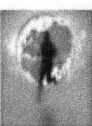 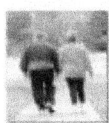 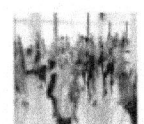 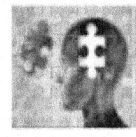  

Brain Mechanisms Associated with Exercise

Cerebral Blood Flow increases to deliver more oxygen and nutrients and remove waste products from brain regions responsible for learning and memory.

Angiogenesis creates new brain blood vessels to help maintain and expand volume in key regions such as the hippocampus that are associated with cognitive function.

Neuroprotection associated with increases in the body's natural antioxidant defense system and other functions to defend brain health.

Neurogenesis spurs the growth of new nerve cells in an important brain memory center called the hippocampus.

Neuroplasticity develops new brain connections by promoting changes in neural pathways and synapses for healthy development, learning, memory, and recovery from brain damage.

Healthy Brain Signals increase levels of (1) brain-derived neurotrophic factor (BDNF), a chemical that improves brain synapses and (2) endorphins that promote a feeling of well-being.

Potential Benefits of Exercise

Helps to slow or reverse shrinkage of key cognitive brain regions such as the hippocampus, important for learning, planning, memory, reasoning and processing speed.

Helps reduce the risk for neurodegenerative diseases.

Helps to manage mood, anxiety and depression, and fosters feelings of well-being.

Case Study #1: Exercise Facilitates Brain Function and Cognition in Children Who Need It the Most

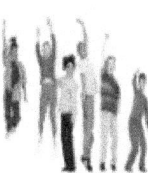

Background:
Despite evidence that physical activity participation is associated with improved cognitive function, academic performance, and overall health in children, there continues to be a decline in the amount of time dedicated to physical activity during the school day. Studies focusing on single bouts of physical activity indicate that increasing the amount of time spent physically active may foster post-exercise cognitive benefits, which can help improve scholastic performance.

Methods:
➢ 40 healthy 8-10 year old children (27 females; 13 males) divided into two groups of 20 high performance and 20 low performance learners engaged in moderate-intensity aerobic activity and were than evaluated for cognitive performance.
➢ These testing sessions were conducted following 20 minutes of either moderate intensity treadmill walking at 60–70% of maximal heart rate, or at quiet rest while seated in a chair that was safely placed on the same treadmill.
➢ Cognitive function was assessed by computer based cognitive testing and neuroelectric assessments.

Results/Conclusions:
➢ Lower-performing students demonstrated an improvement in brain and cognitive function up to a level similar to the high performers after the exercise bout.
➢ Higher-performing students maintained their cognitive performance levels after the exercise bout.
➢ The results suggested that short periods of physical activity during the school day are a means of regulating attention in the classroom, especially among children who need it most.

Case Study #1: Aerobic Exercise and Cognitive Performance in Adults 18 Years or Older

Background:
- One strategy that has gained increased attention is the use of aerobic exercise to improve neurocognitive functioning.
- Although the value of exercise has been critically examined in review articles and meta-analyses, there is still more to be learned about the magnitude of the effect of physical activity on enhanced neurocognitive function.

Methods:
- A systematic literature review was conducted of randomized clinical trails examining the association between aerobic exercise training and neurocognitive performance conducted between January, 1966 and July, 2009.
- Suitable studies were selected for inclusion according to the following criteria: mean age 18 years of age or older, duration of treatment greater than 1 month, incorporated aerobic exercise components, exercise training was supervised, the presence of a non-aerobic-exercise control group.

Results/Conclusions:
- 29 studies met inclusion criteria and were included in the analyses representing data from 2,049 participants.
- Aerobic exercise training demonstrated modest but significant improvements in attention and processing speed, executive function, and memory but the effects of exercise on working memory were less consistent.
- Individuals with mild cognitive impairment tended to demonstrate greater improvements in memory relative to non-cognitive impaired subjects and longer periods of exercise were associated with greater gains in attention and processing speed.

Case Study #1: Aerobic Exercise Increases Size of the Brain Hippocampus Region for Improved Memory in Older Adults

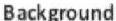

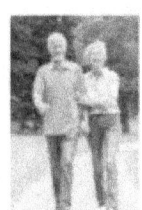

Background:
- As older adults age, they can experience a 1-2% hippocampus shrinkage per year.
- Shrinkage of the brain's hippocampal region precedes and leads to memory impairment in late adulthood and increased risk for dementia.
- Hippocampal and medial temporal lobe volumes are larger in higher-fit adults, and physical activity training increases hippocampal function, but the extent to which aerobic exercise training can modify hippocampal volume in late adulthood needs more research.

Methods:
- 120 older adults (mean age about 65 years) without dementia were randomly assigned to a moderate aerobic exercise group (n = 60) or to a stretching control group (n = 60).
- Magnetic resonance images were collected before the intervention, after 6 mo, and again after 1 year.
- The groups did not differ at baseline in hippocampal volume or attendance rates.

Results/Conclusions:
- Aerobic exercise training increased the size of the hippocampus, leading to a better memory.
- Exercise training increased hippocampal volume by 2%, effectively reversing age-related loss in volume by 1 to 2 years.
- Increased hippocampal volume is associated with greater serum levels of brain-derived neurotrophic factor (BDNF), a mediator of brain neurogenesis.
- Hippocampal volume declined in the control group.
- These findings indicate that aerobic exercise training can reverse hippocampal volume loss in late adulthood and improve memory function.

Case Study #2: Study Suggest that Exercise Helps to Improve Cognitive Function in Teens

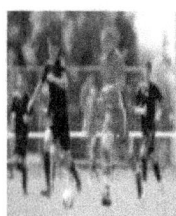

Background: The beneficial effect of aerobic exercise (exercise) on human cognitive functioning and mental well-being has been well documented. Recent findings have suggested that aerobic exercise may have a positive effect on teen brain functioning. Key brain regions affected are the (1) **frontal cortex** - planning complex cognitive behavior, personality expression, decision making, and moderating social behavior and (2) **medial-temporal functions (hippocampus)** - retention of sensory input processing, language comprehension, new memory storage, and emotions.

Methods:
➢ A total of 91 healthy teens (45 regular exercisers and 46 matched sedentary controls) participated in this study. The exercisers were recruited from the Hong Kong Sports Institute where they received intensive training on rowing, swimming, running (>1000 m) or triathlon for at least two months prior to this study. A study design was adopted to compare cognitive functioning associated frontal and temporal brain regions and the serum levels of neurotrophic factors, brain signals known to improve brain function between the two groups.

Results/Conclusions: This study reports preliminary evidence of the beneficial effects of regular aerobic exercise in improving cognitive functions in teens. The exercising teens performed significantly better than the controls on the frontal and temporal functioning parameters, which are associated with the serum levels of neurotrophic factors. In associative learning. The exercisers had a higher memory score and accuracy than sedentary teens. Specifically, adolescent exercisers showed improved memory, inhibitory control, and cognitive flexibility. These findings suggest that chronic exercise would be associated with better performance in associative memory, the ability to learn and remember the relationship between unrelated items such as the name of someone they have just met.

Case Study #2: Moderate Aerobic Exercise Improves Cognitive Function in Young Adults with Intellectual Disabilities

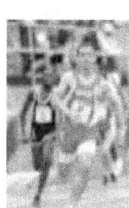

Background:
➢ Intellectual disabilities (IDs) is the most prevalent of all developmental disabilities.
➢ In addition to cognitive impairment, young adults with intellectual disabilities are also more likely to be in poor health. Exercise may help ameliorate both of these deficits.

Methods:
➢ 14 students (averaging about 20 years of age) with mild to moderate IDs participated in an 8-week comprehensive exercise intervention program based on circuit training, aerobic dancing, and adapted sport activities. Sessions lasted 45 minutes, and intensity was maintained at 60–70% of maximum heart rate.
➢ Cognitive improvement was measured before and after the exercise program

Results/Conclusions:
➢ Moderate-intensity exercise training resulted in meaningful improvements in the cognitive functioning and aerobic fitness of young adults with IDs with significant improvements in cognitive processing speed of over 100%.
➢ Aerobic fitness was significantly improved (mean improvement in aerobic fitness was 17.5%).
➢ These effects support the inclusion of exercise into the lives of young adults with ID to promote their physical and cognitive health.

Case Study #2: Moderate Aerobic Exercise Improves Brain Health in Older Adults with Mild Cognitive Impairment

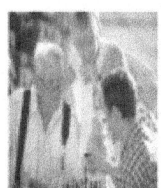

Background:
Evidence from neuropsychological and neuroimaging studies has suggested that mild cognitive impairment (MCI) represents a clinical risk for degenerative dementias such as Alzheimer's disease (AD). Several randomized controlled trials (RCTs) have been conducted to investigate the effects of physical activity on cognitive function in older adults with MCI.

Methods:
- Investigators evaluated 100 older healthy Japanese adults (mean age, 75 years) with MCI.
- The subjects were randomized to either a multi-component aerobic exercise or no exercise control group.
- The moderate aerobic exercise group included 90 minutes a day sessions for 2 days a week or 40 times for 6 months.

Results/Conclusions:
- The aerobic exercise group had significantly better cognition (as measured by the Mini-Mental State Examination) and logical memory scores, and reduced whole brain cortical shrinkage compared to the control group.
- The effects of exercise were most pronounced for logical memory and general cognitive function in older adults with MCI.
- The results suggested that a moderate level of exercise is beneficial for brain health in older adults even if started later in life.

Case Study #3: Aerobic Exercise & Brain Volume in Healthy Middle Aged Adults

Background:
Physical exercise appears to facilitate improved brain function, particularly within the hippocampus, the brain region most critical for memory formation and spatial representation. Better aerobic fitness has been reliably associated with increased hippocampal volume and improved cognitive functioning in children and elderly adults, but until this study almost no data were available concerning this relationship in healthy early to middle aged adults.

Methods:
- 61 healthy adult volunteers (33 males; 28 females) ranging in age from 18 to 45 years from the Boston metropolitan area participated in the neuroimaging study.
- No attempt was made to select participants based on particular physical exercise habits or physical fitness level. The body mass index (BMI) of the sample ranged from 19.2 to 35.
- Upon arrival at the laboratory, participants completed an information questionnaire about their daily routines, which included questions about exercise, diet, height, weight, and sleep habits.
- Structural MRI and brain images were analyzed using voxel-based morphometry for each subject.

Results/Conclusions:
- These findings provide compelling data to suggest that greater levels of physical exercise are associated with larger volume of the hippocampus during the years of early to middle adulthood.
- The relation between increasing physical activity and optimal adult cognition and brain function is rapidly evolving.

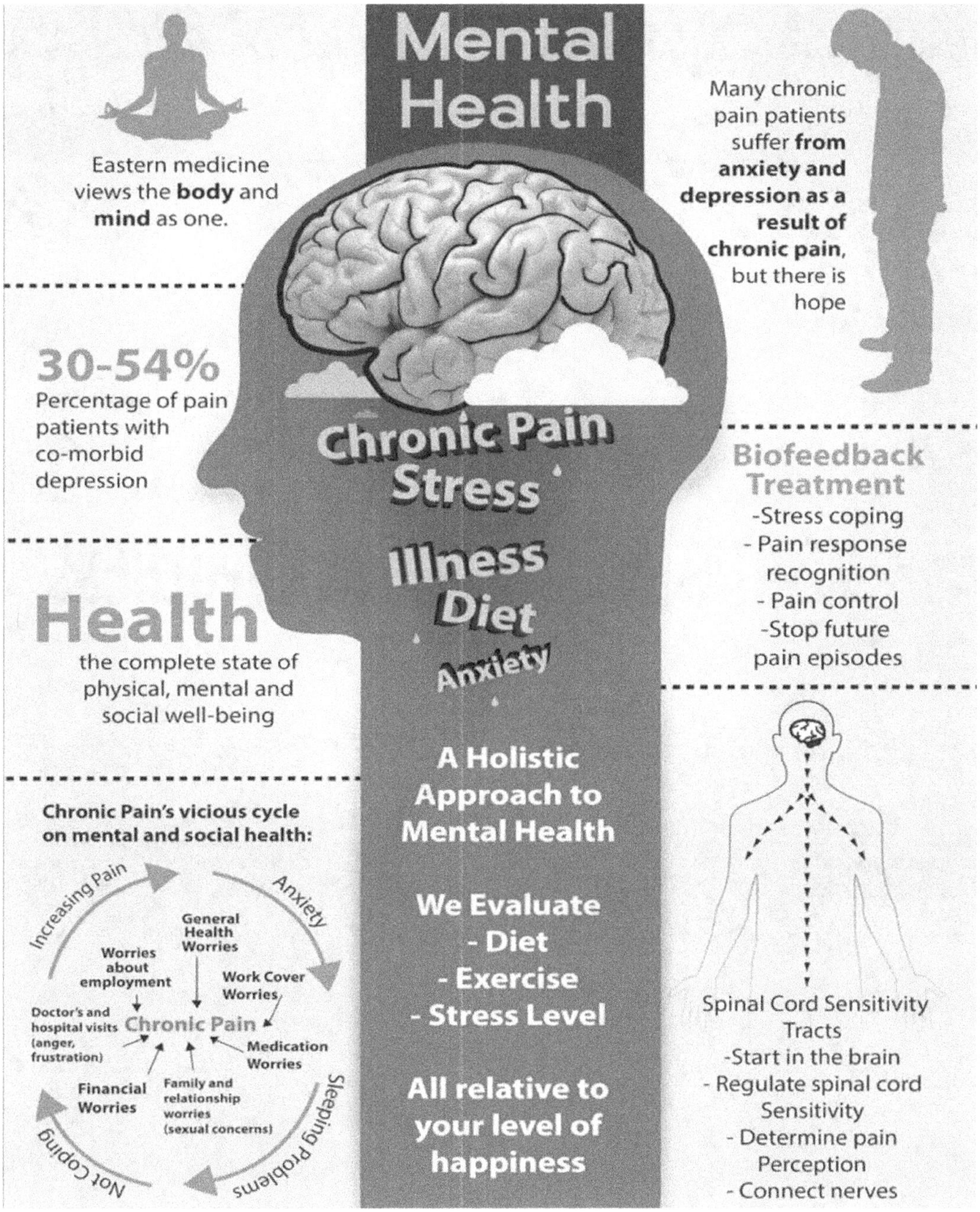

Mental Health

Eastern medicine views the **body** and **mind** as one.

Many chronic pain patients suffer **from anxiety and depression as a result of chronic pain**, but there is hope

30-54% Percentage of pain patients with co-morbid depression

Chronic Pain Stress Illness Diet Anxiety

Health the complete state of physical, mental and social well-being

Biofeedback Treatment
- Stress coping
- Pain response recognition
- Pain control
- Stop future pain episodes

A Holistic Approach to Mental Health

We Evaluate
- Diet
- Exercise
- Stress Level

All relative to your level of happiness

Chronic Pain's vicious cycle on mental and social health:

Increasing Pain — Anxiety — Sleeping Problems — Not Coping

General Health Worries, Worries about employment, Work Cover Worries, Doctor's and hospital visits (anger, frustration), **Chronic Pain**, Medication Worries, Financial Worries, Family and relationship worries (sexual concerns)

Spinal Cord Sensitivity Tracts
- Start in the brain
- Regulate spinal cord Sensitivity
- Determine pain Perception
- Connect nerves

EXERCISE YOUR WAY TO A HEALTHY ... BRAIN?

Fitting in more physical activity; specifically, in the form of walking and running can spur on neurogenesis (new neurons) and increase gray matter volume in several regions of the brain including the prefrontal, temporal, and hippocampal areas. The denser the gray matter tissue is in a particular region of the brain, the higher the intelligence will be relative of the location.

Ways to Increase Neurogenesis

LIFESTYLE

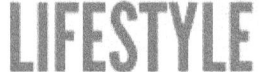 Sunlight

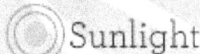 Sex

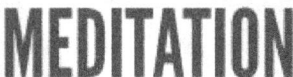 Caloric restriction

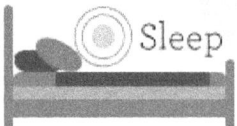 Sleep

DIET

 Omega-3 fatty acids

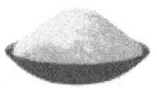
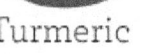 Turmeric

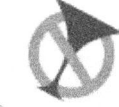
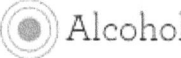 Alcohol

MEDITATION AND MINDFULNESS

Meditation through mindfulness (paying attention to your body's sensations, breath, etc.) has been linked to increased gray matter in the hippocampus.

As it turns out, exercising regularly and eating a healthy diet does more than just help you fit into your skinny jeans. It helps your brain make new neurons, creates more synaptic engagement, increases gray matter density—which can make you smarter—and wards off degenerative brain diseases associated with old age.

Move Something!

What You Eat
What You Drink
Calories In

Body Mass
Resting Energy Expenditure
Programmed Exercise
Aerobic Training
Resistance Training
Physical Activity
Activities of Daily Living
Fidgeting
Calories Out

ENERGY BALANCE = Weight MAINTENANCE

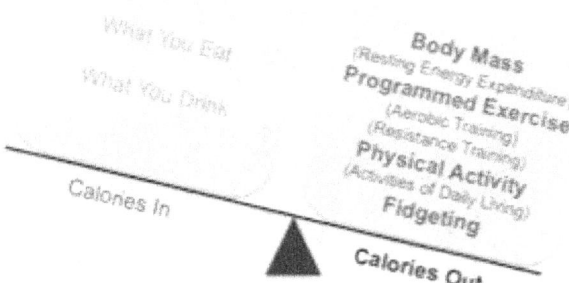

POSITIVE Energy Balance = Weight GAIN

NEGATIVE Energy Balance = Weight LOSS

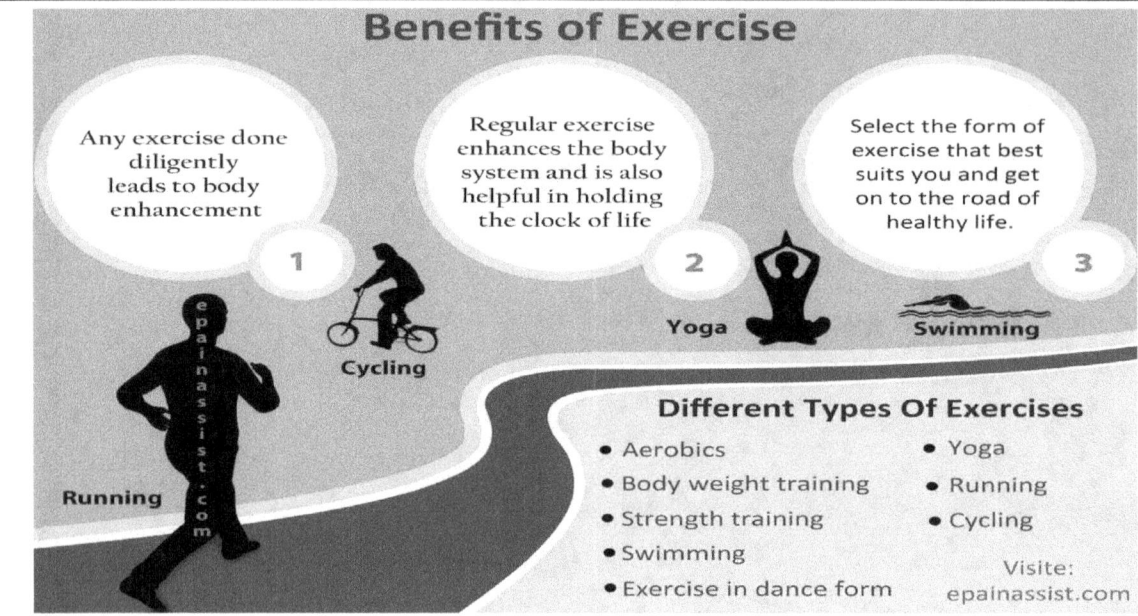
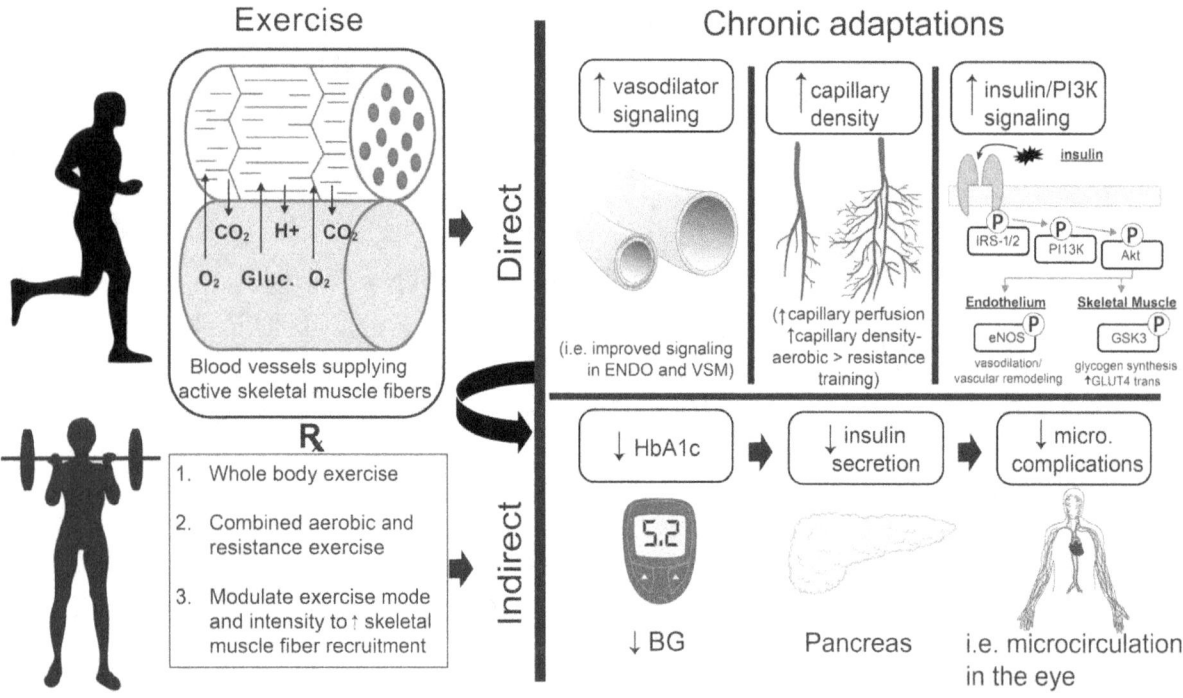

Physical Exercise Appears to Increase the Eating Preference for "Healthier Foods"

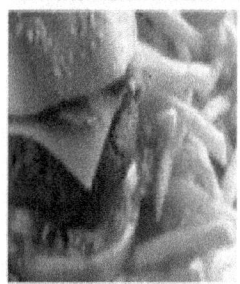

High calorie dense foods (e.g. cheese burgers, ice cream, cake, french fries, candy)

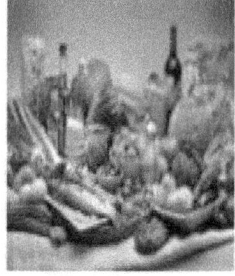

Healthy foods (e.g. fruit, vegetables salads, fish, or whole grain)

Background:
Recent evidence suggests that regular physical exercise may also affect the responsiveness of regions of the brain to food stimuli.

Design:
➢ This study examined whether the total number of minutes of self-reported weekly physical exercise was related to the responsiveness of appetite and food reward-related brain regions to visual presentations of indulgent foods and healthy food images during functional MRI.

➢ While undergoing scanning, 37 healthy adults (15 women and 22 men; average age 30 years) viewed images of Indulgent and low-calorie foods and provided desirability ratings for each food image. The correlation between exercise minutes per week and brain responses to high calorie dense vs healthy foods was evaluated in brain regions previously implicated in responses to food images.

Results:
➢ Higher levels of exercise were significantly correlated with lower brain responsiveness to higher calorie dense foods.

➢ These findings suggest that physical exercise may be associated with reduced activation in food-response and a reduced preference for higher calorie dense foods, particularly those with a savory flavor.

Conclusion:
➢ Physical exercise may confer a secondary health benefit of healthy eating beyond its primary effects on cardiovascular and cognitive fitness and energy expenditure.

➢ More research is needed on the effects of exercise on healthy eating preference to confirm this study.

Exercise

Neurogenesis
Synaptogenesis
Synaptic plasticity
Cognitive function
Motor function
DNA repair
Mitochondrial biogenesis
Reduced inflammation

Decreased resting heart rate
Increased heart rate variability
Decreased blood pressure

Increased insulin sensitivity
Ketone body production

Increased insulin sensitivity

Fatty acid mobilization
Reduced inflammation

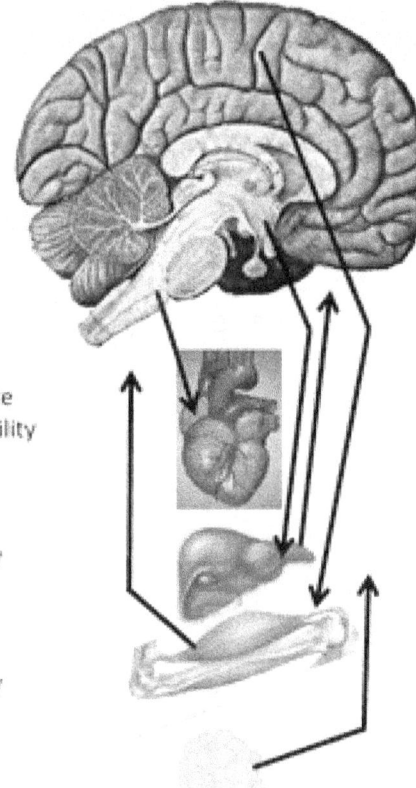

Intermittent Fasting

Neurogenesis
Synaptogenesis
Synaptic plasticity
Cognitive function
Motor function
Reduced inflammation
Enhanced autophagy

Decreased resting heart rate
Increased heart rate variability
Decreased blood pressure

Increased insulin sensitivity
Ketone body production

Increased insulin sensitivity

Fatty acid mobilization
Reduced inflammation

Chapter Six

Eating 2 Live and Exercise!

*****

Poor Diet and Lack of exercise are the #2 Actual Cause of Death. This means that we must address both of these as one and cannot separate them when dealing with your Health and Wellness!

With this chapter, we want to examine How the Combination of Good Diet and Exercise Unleashes Tons of Positive Benefits For You!

What happens in your body when you combine whole-effort exercise with whole-food nutrition? You get a whole-new you!

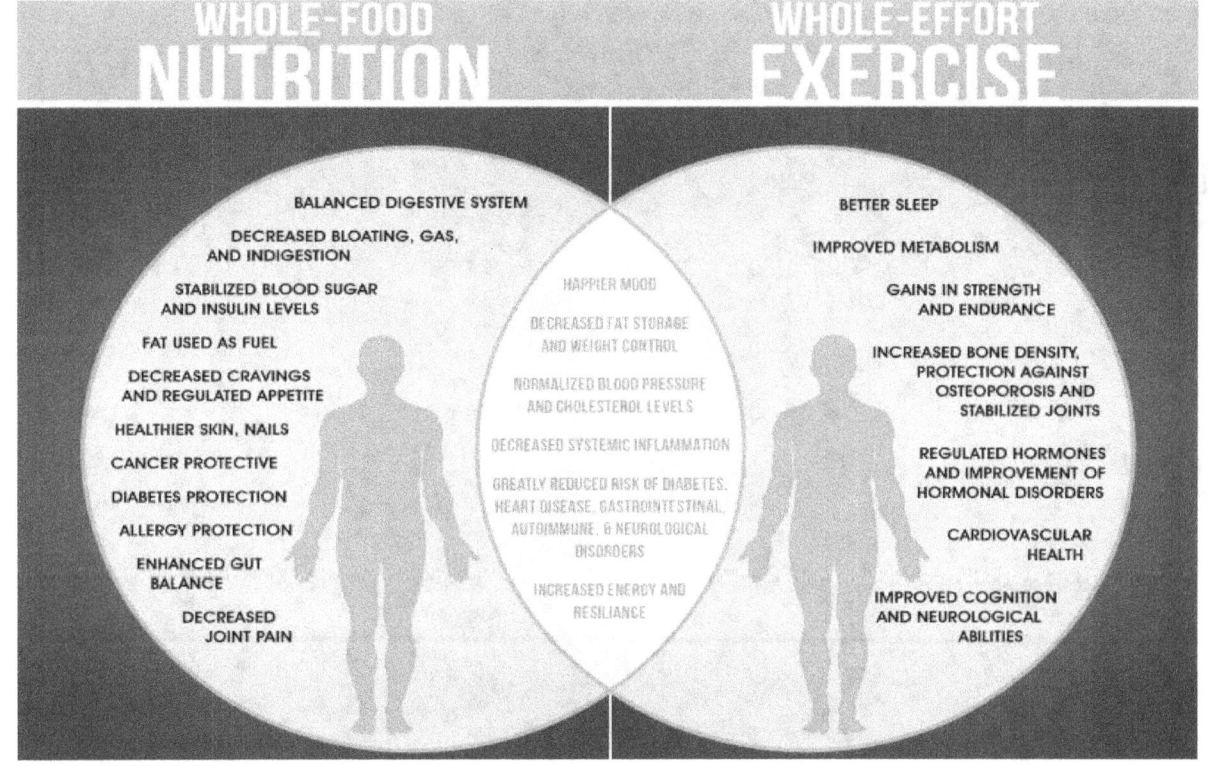

Eating right and exercising regularly can help you avoid excess weight gain and maintain a healthy weight. According to the Mayo Clinic, being physically active is essential to reaching your weight-loss goals. Even if you're not trying to lose weight, regular exercise can improve cardiovascular health, boost your immune system, and increase your energy level.

Plan for at least 300 - 420 minutes of moderate physical activity every week. If you can't devote this amount of time to exercise, look for simple ways to increase activity throughout the day. For example, try walking instead of driving, take the stairs instead of the elevator, or pace while you're talking on the phone.

Applying the Science of Eating To Live is the foundation for your physical Health and Wellness – to ensure that you are Energy and Nutritionally Balanced. When you start the day without food, you avoid becoming overly hungry later, which could send you running to get fast food before lunch.

Incorporate fresh fruits and vegetables into your diet when you do eat your meal. These foods, which are low in calories and high in nutrients, help with weight control. Limit consumption of sugary beverages, such as sodas and fruit juices.

Growing you own food is the best way to ensure that you are getting Nutritionally dense Fruits and Veggies.

Eliminate all animal meats and processed or manufactured food-like items.

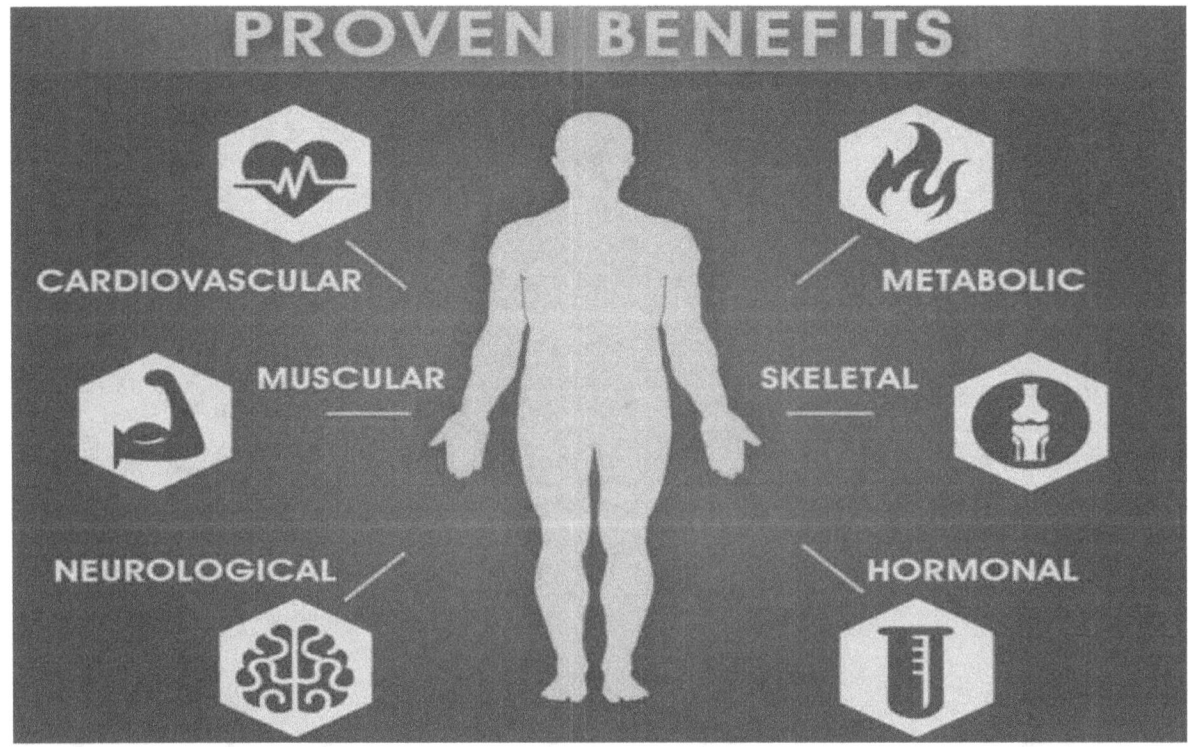

Benefits of Exercise

Performing just one single bout of exercise triggers a cascade of **hormonal**, **cardiovascular**, **physiological**, **neurological**, **endocrinological** and **biological** benefits in you. Muscles have been called the windows to every system of the body. If you start with this premise, you can see how transformative whole effort exercise (exercise which delivers immediate effects as well as longer term benefits that force your body to make positive adaptations) can be so meaningful.

Doing right by your body pays off for your mind as well. The Mayo Clinic notes that physical activity stimulates the production of endorphins.

Endorphins are your brain chemicals that leave you feeling happier and more relaxed. Eating a healthy diet as well as exercising can lead to a better physique.

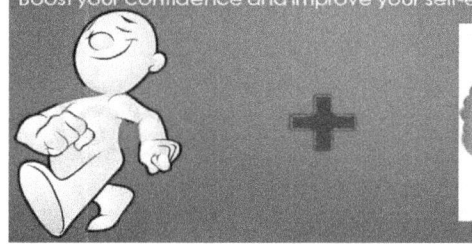

Exercise combats bad health conditions and diseases

Being active, boosts high-density lipoprotein (HDL)
Decreases unhealthy triglycerides (keep your blood flowing smoothly)
decreases your risk of heart diseases
Regular exercise = prevent a wide range of health problems

Exercise improves mood

30-minute walk can help your emotional health
Physical activity triggers brain chemicals that make you feel happier and more relaxed
Boost your confidence and improve your self-esteem

You'll feel better about your appearance, which can boost your confidence and self-esteem. Short-term benefits of exercise include decreased stress and improved cognitive function.

It's not just diet and exercise that lead to improved mood. Another healthy habit that leads to better mental health is making social connections. Whether it's volunteering, joining a club, or attending a movie, communal activities help improve mood and mental functioning by keeping the mind active and serotonin levels balanced.

Combats diseases

Healthy habits help prevent certain health conditions, such as heart disease, stroke, and high blood pressure. If you take care of yourself, you can keep your cholesterol and blood pressure within a safe range.

This keeps your blood flowing smoothly, decreasing your risk of cardiovascular diseases.

If you Eat To Live and Move YourSelf you will NEVER get sick!

Regular physical activity and proper diet can also prevent or help you manage a wide range of health problems, including:

- **metabolic syndrome**
- **diabetes**
- **depression**
- **certain types of cancer**
- **arthritis**

Make sure you schedule a physical exam every year. Your doctor will check your weight, heartbeat, and blood pressure, as well as take a urine and blood sample. This appointment can reveal a lot about your health. It's important to follow up with your doctor and listen to any recommendations to improve your health.

Boosts Energy

We've all experienced a lethargic feeling after eating too much unhealthy food. When you eat a balanced diet your body receives the fuel it needs to manage your energy level. A healthy diet includes:

- **whole grains**
- **low-fat dairy products**
- **fruit**
- **vegetables**

BOOST IN ENERGY LEVEL

Exercise improves the blood flow in the body and promotes better sleep, both of which boost energy. A regular exercise program, especially in the mornings, will give you energy and drive for the rest of the day. This effect is related to the increased metabolism associated with a fitter body.

Regular physical exercise also improves your muscle strength and boosts endurance, giving you more energy, says the Mayo Clinic.

Exercise helps deliver oxygen and nutrients to your tissues and gets your cardiovascular system working more efficiently so that you have more energy to go about your daily activities. It also helps boost energy by promoting better sleep.

This creates the conditions inside of you – Mentally and Physically that helps you fall asleep faster and get a deeper sleep.

Our chosen benefits of physical activity
- It controls weight
- Exercise combats health conditions and diseases
- Exercise improves mood
- Exercise boost energy and maintains your fitness level
- Exercise promotes better sleep

Your Healing, Restoration, Rejuvenation and Growth Hormones happens when you are RESTING!

Insufficient sleep can trigger a variety of problems. It creates a Stress in and on your Mind and Body.

Aside from feeling tired and sluggish, you may also feel irritable and moody if you don't get enough sleep. What's more, poor sleep quality may be responsible for high blood pressure, diabetes, and heart disease, and it can also lower your life expectancy.

To improve sleep quality, stick to a schedule where you wake up and go to bed at the same time every night.

Reduce your caffeine intake, limit napping, and create a comfortable sleep environment.

Turn off lights and the television, if any light touches any part of your body it prevents your body from producing and secreting Melatonin. Also maintain a cool room temperature.

Improves longevity

When you practice healthy habits, you boost your chances of a longer life. The American Council on Exercise reported on an eight-year study of 13,000 people. The study showed that those who walked just 30 minutes each day significantly reduced their chances of dying prematurely, compared with those who exercised infrequently.

Looking forward to more time with loved ones is reason enough to keep walking.

Start with short five-minute walks and gradually increase the time until you're up to 30 minutes.

Exercise Benefits

The health benefits of regular exercise and physical activity are hard to ignore, regardless of your age, sex or physical ability:

Exercise controls weight

Exercise combats health conditions and diseases

Exercise improves mood

Exercise boosts energy

Exercise promotes better sleep

Exercise puts the spark back into your sex life

Exercise can be fun

As Your Muscle Quality Improves So Improves:

- Neurological activity and motor unit recruitment (the greater the ability to recruit muscle fibers). This means you can use more muscle fibers which in turn leads to greater capacity for increased muscular growth (density/quality) and a greater ability to improve your glucose metabolism.

- Your body's ability to lose fat and reduce the risk of obesity and type II diabetes by improving glucose metabolism and insulin sensitivity.

- Cardiovascular function and oxygen uptake in your body. This enhancement leads to lower blood pressure and takes stress off your heart. This also eases the burden of your lungs to ensure oxygen is delivered in your body.

- Your skeletal system because demanding greater load on your muscles leads to stronger tendons and stronger bones.

- Your gastrointestinal tract and its ability to digest food and filter out the nutrition while helping the waste exit your body.

- Your endocrine system and its ability to properly balance the production and release of your anabolic and catabolic hormones (stress, cortisol, HGH and its impact on the thyroid).

- Your body's ability to deal with inflammation and the host of chronic disease that begins with cellular inflammation.

- Your body's ability to actually slow down and in some cases reverse your aging process as well as keep you living a fully functional life.

Benefits of Whole-Food Nutrition

Your body experiences lots of positive metabolic changes when you improve your diet. These changes greatly impact your overall health and wellbeing. When you make the switch to a whole-food diet, look for changes in your body like improved focus and mood, decreased sugar cravings, energy stabilization, better sleep, reduction in allergies and more.

For those willing to make positive changes towards regular, meaningful and appropriately challenging exercise – Move YourSelf and Eating To Live are the Foundation to Your Health, Wellness and Abundant Life!

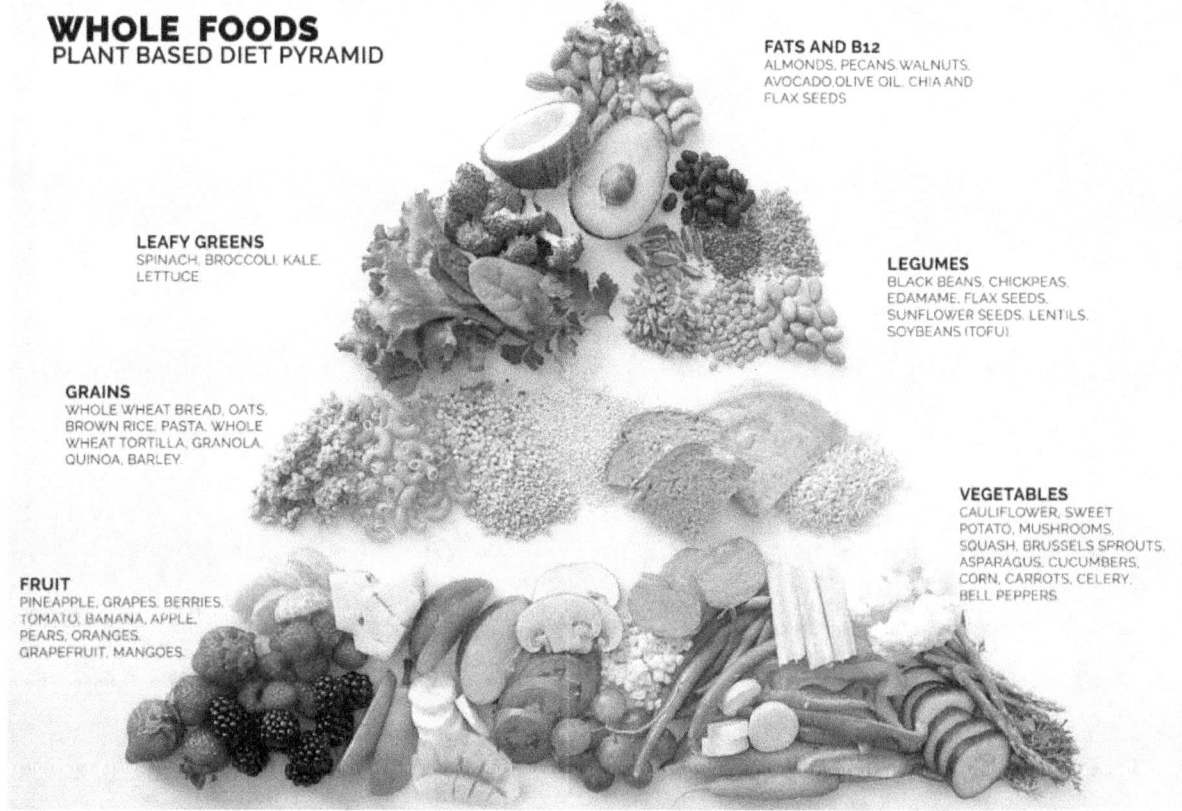

HEALTHY EATING vs UNHEALTHY EATING

 2 MILLION
Americans live 20 miles or more from a supermarket

 2.7 MILLION+
people die per year due to not getting enough fresh fruits and vegetables

 40%
increased inflation price of fresh produce in recent decades

 27 MINUTES
the average time an American spends cooking daily

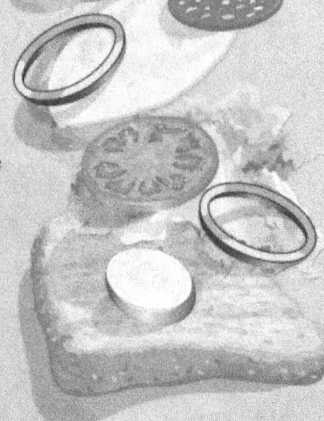

 5
fast food restaurants for every supermarket

 2.6 MILLION
deaths per year due to obesity-related illnesses

 40%
of cancers are due, in part, to an unhealthy diet

POLYDIMETHYLSILOXANE
an anti-foaming agent found in McDonald's Chicken McNuggets that is also found in Silly Putty

EFFECTS

- **Healthy Body**
  Healthy food provides a substantial amount of essential nutrients.

- **Happier Life**
  Amino acids and Vitamin B found in fruits and vegetables trigger the serotonin which is the body's "feel good" neurotransmitter.

EFFECTS

- **Diabetes**
  25.8 million Americans suffer from diabetes.

- **Depression**
  consuming trans-fats, saturated fats, and processed foods increases the chances of depression by 58%.

The Risks of Poor Fitness*

PREMATURE DEATH	**52%** higher risk
DIABETES	**39%** greater chance of developing diabetes
HEART DISEASE	**26%** higher risk

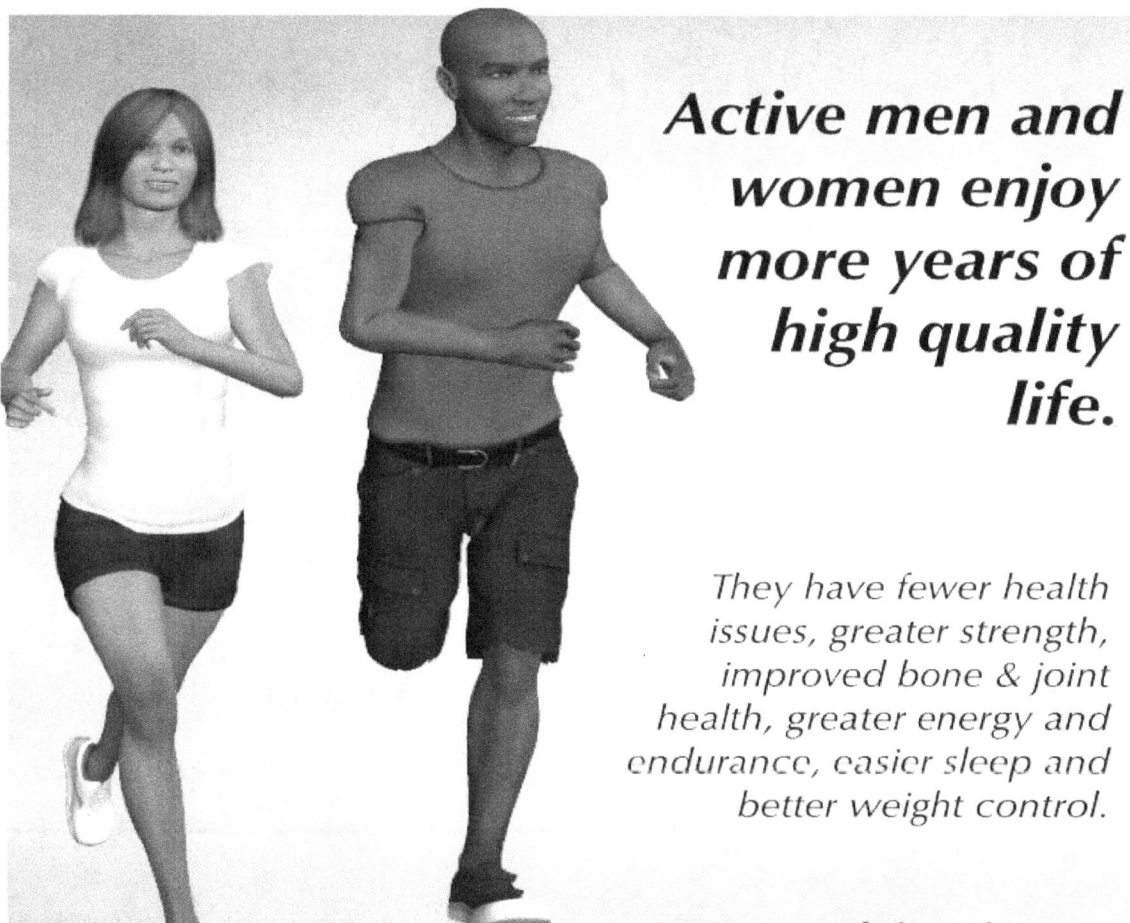

Active men and women enjoy more years of high quality life.

They have fewer health issues, greater strength, improved bone & joint health, greater energy and endurance, easier sleep and better weight control.

whyiexercise.com

Move Something!

Chapter Seven

Are You Fit ... Check YourSelf

*****

You know your physical health status better than anyone else ..... It's Your Body and you know how much you Move it and what you put In it.

With this chapter, you will easily access yourself so that you can have a clear picture of your current health status as well as where you want or need improvement at. Regardless to your status, it is always important to have a current update.

Before we begin, remember that there are no right or wrong answers. The questions are easy and cover the categories of health and fitness. The more honest you are = the better results for improving your health and wellness.

#1 Your Cardio Endurance

How long are you able to exercise vigorously without stopping?

5	I do this very easily.
4	It takes some effort, but I do this without any problems.
3	I have some difficulty, but I can do this most of the time.
2	Often I have difficulty doing this.
1	I can't do this at all

This category depends on your heart's ability to supply blood to your working muscles and your muscles' ability to use the oxygen in your blood.

As you can see in the below picture, many everyday activities depend on you having a fit and fully functional cardiovascular system.

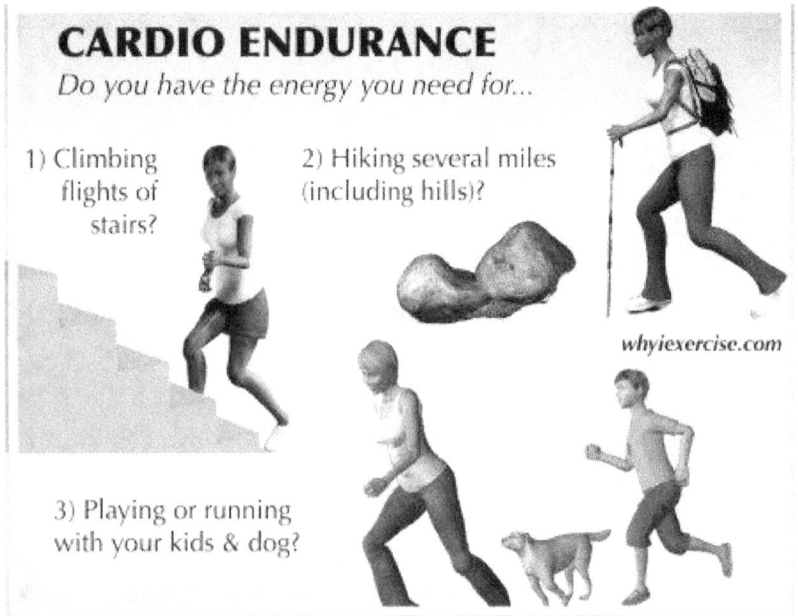

Your Cardio Goals: Work toward being able to exercise vigorously for at least 30 minutes, and reach at least an average level of cardio fitness for your age

#2 Your Muscular Performance (strength and muscular endurance)

<u>How easy is it for you to push, pull or lift heavy objects?</u>

<u>How well are you able to resist fatigue and participate fully in sports and active hobbies like dancing?</u>

5	I do this very easily.
4	It takes some effort, but I do this without any problems.
3	I have some difficulty, but I can do this most of the time.
2	Often I have difficulty doing this.
1	I can't do this at all

The level of Your Strength requires powerful muscular contractions and good coordination between your muscle groups.

The success of Good muscular performance also includes your bodies ability to work consistently over a period of time.

The following pictures are examples of everyday activities that involve and use your Muscular Strength and your Muscular Endurance.

These are some of the first activities that we LOSE our abilities to successfully complete or perform and underscores the value and importance of Moving YourSelf.

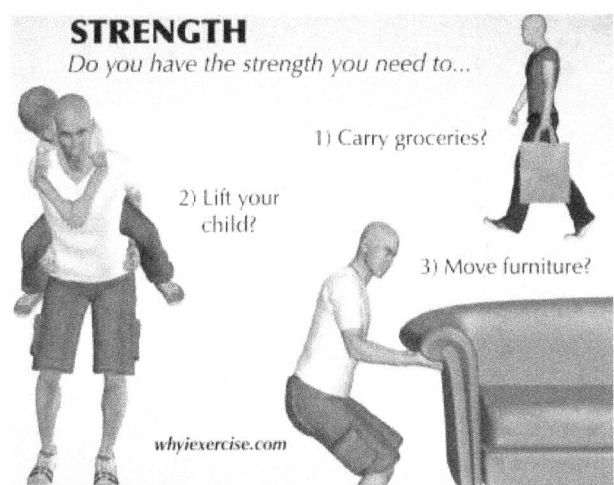

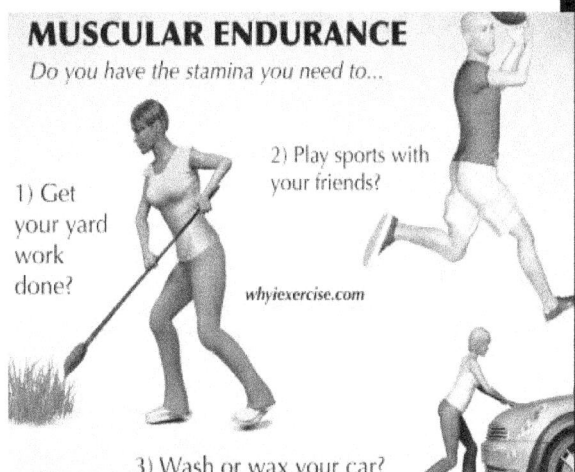

Your Strength Goal: Aim for average strength or greater for your age group. Find out how you measure up with the fitness tests below.

#3 Your Flexibility

<u>*How would you rate your ability to move your joints freely without strain?*</u>

5	I do this very easily.
4	It takes some effort, but I do this without any problems.
3	I have some difficulty, but I can do this most of the time.
2	Often I have difficulty doing this.
1	I can't do this at all

Having Good flexibility is helpful in all activities that you can perform.

It allows you to squat, bend, and reach, with a full range of motion.

Maintaining and improving your flexibility is helpful for the level and quality of your muscular performance as well as injury prevention.

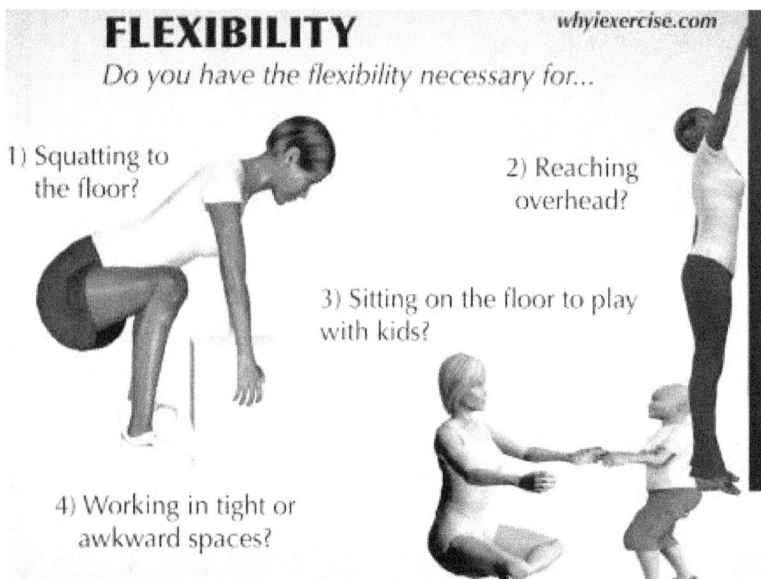

Your Flexibility Goal: The more flexible you are = the better movement you can perform. Lifestyles that require a lot of sitting have been shown to cause the tightening up of muscles in the majority of teens and adults. This is why being sedentary is dangerous to your health and wellness. You LOSE your ability to control and move your body as you want or need.

#4 Freedom from pain

Pain is common - but it is NOT normal.

How much does pain affect your work day, hobbies, family time and restfulness?

First of all, please see your health care provider and follow their instructions if you have significant pain, an injury or any medical condition.

Physical therapy exercises and lower back exercise may be helpful if you have issues with your muscles and joints.

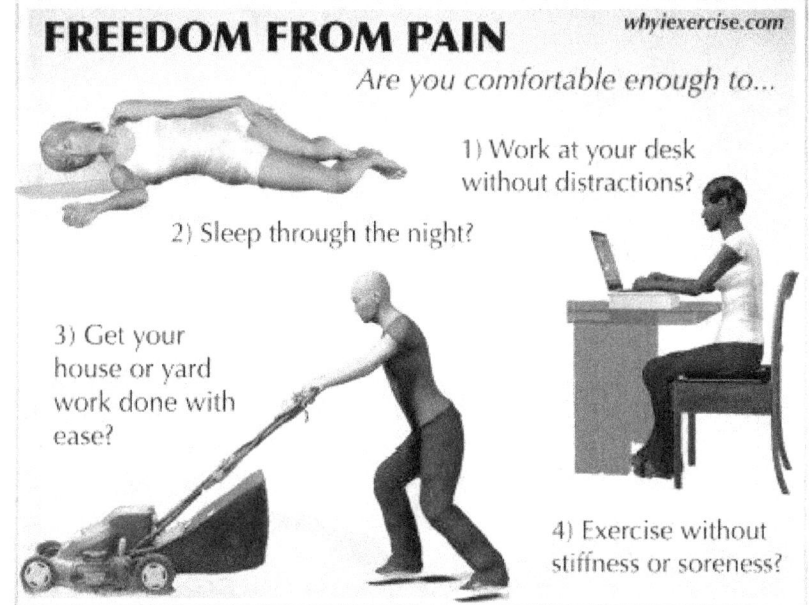

Why it's worth your time and effort to become more fit.

Just as it's hard to put a value on your time, it's also hard to overstate the benefits of physical fitness. Your well-being affects your decisions, activities, opportunities, relationships...nearly every part of your life.

Personal health and fitness directly relates to your quality of life and are the major contributing factors for you to Successfully Enjoy your Abundant Life.

Here are 4 great reasons to make daily exercise a priority.

#1 Consistency pays off quickly.

Do you feel like there's too much work ahead of you to become physically fit? If you are new to exercise or 'out of shape', you actually have an advantage. Though it may be tough at first, be consistent with exercise, and your body will adapt to these new physical activities. You will make progress every week, and your quality of life will change even quicker, usually within a month's time.

Your Increased muscular strength will make it easier to lift children, groceries or everything else.

A lower body fat percentage will show in the mirror which will put a Smile on Your Face!

Weight loss and improved endurance will help you Move YourSelf with much less effort.

#2 Health benefits last for a lifetime.

Do you like the idea of looking better and being more physically capable?

Your own benefits of physical fitness will include a *significantly reduced risk of death from all causes, cardiovascular disease, cancer, diabetes, and osteoporosis.*

Add the Science of Eating To Live to an active lifestyle and you'll have a powerful combination for building your Supreme Health and Fitness!

#3 It's simply too deadly to be out of shape.

Lack of physical activity tends to make people feel sluggish, and when you combine that with mental fatigue from a long day at work or school, it's natural to want to rest in front of the TV at the end of the day. But studies show that diabetes and obesity are linked with TV time.

While watching TV or video content (i. e. video on internet), you burn no more energy than we do at complete rest, and we're also bombarding ourselves with fast food commercials compelling us to eat! So even in those who are otherwise physically active, excessive TV time may pose a health risk.

Researchers recommend less than 10 hours of TV per week. They estimate that 30% of new obesity cases and 43% of new diabetes cases can be prevented through watching less than 10 hours of TV / week and walking briskly for at least 60 minutes per day. The average American watches over 35 hours of video content per week according to Neilsen.

There is one thing that is for sure …. That It's Never Too Late to start an exercise program and that as soon as you Start it = You automatically Improve the quality of your Health and Life!

It's FUN and EASY …. All You Have To Do Is …..

Move SomeThing!

What are You Moving?

YourSelf!

Where are You Going?

Abundant Life!

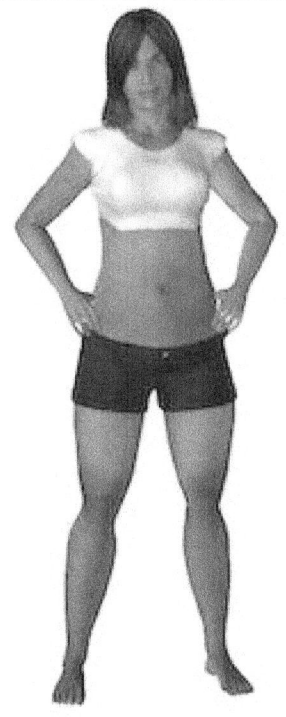 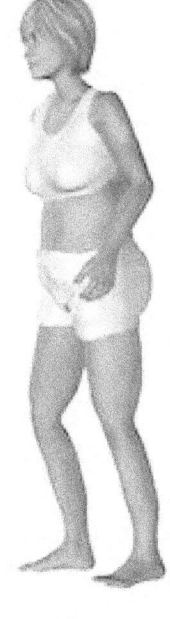

The average US female (5'4" 165 lbs) needs to lose 25 lbs* to lower her risk for health problems.

What is your weight loss goal?

The average US male (5'9" 190 lbs) needs to lose about 25 lbs* to have a healthy body weight.

How much weight do you need to lose?

whyiexercise.com

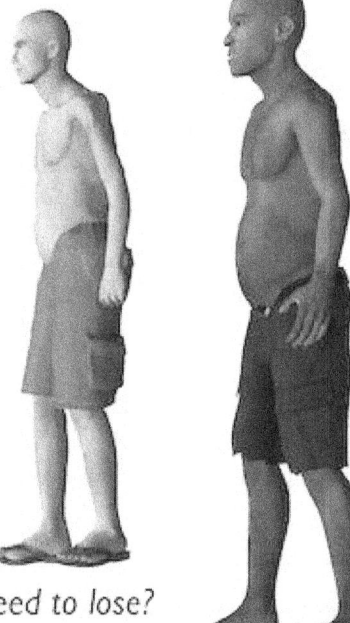

Move Something!

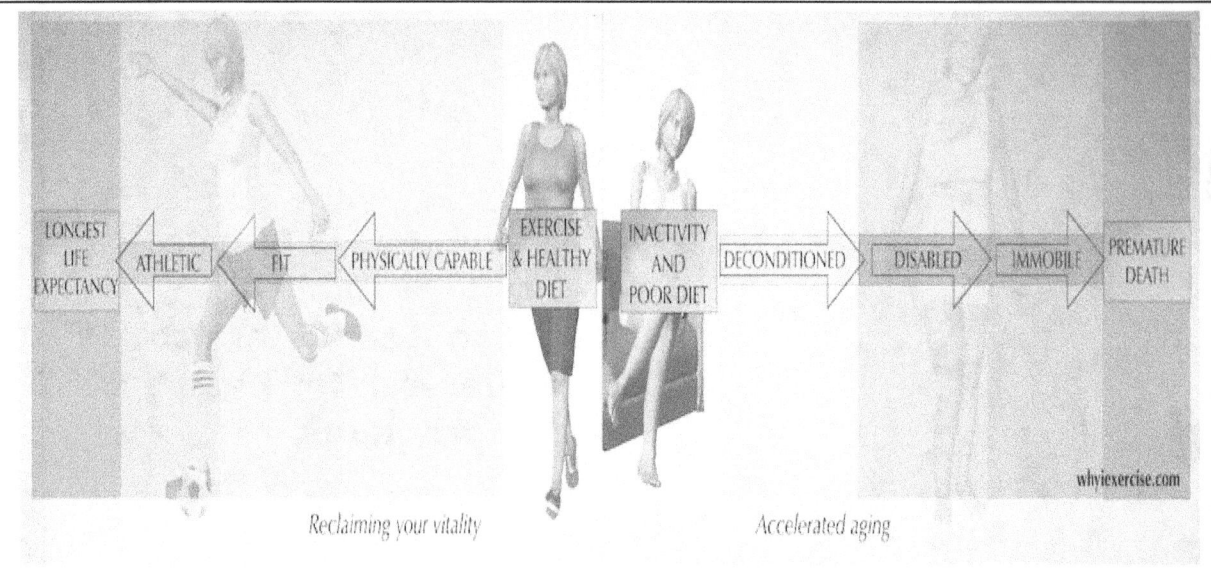

Reclaiming your vitality   Accelerated aging

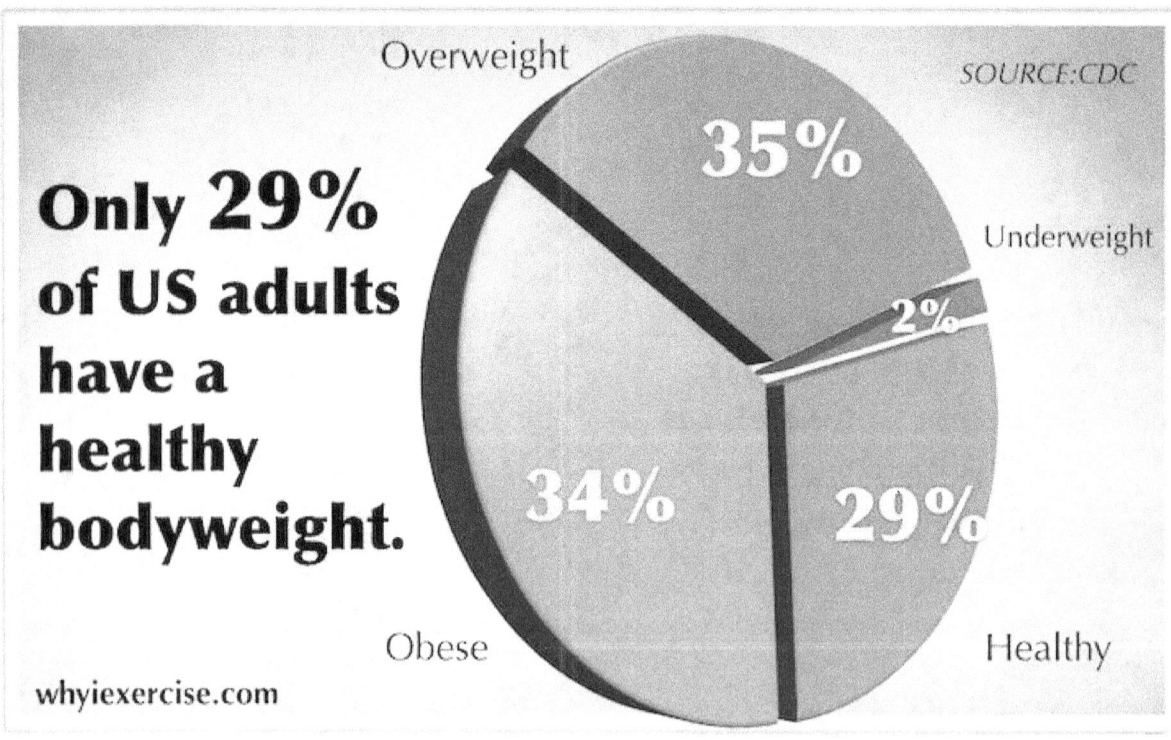

Only 29% of US adults have a healthy bodyweight.

whyiexercise.com

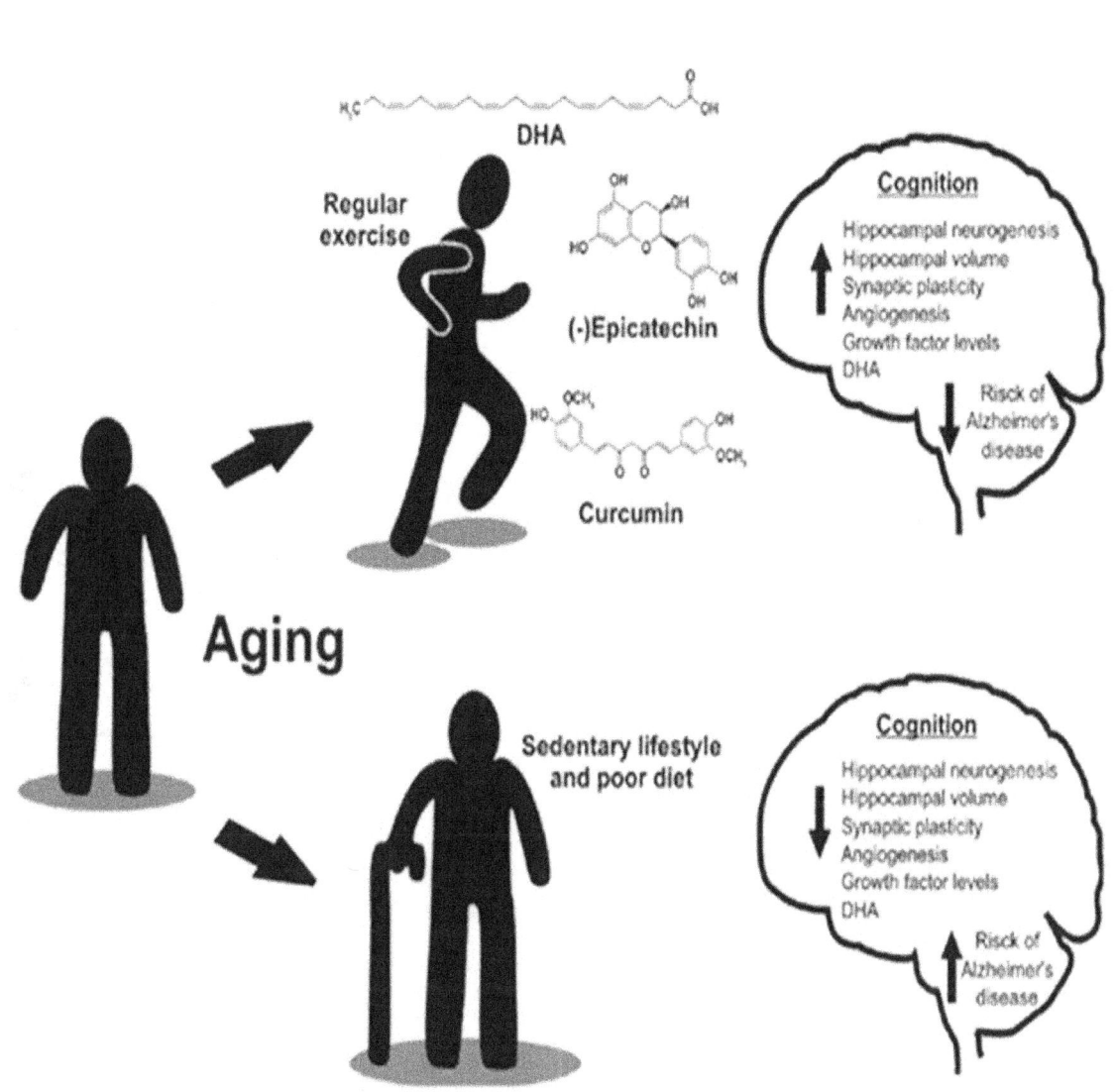

Move Something!

Chapter Eight

It's NEVER Too Late!

*****

The older I get, the more I realize how important weight training is. It now makes up about half of my workouts, and if you're middle-aged or beyond, I encourage you to make this a regular part of your exercise routine.

The fact is, even though you might not care as much about how your muscles *look* as you did in your 20s (but then again, you might!), you certainly care about how your muscles *function*.

You need your body to be able to carry you into the Enjoyment of Your Abundant Life!

Your Body is the vehicle the houses the Awesome Power that is YOU!

So that you can Say BE and your Body WILL Work to make it BECOME!

You Body will be Strong enough to make manifest the Force and Power of God that You ARE!

The better condition that your Body the Greater Works you can accomplish with the Greatest being you Successfully Enjoying Abundant Life!

Without weight training, your muscles will atrophy and lose mass. Age-related loss of muscle mass is known as sarcopenia, and if you don't do anything to stop it you can expect to lose about 15 percent of your muscle mass between your 30s and your 80s.

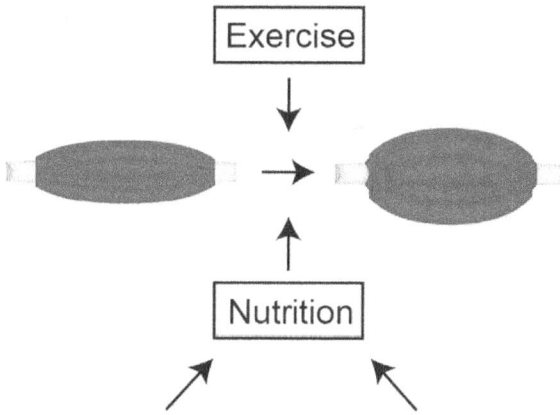

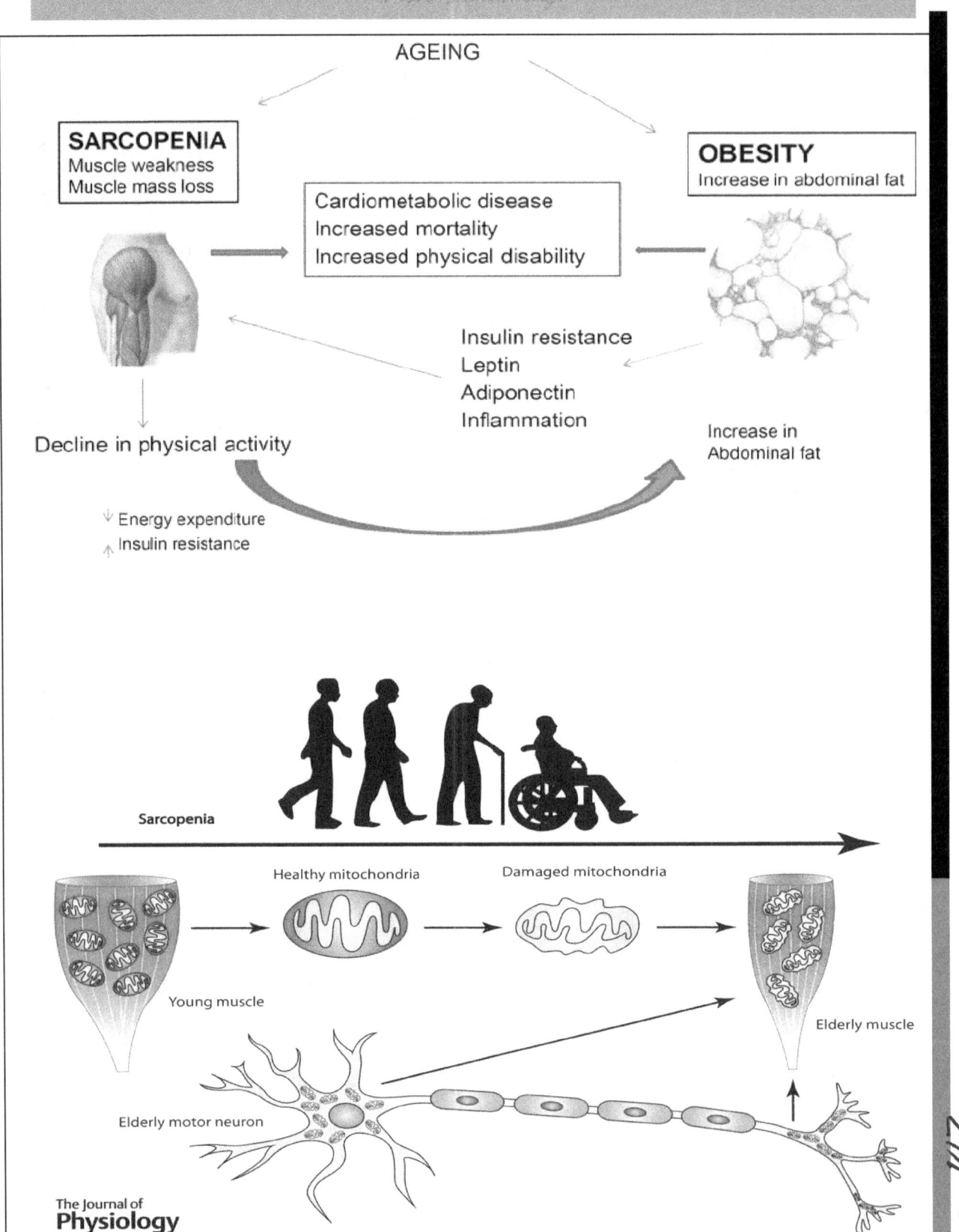

Slow Down Muscle Loss and Boost Your Strength Three-Fold

Muscle loss happens gradually, so you probably won't notice it occurring at first. But by the time you're in your 70s, when sarcopenia tends to accelerate, you might start to feel weaker and find you can't do things, physically, that you used to do.

PLEASE UNDERSTAND: *Sarcopenia is Nutrition and Exercise based ... meaning that HOW and WHAT you choose to Eat and the amount of Exercise will keep you Grow YOUNG or Cause you to Grow OLD!*

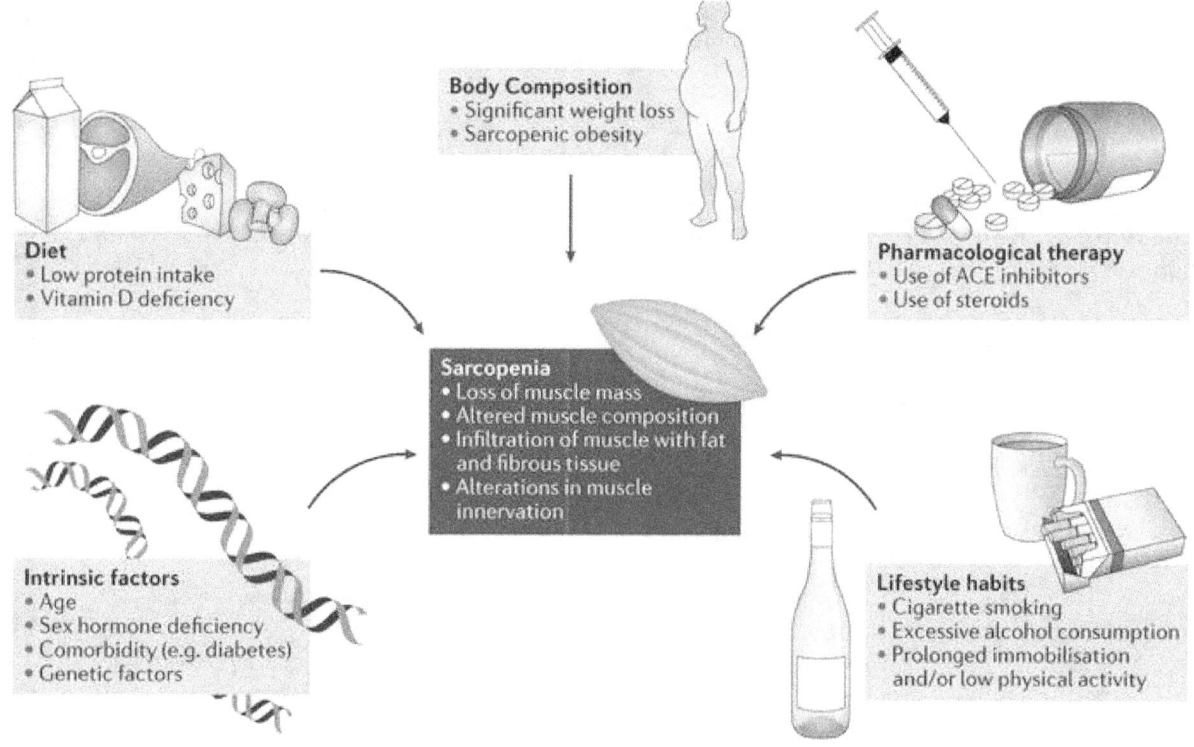

According to the American College of Sports Medicine (ACSM):

"A gradual loss in muscle cross-sectional area is consistently found with advancing age; by age 50, about ten percent of muscle area is gone. After 50 years of age, the rate of loss accelerates significantly.

Muscle strength declines by approximately 15 percent per decade in the sixties and seventies and by about 30 percent thereafter. Although intrinsic muscle function is reduced with advancing age, age-related decrease in muscle mass is responsible for almost all loss of strength in the older adult."

By helping you maintain your muscle mass and strength, strength training can, quite literally, give you the ability to keep on living.

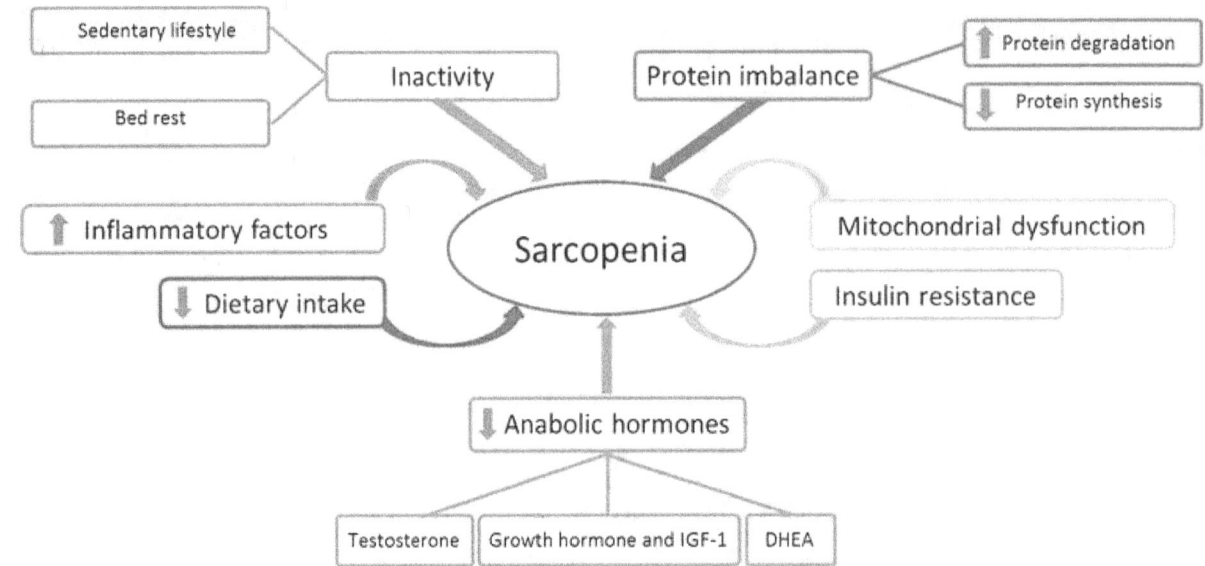

On the contrary, if you stop working your muscles, the consequences of sarcopenia are steep and include:

- *Increased risk of falls and fractures*
- *Impaired ability to regulate body temperature*
- *Slower metabolism*
- *Loss in the ability to perform everyday tasks*

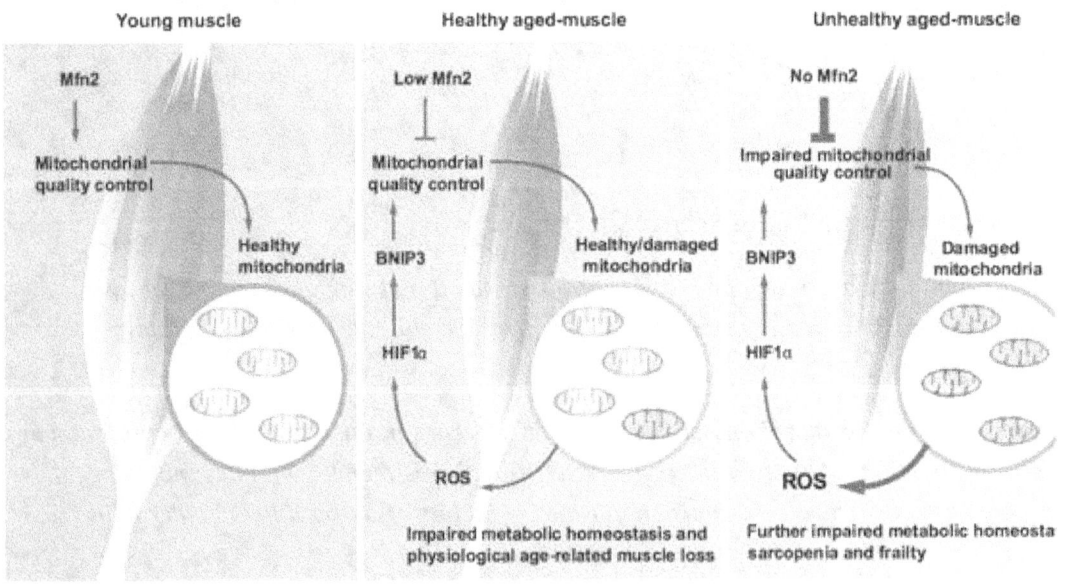

Now, what do you have to *gain* by starting weight training – even if you're already "older?" As ACSM explains:

"Given an adequate training stimulus, older adults can make significant gains in strength. A two- to three-fold increase in strength can be accomplished in three to four months in fibers recruited during training in older adults. With more prolonged resistance training, even a modest increase in muscle size is possible.

…With increasing muscle strength come increased levels of spontaneous activity in both healthy, independent older adults and very old and frail men and women. Strength training, in addition to its possible effects on insulin action, bone density, energy metabolism, and functional status, is also an important way to increase levels of physical activity in the older adult."

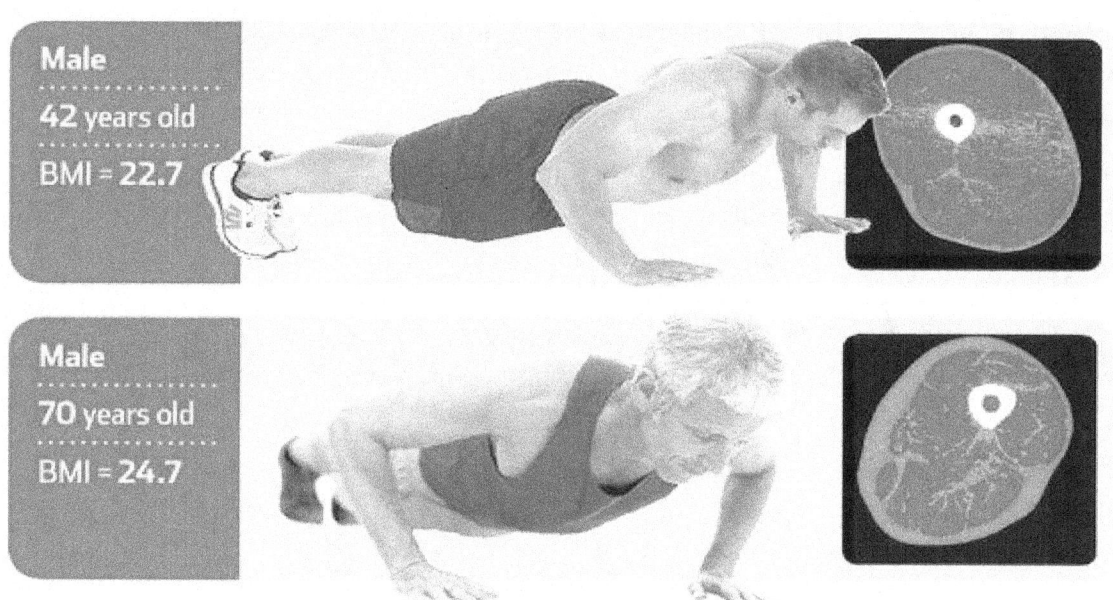

Critical Mass | How muscles decline as we age

These cross-section scans of thighs of men of similar body-mass index show typical loss of muscle quantity and quality with age. Normal-density muscle, shown in blue, gives way to low-density muscle, the green marbling, and fat, in red and orange.

Male — 42 years old — BMI = 22.7

Male — 70 years old — BMI = 24.7

The Many Benefits of Weight Training for Older Adults

Weight training is important throughout your life, but in many ways it becomes even more important as you age. Even if you're in your 90s, it's *not too late.* One study found a group of nursing home residents with an average age of 90 improved their strength between 167 and 180 percent after just eight weeks of weight training.

What are some of the other benefits?

- **Improved walking ability:** After 12 weeks of weight training, seniors aged 65 and over improved both their leg strength and endurance and were able to walk nearly 40 percent farther without resting.

- **Improved ability to perform daily tasks:** After 16 weeks of "total body" weight training, women aged 60 to 77 years "substantially increased strength" and had improvements in walking velocity and the ability to carry out daily tasks, such as rising from a chair or carrying a box of groceries.

- **Decreased risk of falls:** Women between the ages of 75 and 85, all of whom had reduced bone mass or full-blown osteoporosis, were able to lower their fall risk with weight training and agility activities.

- **Relief from joint pain:** Weight training strengthens the muscles, tendons and ligaments around your joints, which takes stress off the joint and helps ease pain. It can also help increase your range of motion.

- **Improved blood sugar control:** Weight training helps to control blood sugar levels in people with type 2 diabetes. It can also reduce your type 2 diabetes risk; strength training for at least 150 minutes a week lowered diabetes risk by 34 percent compared to being sedentary.

Weight training can also go a long way to prevent brittle bone formation and can help reverse the damage already done. For example, a walking lunge exercise is a great way to build bone density in your hips, even without any additional weights. Strength training also increases your body's production of growth factors, which are responsible for cellular growth, proliferation, and differentiation. Some of these growth factors also promote the growth, differentiation, and survival of your *neurons*, which helps explain why working your muscles also benefits your brain and helps prevent dementia.

Super-Slow Weight Training Best if You're Older

By slowing your movements down, it turns your weight-training session into high-intensity exercise. The super-slow movement allows your muscle, at the microscopic level, to access the maximum number of cross-bridges between the protein filaments that produce movement in the muscle.

This is a beneficial and safe way to incorporate high-intensity exercise into your workouts if you're older and have trouble getting around. You only need about 12 to 15 minutes of super-slow strength training once a week to achieve the same human growth hormone (HGH) production as you would from 20 minutes of Peak Fitness sprints, which is why fitness experts like Dr. Doug McGuff are such avid proponents of this technique.

The fact that super-slow weight training gives you an excellent boost in human growth hormone (HGH), otherwise known as the "fitness hormone," is another reason why it's so beneficial if you're older.

As you reach your 30s and beyond, you enter what's called "somatopause," when your levels of HGH begin to drop off quite dramatically. This is part of what drives your aging process. According to Dr. McGuff, there's also a strong correlation between somatopause and age-related sarcopenia.

HGH is needed to sustain your fast-twitch muscle fibers, which produce a lot of power. It's also needed to stimulate those muscles.

"What seems to be evident is that a high-intensity exercise stimulus is what triggers the body to make an adaptive response to hold on to muscle," Dr. McGuff says. *"We have to remember that muscle is a very metabolically expensive tissue… If you become sedentary and send your body a signal that this tissue is not being used, then that tissue is metabolically expensive. The adaptation is to deconstruct that tissue…"*

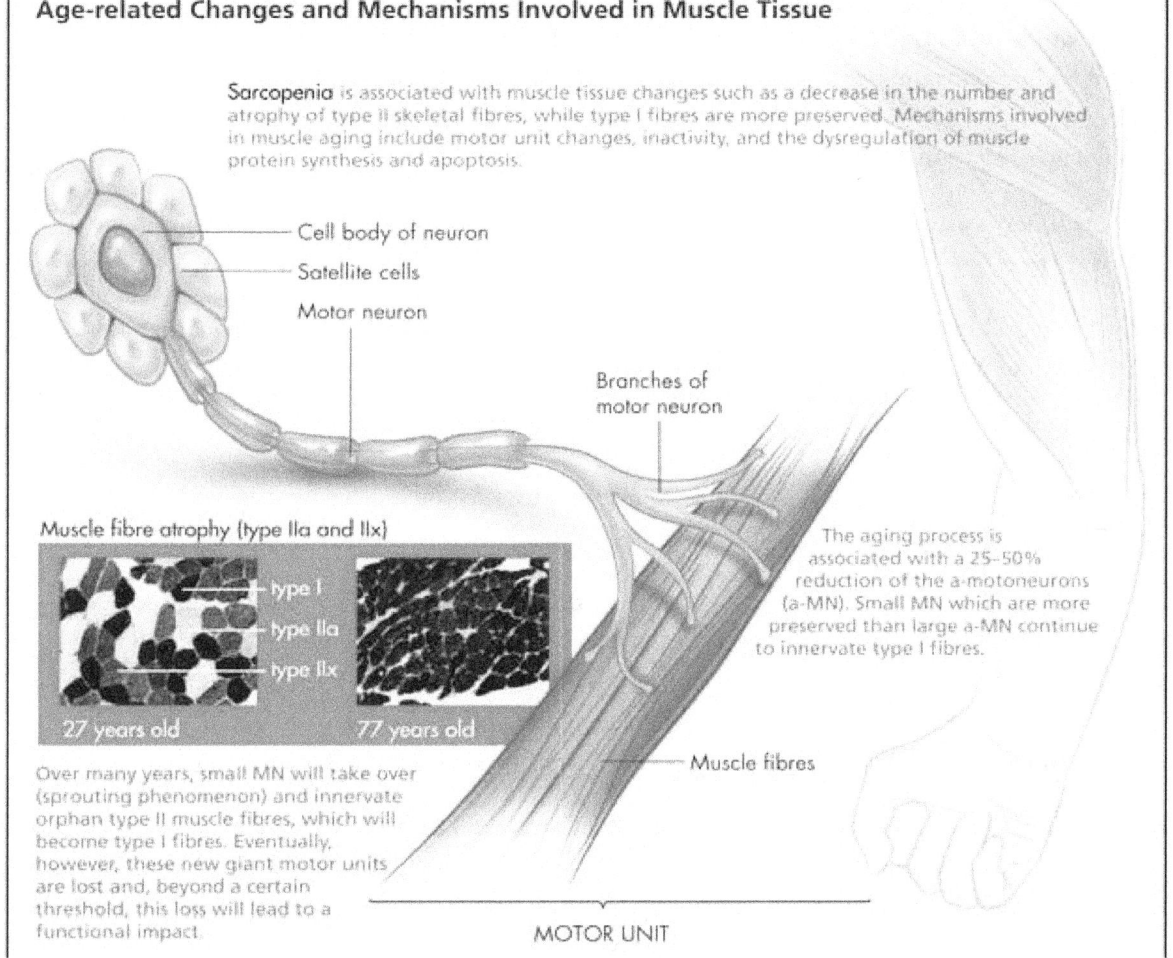

People of all ages can and also do benefit from super-slow weight training, but this is definitely a method to consider if you're middle-aged or older.

I recommend using four or five basic compound movements for your super-slow (high intensity) exercise set. Compound movements are movements that require the coordination of several muscle groups—for example, squats, chest presses and compound rows.

Here is my version of the technique.

- **Begin by lifting the weight *as slowly and gradually as you can*. You perform this by doing a four-second positive and a four-second negative, meaning it takes four seconds, or a slow count to four, to bring the weight up, and another four seconds to lower it. (When pushing, stop about 10 to 15 degrees before your limb is fully straightened; smoothly reverse direction)**
- *Slowly* lower the weight back down to the slow count of four
- **Repeat until exhaustion, which should be around four to eight reps. Once you reach exhaustion, don't try to heave or jerk the weight to get one last repetition in. Instead, just keep trying to produce the movement, even if it's not "going" anywhere, for another five seconds or so. If you're using the appropriate amount of weight or resistance, you'll be able to perform eight to 10 reps**
- **Immediately switch to the next exercise for the next target muscle group, and repeat the first three steps**

Whether you've never exercised before or have simply fallen off track, today is the day you can renew your commitment to physical activity.

Remember, you are never too old to start exercising.

I'm hoping that the information in this chapter and book will Inspire you to get active as well, no matter what your age.

If you're just starting out, consult with a personal fitness trainer who can instruct you about proper form and technique. He or she can also help you develop a plan based on your unique fitness goals and one that is safe for any medical conditions you may have. Just keep in mind that while you need to use caution, you *do* need to exercise at a level that is challenging to your body. Many make the mistake of exercising with not enough intensity, and this will result in many of your benefits being forfeited.

It's important that before you start to adjust your *mindset* as well. You have to have the proper level of Motivation, Purpose and Focus to Visualize your Health Needs and Goals and the Power to begin and to Successfully Complete your program to Get Healthy!

As soon as you become open and prepare yourself mentally to becoming fit and strong, your body will follow suit.

Do start slowly and gradually increase your intensity while listening to your body. And be sure to give your body ample time for recovery, as well as the proper nourishment to help build your muscles.

Amino acids are extremely important as they form the building blocks for muscle. Leucine is a powerful muscle builder. However, you should avoid amino acid isolates of leucine because, in its free form, it's been shown to contribute to insulin resistance and may lead to muscle wasting. It's far better to get leucine from whole foods, and the best source is a high-quality whey protein.

Applying the Sciences of Eating To Live and Moving YourSelf is the Foundation for creating your Health and Wellness!

And its as Easy as Moving Something!

Move Something!

WHAT Are YOU Moving?

YourSelf!

WHERE Are YOU Going?

Abundant LIFE!

Energy Balance Scales – Weight Gain

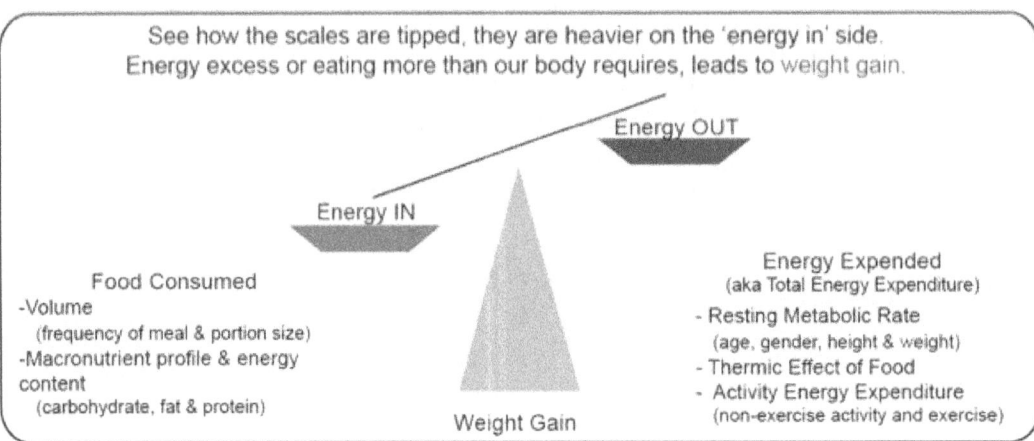

Fig. 2b Energy imbalance - scales are tipped to weight gain

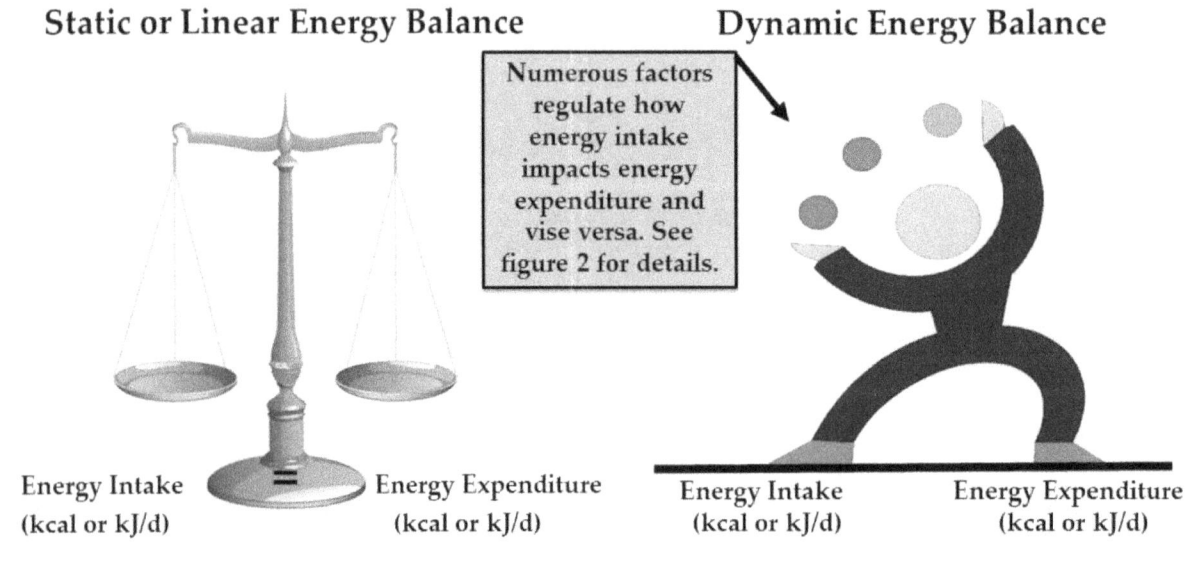

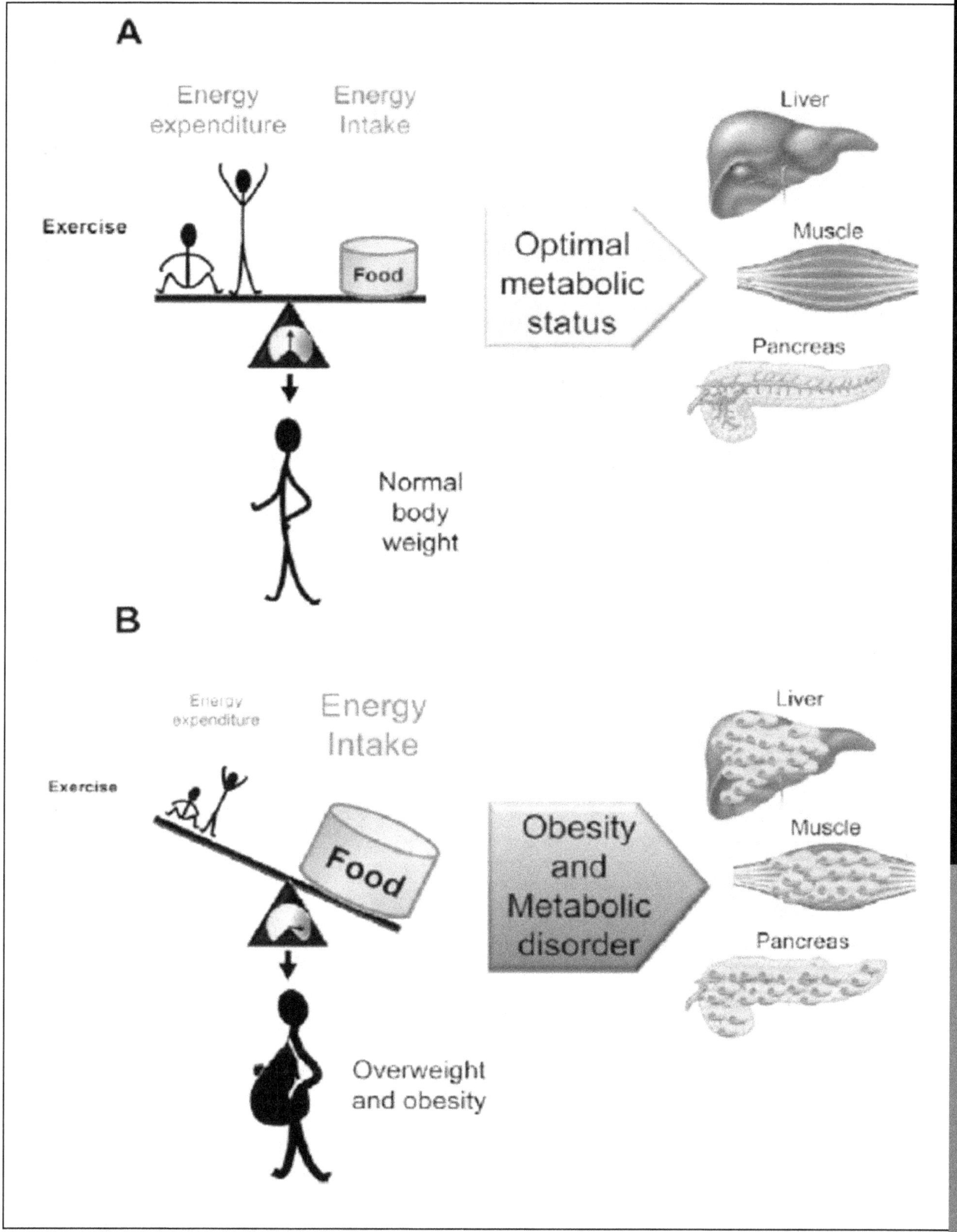

Move SomeThing!

A

Energy expenditure | Energy Intake

Exercise

Food

Optimal metabolic status

Liver
Muscle
Pancreas

Normal body weight

B

Energy expenditure | Energy Intake

Exercise

Food

Obesity and Metabolic disorder

Liver
Muscle
Pancreas

Overweight and obesity

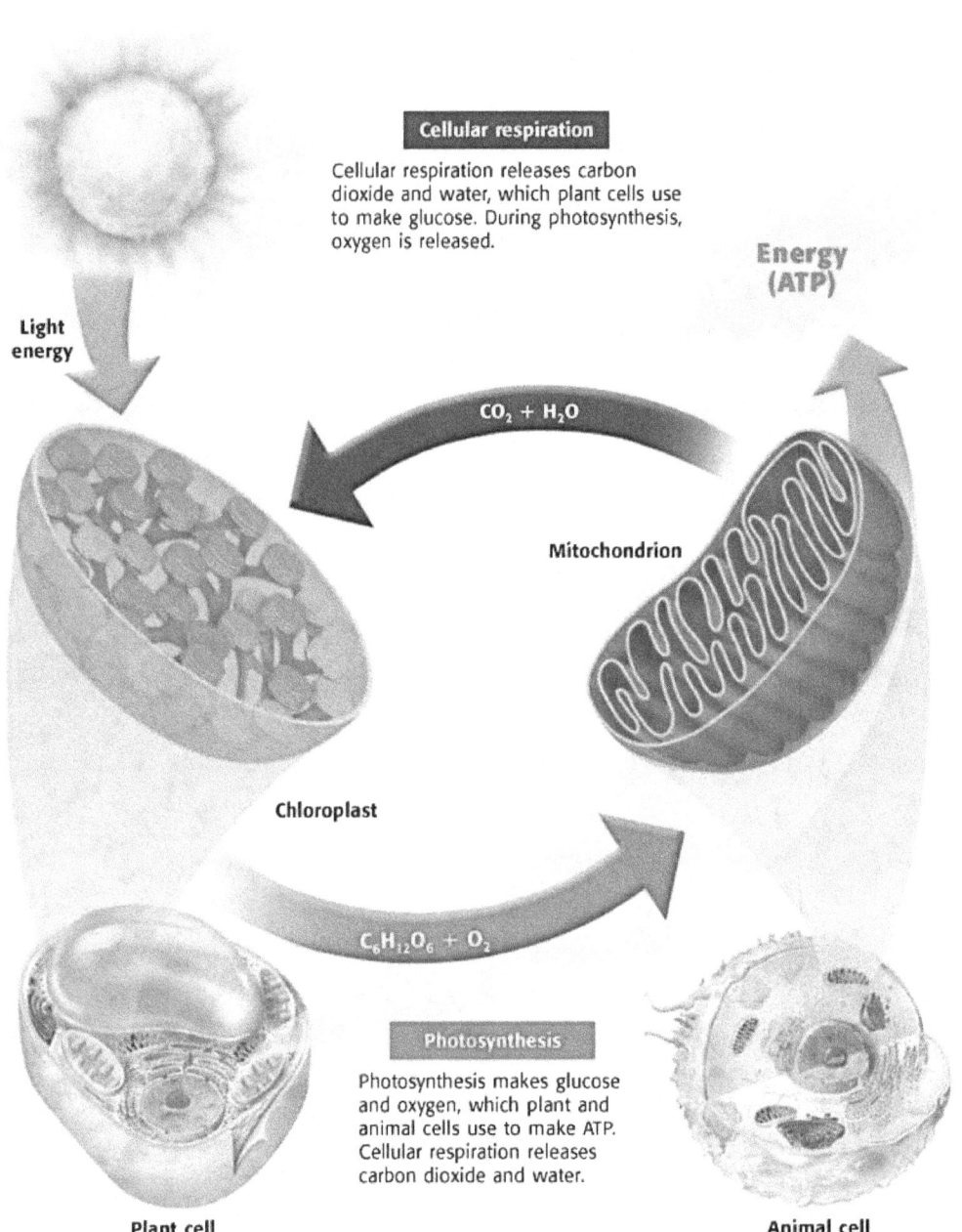

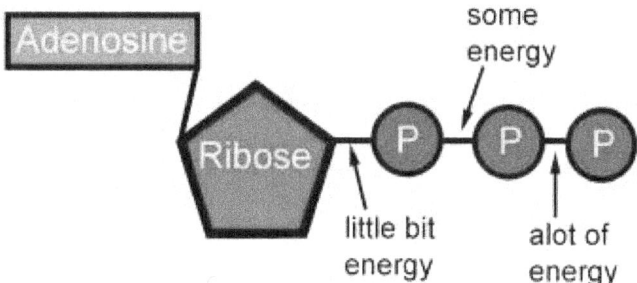

Notice that an ATP molecule has three main parts—a nitrogenous base (called adenine, colored orange in the diagram above), a sugar named ribose (the blue hexagon in the diagram above), and three phosphate groups (labeled "P" in the diagram, and are the three purple circles).

Sources of ATP for Muscle Contraction
It is evident that ATP availability is critical for muscle contraction. For example, during the onset of exercise, the muscle's ATP needs are increased. The basal level of ATP is not sufficient to meet the increased energy needs for muscle contraction. Depending on the intensity and the duration of exercise, the muscle's energy needs are met by the following sources:

1. **Short-term/immediate source:** As ATP gets utilized during the onset of exercise, ADP accumulates. The **Phosphagen System** serves a reserve of inorganic phosphate that can be quickly utilized to re-phosphorylate ADP to regenerate ATP. This is an **anaerobic system** for ATP production. The sources of phosphate in the phosphagen system are:
    - Creatine phosphate
    - ADP (adenosine-di-phosphate)

2. **Intermediate source: Anerobic glycolysis** serves as an important intermediate source of ATP production to meet the muscle's energy needs. The process also does not depend on oxygen availability. **Glucose** is the substrate for anaerobic glycolysis and glucose is derived from:
    - Muscle glycogenolysis : major source
    - Blood glucose: a very minor source

3. **Longer-term source**: Mitochondrial respiration can serve as a long term source of ATP during muscle contraction. This process requires **oxygen** and is therefore an **aerobic process**. The substrates for ATP production are:
    - Fatty acids
    - Glucose

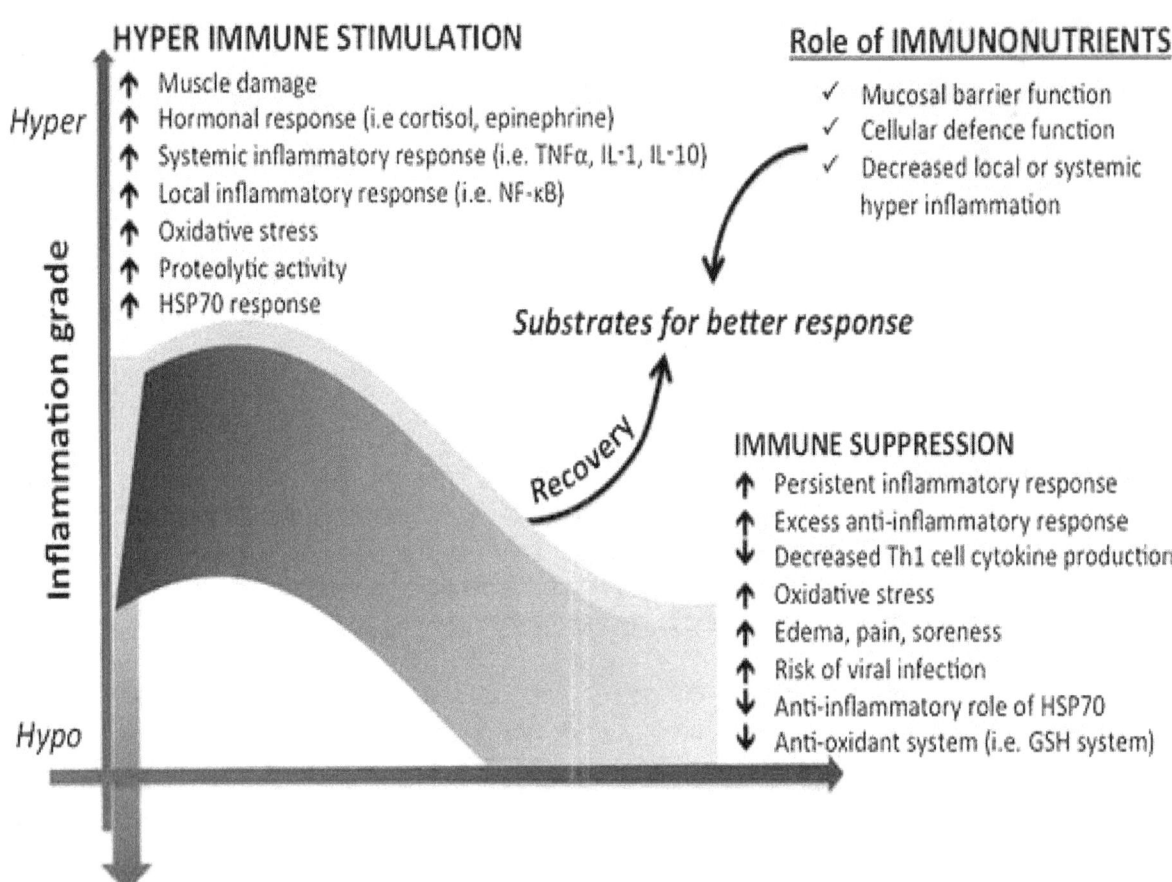

Chapter Eight

Your Energy & Work

*****

Everything IS Energy!

Energy is what makes your body go. There are several kinds of energy exist in your biological system/body: **electrical** energy in your nerves and muscles, **chemical** energy in the synthesis of your molecules, **mechanical** energy in the contraction of your muscle and **thermal** energy that is derived from all of these processes and helps maintain your body temperature.

The ultimate source of this Energy found in your external and internal biological systems is the Sun.

What I call Life Energy.

The **Radiant** Life Energy from the Sun is captured by plants and used to convert simple atoms and molecules into carbohydrates, fats and proteins.

The Sun's Life Energy is trapped within the chemical bonds of these food molecules.

Photosynthesis
carbon dioxide + water + light energy ⟶ sugar + oxygen

Cell respiration
sugar + oxygen ⟶ carbon dioxide + water + energy

The chloroplasts that trap the sun's energy in plants, and the mitochondria that release that energy in almost all cells are both descended from ancient bacteria. The bacteria were swallowed by our single-celled ancestors hundreds of millions of years ago, and they've been slaving away capturing (photosynthesis) and releasing (respiration) energy for their 'host' cells ever since. Life never would've left the pond without them.

For your cells to use this Life Energy, they must first break-down the foodstuffs in a manner that conserves most of the Life Energy contained in the bonds of the carbohydrates, fats, and proteins. In addition, the final product of the break-down must be a molecule your cell can use — **Adenosine Triphosphate** (ATP).

Chemical Energy and ATP

Organisms break down carbon-based molecules to produce ATP.

- Carbohydrates are the molecules most commonly broken down to make ATP.
  - not stored in large amounts
  - up to 36 ATP from one glucose molecule

Essentially, your body converts the Life Energy of the Sun that contained IN the Bonds of the Molecules of your Food and TRANSFERS it into the BONDS of the ATP Molecule.

This goes into the Importance of applying the Science of Eating To Live which involves knowing WHY you are eating, WHEN to eat, as well as HOW to eat.

Your Cells use ATP as the primary Life Energy source for your biological work, whether this work is electrical, mechanical, or chemical.

In ATP, there are 3 phosphates that are linked by **high-energy bonds**. When a bond between the phosphates is broken, energy is released and may be used by the cell. At this point the ATP has been reduced to a lower energy state, becoming adenosine diphosphate (ADP) and inorganic phosphate (P_i).

ATP and ADP

Act as chemical batteries
Carry and release small amounts of energy

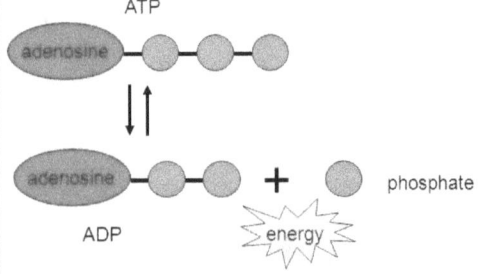

During your muscular activity, ATP is constantly converted to ADP and P_i in order to provide the energy needed for your work. The ATP must be replaced as fast as it is used if your muscle is to continue to generate force.

Your muscle cell has a great capacity to replace ATP under a variety of work circumstances, from a short dash to a marathon.

Edington and Edgerton devised a logical approach to help us understand how energy is supplied for muscle contraction — they divided the energy sources (ATP sources) into **immediate**, **short-term** and **long-term**.

Understanding the Science of your Life Energy Source allows you to accurately calculate and formulate the exact amount of Life Energy you need to constantly and consistently Move YourSelf into the Successfully Enjoyment of your Abundant Life!

The Life Energy of the ATP is essentially and literally SUN-LIGHT!

This means that you can SKIP the Eating process - GO STAND IN THE SUN and get the LIFE ENERGY DIRECTLY FROM THE SUN!

YOU BODY WILL CONVERT AND STORE IT DIRECTLY IN THE BONDS OF ATP …. WITHOUT WEAR ON YOUR DIGESTIVE SYSTEM!

Chemical Energy and ATP

Cellular respiration is like a mirror image of photosynthesis.

- The Krebs cycle transfers energy to an electron transport chain.
  - takes place in mitochondrial matrix
  - breaks down three-carbon molecules from glycolysis
  - makes a small amount of ATP
  - releases carbon dioxide
  - transfers energy-carrying molecules

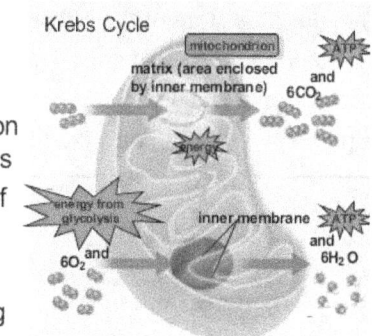

Your Immediate Sources of Energy

The very limited amount of ATP stored in your muscles might meet the energy demands of a maximal effort lasting about **1 second**.

Phosphocreatine (PC), another **high-energy** phosphate molecule stored in your muscle, is your most important immediate source of Energy. The PC molecule can donate its phosphate molecule (and the energy therein) to ADP in order to make ATP, allowing your muscle to continue producing force.

This means that you can keep and maintain you Motion of Life!

Your body will do and create what it needs for you to Successfully Move YourSelf INTO the enjoyment of your Abundant Life!

$$PC + ADP \rightarrow ATP + C = ENERGY$$

This reaction takes place as fast as your muscle forms ADP. Unfortunately, the PC store in your muscle lasts only **3 to 5 seconds** when your muscle is working at its maximal effort. This process also does not require Oxygen and is one of your **anaerobic energy** (without oxygen) mechanisms for producing your ATP.

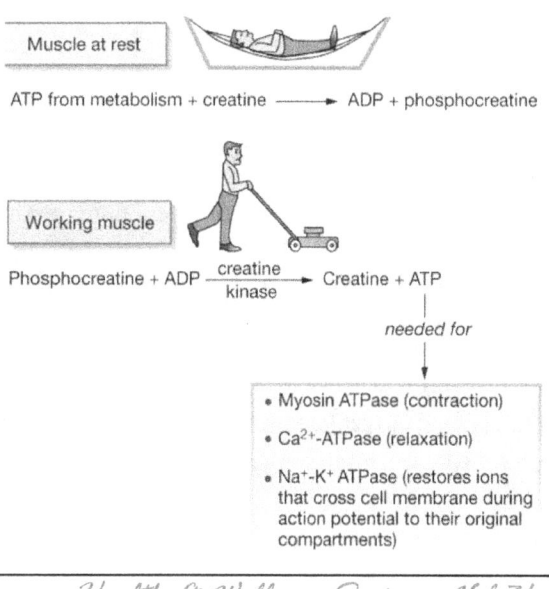

The PC molecule is the primary source of ATP during an activity or exercise like shot put, a vertical jump, or the first seconds of a sprint.

Your Short-Term Sources of Energy

As the muscle's store of the PC molecule decreases, your muscle fibers break down glucose (a simple sugar) to produce ATP at a high rate. The glucose is obtained from your blood or your muscle's glycogen store. The multi-enzyme pathway for glucose metabolism is called **glycolysis**, and it does not require oxygen to function (like the breakdown of PC, it too is an anaerobic process).

$$\text{Glucose} \rightarrow 2\ \text{Pyruvic Acid} + 2\ \text{ATP} = \text{ENERGY}$$

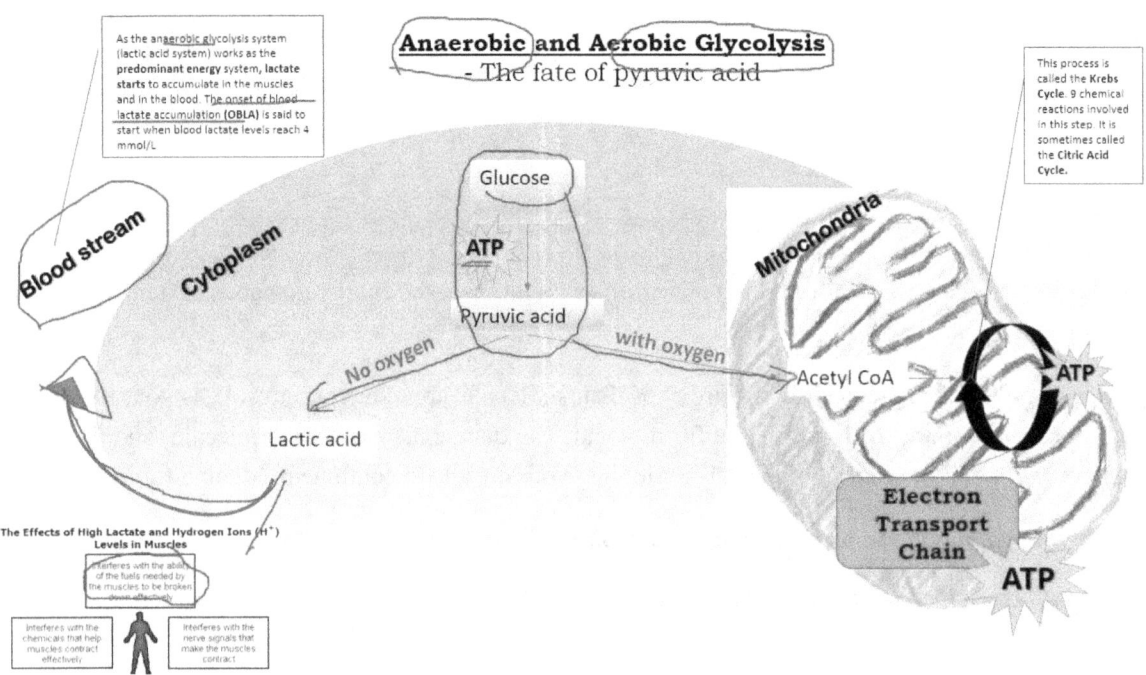

In glycolysis, glucose is broken down into two molecules of pyruvic acid; in the process, ADP is converted to ATP, allowing your muscle to maintain a high rate of work.

However, glycolysis can only continue for a limited time.

When glycolysis operates at high speed, pyruvic acid is converted to **lactic acid** and lactic acid (lactate) accumulates in your muscle and your blood. This accumulation of lactic acid in your muscles actually **slows** the rate of glycogen metabolism and may interfere with the mechanism involved in your muscle contractions – potentially impairing your ability to Successfully Move YourSelf or to maintain your Motion.

Supplying ATP via glycolysis has its shortcomings, but it does allow a person to run at fast speeds for short distances. This short-term energy source is of primary importance in events involving maximal work lasting about **2 minutes**.

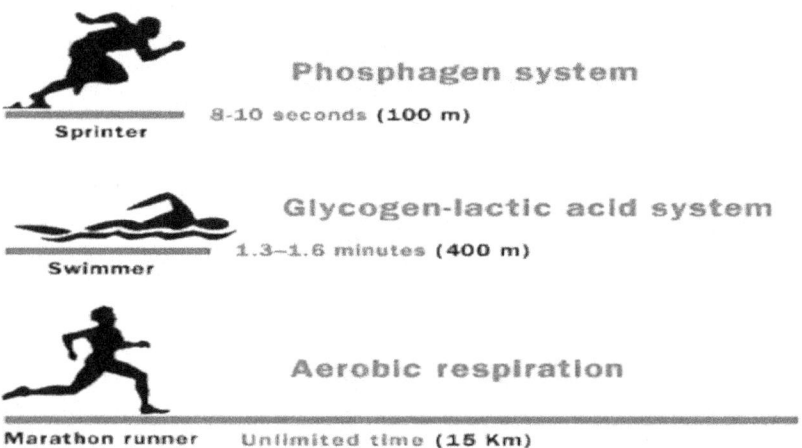

Long-Term Sources of Energy

Your **Long-term** sources of Energy involve the production of ATP from a variety of fuels, but this method requires the utilization of Oxygen — in other words, it is **aerobic energy**.

Your primary fuels include muscle glycogen, blood glucose, plasma free fatty acids and intramuscular fats.

Protein provides only a **small** percentage of energy for your muscle contraction, so the focus is on **carbohydrate** and **fat** intake, with the main element being carbohydrate. Glucose is broken down in glycolysis (as described previously), but

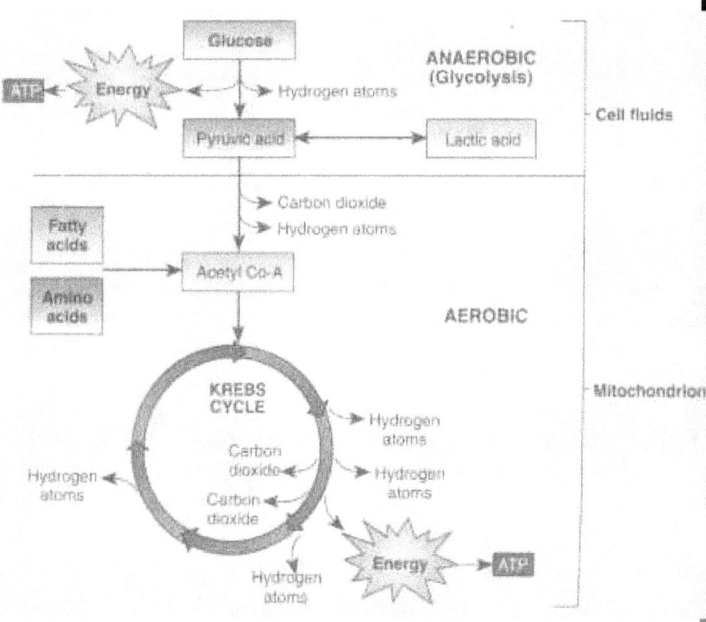

in this case the pyruvic acid is taken into the **mitochondria** of your cell, where it is converted to a 2-carbon fragment (acetyl CoA) that enters the Krebs cycle.

Fats are taken into your mitochondria, where they are also broken down into acetyl CoA, which again enters the Krebs cycle. The energy originally contained in the glucose and fats is extracted from the acetyl CoA and is used to generate ATP in the electron transport chain in a process called *oxidative phosphorylation*, which requires oxygen.

Carbohydrate and Fat + O_2 → ATP = ENERGY

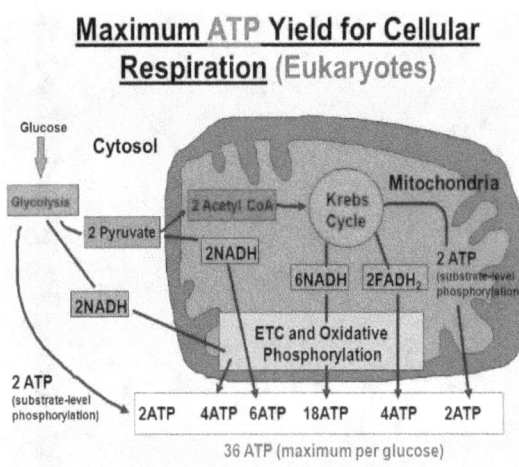

Maximum ATP Yield for Cellular Respiration (Eukaryotes)

ATP production via aerobic mechanisms is slower than production from immediate and short-term sources of energy and during submaximal work it may be **2 or 3 minutes** before the ATP needs of your cells are met completely by this aerobic process.

One reason for this lag is the time it takes for your heart to increase the delivery of oxygen-enriched blood to your muscles at the rate needed to meet the ATP demands of your muscle.

Another is the time it takes for oxidative phosphorylation to increase its rate of ATP production from resting levels to that needed to meet the exercise demand. Aerobic production of ATP is the primary means of supplying energy to your muscle in maximal work lasting **more than 2 minutes** and in all your submaximal work.

Interaction of Your Exercise Intensity, Exercise Duration & Energy Production

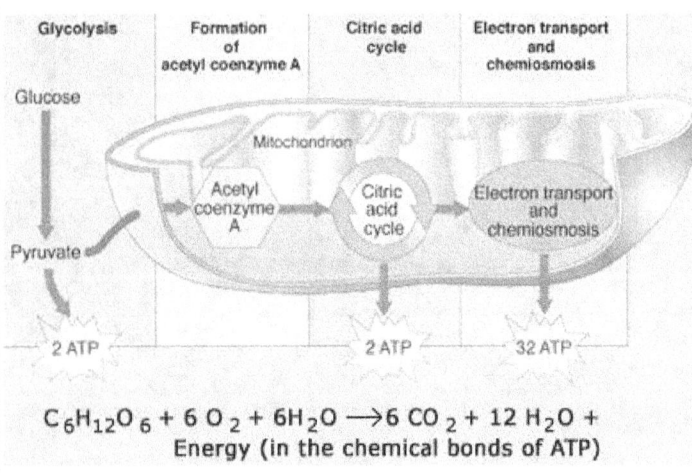

$C_6H_{12}O_6 + 6 O_2 + 6H_2O \rightarrow 6 CO_2 + 12 H_2O +$ Energy (in the chemical bonds of ATP)

The proportion of energy coming from anaerobic sources (immediate and short-term energy) is influenced by the intensity and duration of the activity that you are performing.

During an all-out activity lasting **less than 1 minutes** (e.g., a 400 m dash), your muscles obtain most of their ATP from anaerobic sources.

In a **2 to 3 minute maximal effort**, approximately **50%** of your energy comes from anaerobic sources and 50% comes from aerobic sources.

In a **10 minute maximal effort**, the anaerobic component drops to **15%**.

For a **30 minute all-out effort**, the anaerobic component is about **5%,** and it is even smaller in a typical submaximal 30 minute training session.

You can know the exact Energy requirements that you need to complete any task or operation.

Knowing how your body forms and uses Energy to move gives you the understanding of what you need to eat to supply your body with the necessary elements it needs to create the Energy to Successfully Move YourSelf into the Enjoyment of your Abundant Life!

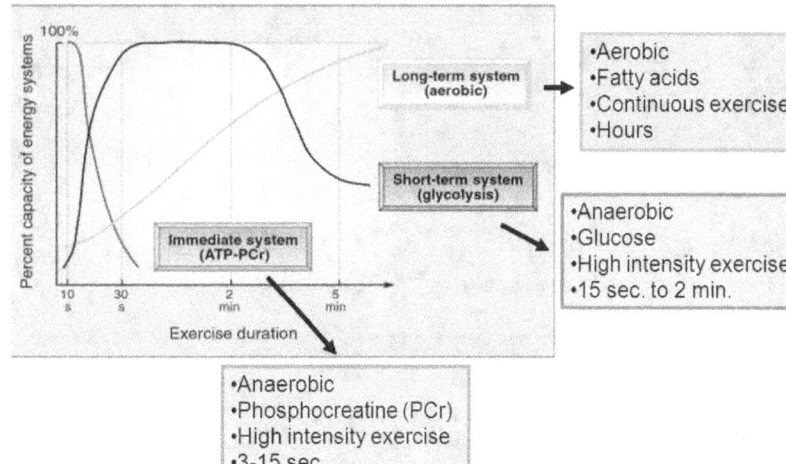

By constantly and consistently Moving YourSelf, you Increase your bodies ability to create and maintain your Energy production!

Your Muscle Fiber Types and Performance

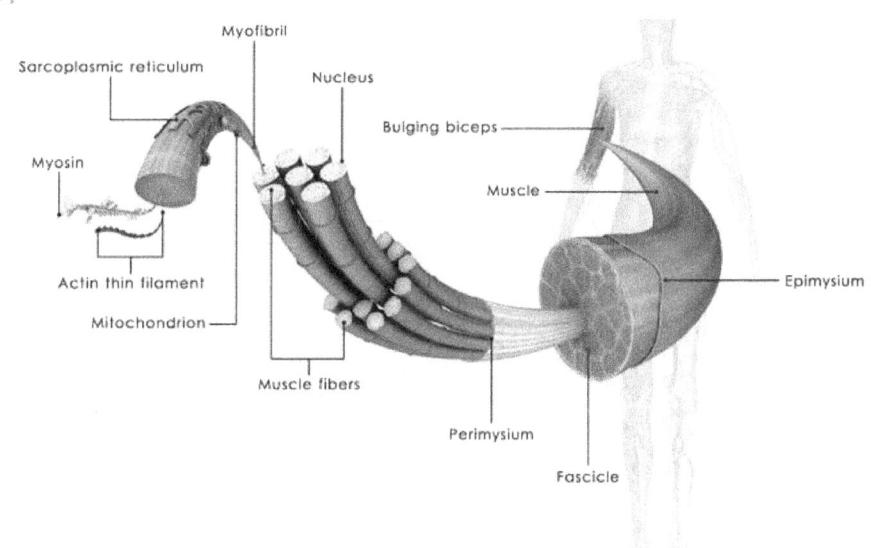

Muscle fibers vary in their abilities to produce ATP by the aerobic and anaerobic mechanisms described earlier in the chapter. Some of your muscle fibers contract quickly and have an innate capacity to produce great force, but they fatigue quickly. These muscle fibers produce most of their ATP by PC breakdown and glycolysis, and they are called **fast glycolytic fibers** or **type IIx fibers.**

You have other muscle fibers that contract slowly and produce little force, but they have great resistance to fatigue.

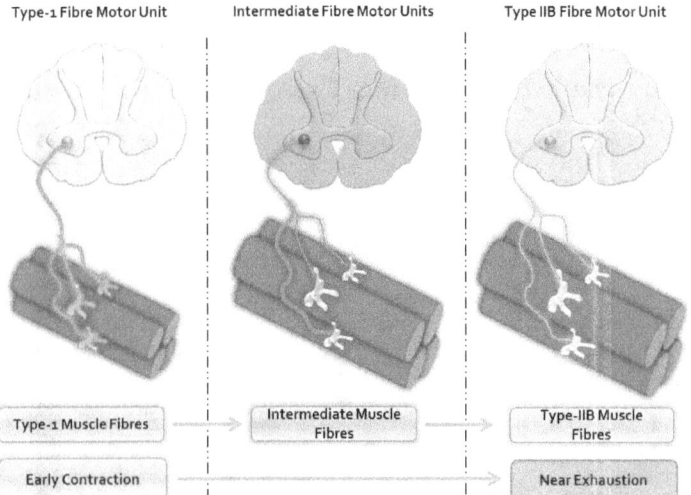

These fibers produce most of their ATP aerobically in the mitochondria and are called **slow oxidative fibers** or **type I fibers.** These fibers have many mitochondria and a relatively large number of capillaries helping to deliver oxygen to the mitochondria.

Last, you have a fiber with both type I and type IIx characteristics. It is a fast-contracting muscle fiber that not only produces great force when stimulated but also resists fatigue because of its large number of mitochondria and capillaries.

These fibers are called **fast oxidative glycolytic fibers** or **type IIa fibers.**

Your Muscle fibers differ in speed of **contraction**, **force**, and **resistance** to fatigue. Your Type I fibers are slow, generate low force and resist fatigue. Your Type IIa fibers are fast, generate high force and resist fatigue.

Your Type IIx fibers are fast, generate high force, and easily fatigue.

Tension (Force) Development in your Muscle

The tension, or force, generated by a muscle depends on more than the fiber type. When a single threshold-level stimulus excites a muscle fiber, a single, low-tension twitch results—a brief contraction followed by relaxation. If the frequency of stimulation increases, the muscle fiber can't relax between stimuli and the tension of one contraction adds to tension from the previous one.

This addition process is called **summation.** A further increase in the frequency of stimulation results in the contractions fusing together into a smooth, sustained, high-tension contraction called **tetanus.**

Your Thoughts are the Action Potential, or stimulation for your muscle contractions. Producing thoughts of Healing, Health, Life and Power causes a Stimulation that corresponds to their specific frequency.

This means that with a Thought of your Healing – you can cause your muscles to contract and Move To HEAL …. Which is the Summation process.

Now, if you increase that Thought pattern with Focused Concentration – you can increase the frequency, intensity and duration of the contraction of your muscles to continuously MOVE TO HEAL!

The same with creating the Thought that is the Action Potential that causes your Muscles and Body to MOVE TO YOUR POWER!

Tension in a Muscle

- Applying increased numbers of action potentials to a muscle fiber (or a fascicle, a muscle, or a muscle group) results in fusion of contractions (tetanus) and the performance of **useful work**

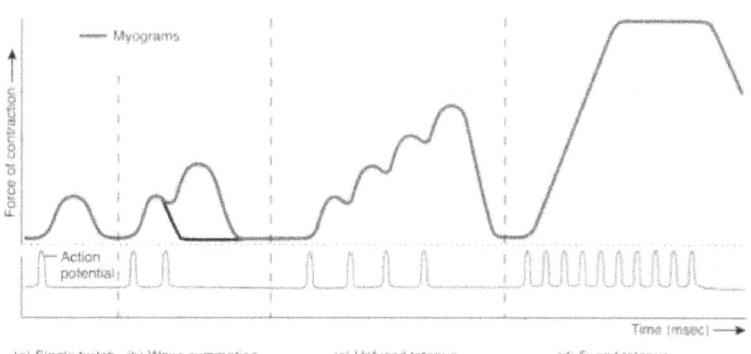

(a) Single twitch (b) Wave summation (c) Unfused tetanus (d) Fused tetanus

This means that you can Successfully Move YourSelf into the Enjoyment of Your Abundant Life!

Your Muscle fibers typically develop tension through tetanic contractions. In addition to the frequency of stimulation, the force of contraction depends on the degree to which the muscle fibers contract simultaneously (synchronous firing) and the number of muscle fibers recruited for the contraction. The latter factor, muscle fiber recruitment, is the most important.

The more your Thought is Focused and Concentrated = the Greater the Action Potential = the More Muscle Fibers recruited = Total Body MoveMent to Your Healing, Your Health, Your Power and Your Abundant Life!

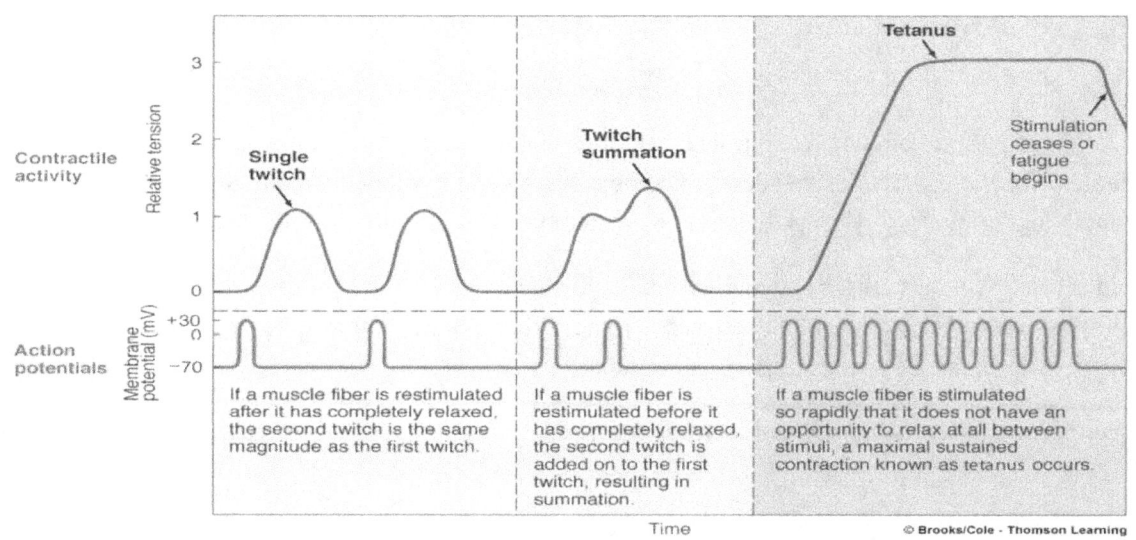

Your Muscle tension depends on the frequency of the stimulation of your Thought that leads to a tetanus contraction, the synchronous firing of muscle fibers and the recruitment of muscle fibers.

The order of recruitment of muscle fibers is from the most to the least oxidative.

Light to moderate exercise uses you Type I muscle fibers, whereas moderate to vigorous exercise requires your Type IIa fibers.

Both of your muscle types favor the **aerobic metabolism** of **carbohydrate** and underscores the importance of Breathing according to your anatomical structure and function, as well as applying the Science of Eating To Live!

Heavy exercise requires type IIx fibers that favor anaerobic glycolysis, which increases the likelihood of lactate production.

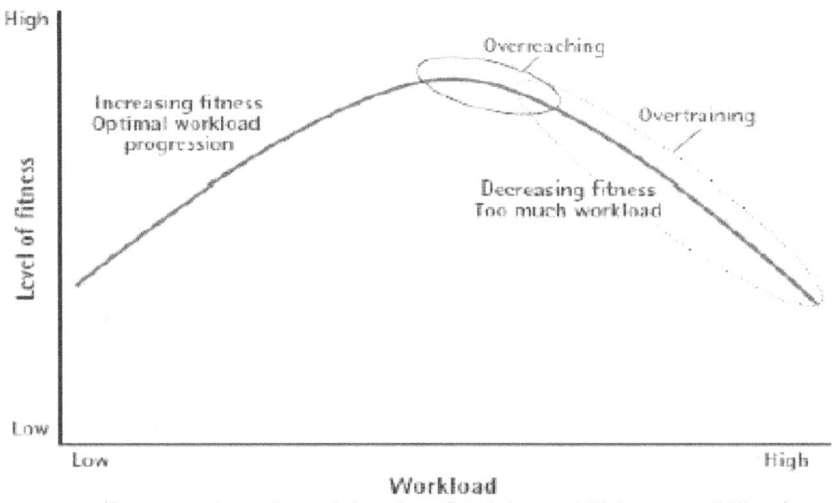

Your Metabolic, Cardiovascular & Respiratory Responses to Exercise

A primary task is to perform or complete physical activities that increase or maintain your cardiorespiratory function. Activities that demand aerobic energy (ATP) production automatically cause your circulatory and respiratory systems to deliver oxygen to your muscles to meet the demand.

The selected aerobic activities must be strenuous enough to challenge and thus improve your cardiorespiratory system. This crucial link between aerobic activities and cardiorespiratory function provides the basis for much of your exercise programming.

You need your Heart to beat you into your Abundant Life!

Measuring Your Oxygen Uptake

How does oxygen get to the mitochondria? First, oxygen enters your lungs during inhalation; it then diffuses from your alveoli of your lungs into your blood.

Oxygen is bound to the hemoglobin in your red blood cells and your heart delivers the oxygen-enriched blood to your muscles. Oxygen then diffuses into your muscle cells and reaches the mitochondria, where it is used (consumed) in the production of your ATP.

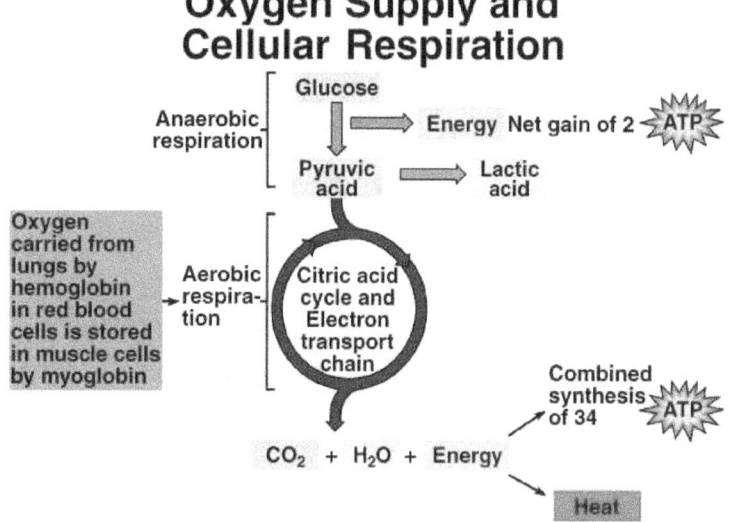

The more Oxygen you have – the more proficient your body is at creating ATP, which allows you to keep yourself in perpetual Motion of LIFE!

Oxygen consumption (VO₂) during exercise is measured by subtracting the volume of oxygen exhaled from the volume of oxygen inhaled.

$$VO_2 = \text{volume } O_2 \text{ inhaled} - \text{volume } O_2 \text{ exhaled.}$$

Oxygen consumption (uptake) is calculated by multiplying the volume of air breathed by the percentage of oxygen extracted. Oxygen extraction is the percentage of oxygen extracted from the inhaled air, the difference between the 20.93% of O_2 in room air and the percentage of O_2 in exhaled air.

CO_2 is produced in your mitochondria and diffuses out of your muscle into your venous blood, where it is carried back to your lungs. There it diffuses into your alveoli and is exhaled. CO_2 production (VCO_2) can be calculated as described for the VO_2.

The ratio of CO_2 production (VCO_2) to oxygen consumption (VO_2) at the cell is called the **respiratory quotient (*RQ*)**.

Because VCO_2 and VO_2 are measured at the mouth rather than at the tissue, this ratio is called the **respiratory exchange ratio (*R*).**

This ratio tells us what type of fuel is being used during exercise.

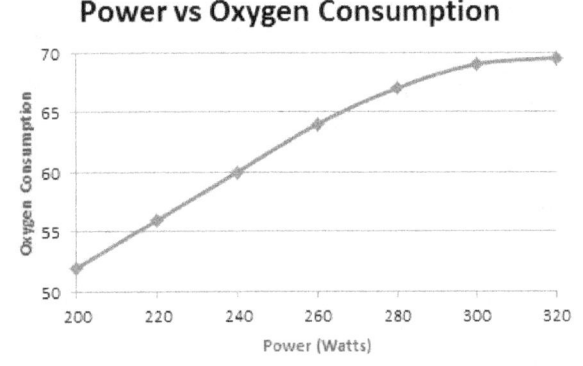
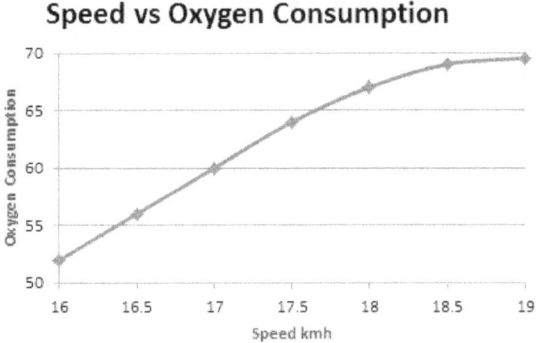
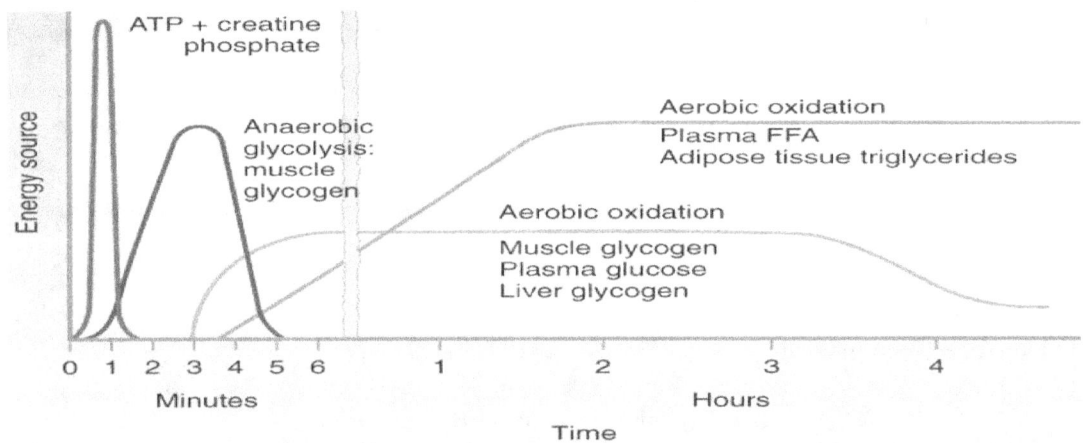

Your Fuel Utilization During Exercise

In general, protein contributes **less than 5%** to your total energy production during exercise, and for the purpose of our discussion it will be ignored. Ignoring protein leaves us to focus on your other 2 macronutrients - **carbohydrate** (muscle glycogen and blood glucose, which is derived from liver glycogen) and **fat** (adipose tissue and intramuscular fat) as your primary fuels for exercise.

The ability of your respiratory exchange ratio (R) to provide good information about the metabolism of fat and carbohydrate during exercise stems from the following observations about the metabolism of fat and glucose.

When $R = 1.0$ it means that **100%** of your energy is derived from **carbohydrate**, with **0%** from your **fat** tissue; when $R = 0.7$, the **reverse** is true.

When $R = 0.85$, approximately **50%** of your energy comes from **carbohydrate** and **50%** comes from **fat** tissue.

Carbohydrate fuels for muscular exercise include both **muscle glycogen** and **liver glycogen**, which maintains your blood glucose concentration. Muscle glycogen is your primary carbohydrate fuel for heavy exercise lasting less than 2 hours and having an inadequate supply of muscle glycogen results in premature fatigue.

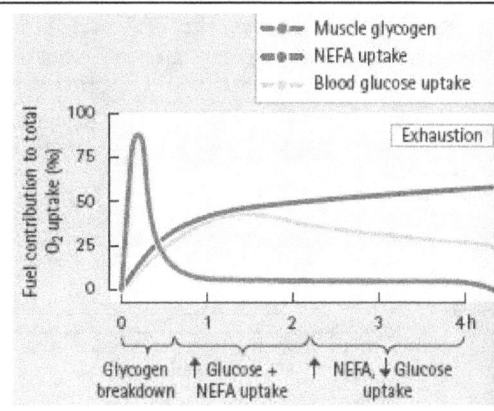

As your muscle glycogen is depleted during prolonged heavy exercise, your blood glucose becomes more important in supplying the carbohydrate fuel. Toward the end of heavy exercise lasting 3 hours or more, your blood glucose provides almost all the carbohydrate used by your muscles.

Therefore, heavy exercise is limited by the availability of carbohydrate fuels, which must be either stored in abundance before exercise (muscle glycogen) or replaced through the ingestion of carbohydrate during exercise (blood glucose).

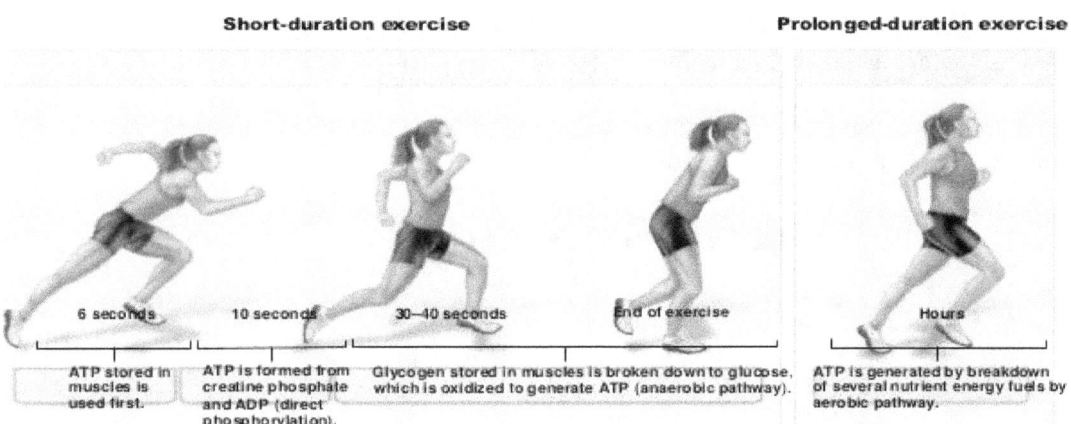

Comparison of energy sources used during short-duration exercise and prolonged-duration exercise.

Effect of Exercise Duration on Your Fuel Utilization

R changes during a 90 minute exercise performed at 65% of your VO_2max. R decreases over time, indicating a greater reliance on your **fat** tissue as a fuel.

The fat is derived from both your **intramuscular** fat stores and **adipose** tissue, which releases free fatty acids into your blood to be carried to your muscle.

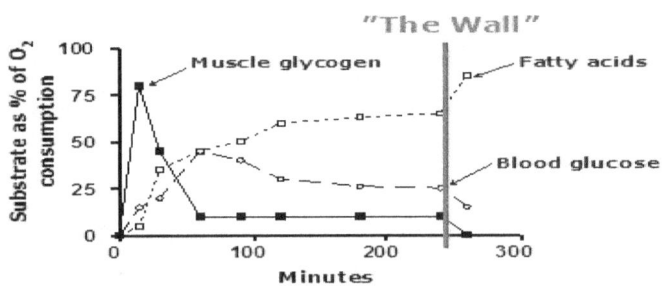

Using more fat spares the remaining carbohydrate stores and extends the time to exhaustion.

Also, you LOSE the potentially dangerous FAT tissue – LOSING Weight and Becoming HEALTHIER!

Effect of Diet and Training on Your Fuel Utilization

The type of fuel used during exercise directly depends on and is determined by your diet. It has been demonstrated clearly that a diet high in carbohydrate (versus an average diet) increases your muscle glycogen content and extends the time to your exhaustion.

This underlines the Importance of applying the Science of Eating To Live!

Further, your muscle gains a greater capacity to increase its glycogen store if you perform your strenuous exercise **before** eating high-carbohydrate meals.

Finally, during prolonged heavy exercise, carbohydrate drinks help to maintain your blood glucose concentration and extend the time to your fatigue.

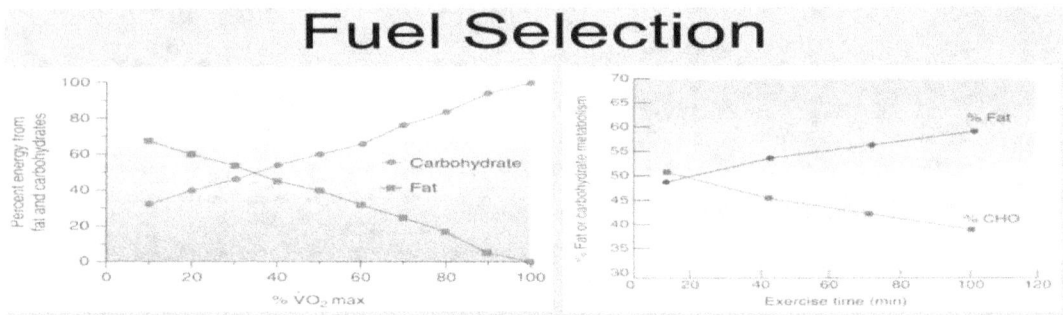

From: Powers & Howley. (2007). **Exercise Physiology**. McGraw-Hill.

- As intensity increases carbohydrate use increases, fat use decreases
- As duration increase, fat use increases, carb use decreases

Endurance training increases the number of mitochondria in your muscles involved in your training program. Having more mitochondria increases the ability of your muscles to use your fat as your fuel and to process the available carbohydrate aerobically.

During prolonged moderately strenuous exercise, R decreases over time, indicating that fat is being used more.

This ability spares your carbohydrate store and reduces lactate production, both of which favorably influence your performance – allowing you to Move LONGER, STRONGER and FASTER!

You can use your excess fat tissue for Energy, while conserving the Carbohydrates that you ate for future use so that you won't become fatigued or exhausted. This means you can Successfully Move YourSelf into the Enjoyment of your Abundant Life!

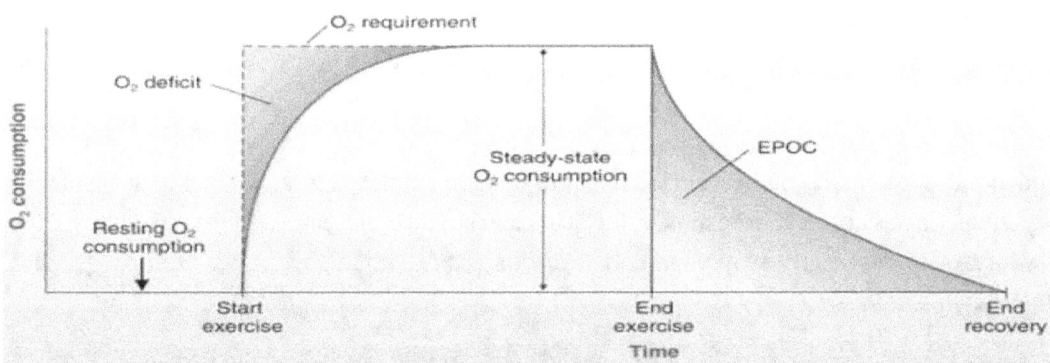

Your Transition From At-Rest to Steady-State Work

It may seem that your immediate, short-term, and long-term sources of energy (ATP) are used in distinct activities and do not work together to allow the body to make the transition from rest to exercise, but they all often work together versus operating with just their specific energy system.

Your cardiovascular and respiratory systems cannot instantaneously increase the delivery of oxygen to your muscles to completely meet the ATP demands of aerobic processes.

For an example, in the interval between the time you would step on a treadmill and the time your cardiovascular and respiratory systems deliver the required oxygen, your immediate and short-term sources of energy would supply the needed ATP for you to successfully complete the exercise.

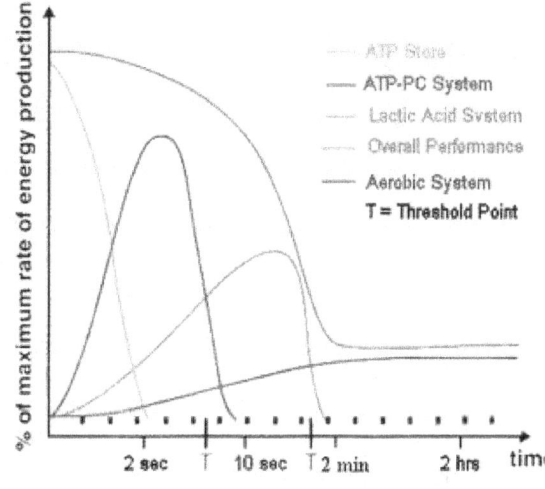

The volume of oxygen missing in the first few minutes of work is your **oxygen deficit**. PC supplies some of your needed ATP, and the anaerobic breakdown of glycogen to lactic acid provides the rest until your oxidative mechanisms meet your ATP requirement.

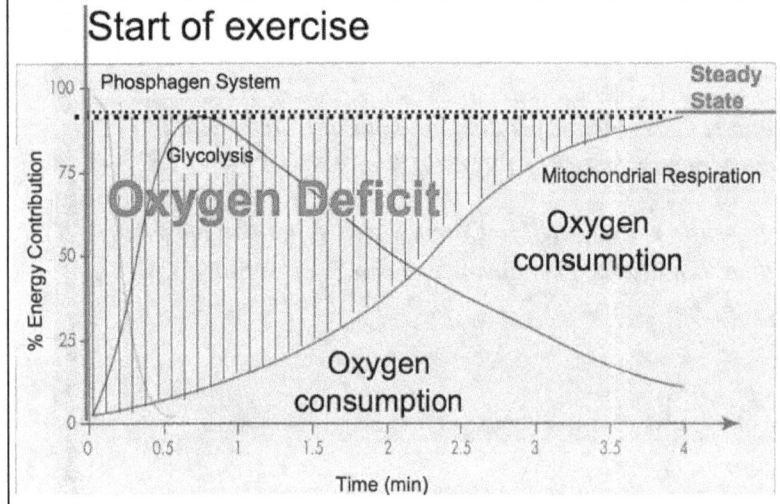

When your uptake of oxygen levels off during submaximal work, your oxygen uptake value represents your **steady-state oxygen requirement** for the activity. At this point, the ATP need of your cell is being met by the aerobic production of ATP in the mitochondria of your muscle on a pay-as-you-go basis.

When you stop running and step off the treadmill, the ATP need of your muscles that were involved in the activity suddenly drops toward your resting value. Your oxygen uptake decreases quickly at first and then more gradually approaches your resting value. This elevated oxygen uptake during recovery from exercise is your **excess post-exercise oxygen consumption (EPOC)**; it also is called your *oxygen debt* and *oxygen repayment*.

In part, your elevated oxygen uptake is used to make additional ATP to bring the PC store of your muscle back to normal (remember that it was depleted somewhat at the onset of work). Some of the extra oxygen taken in during recovery is used to pay your ATP requirement for the higher Heart Rate (HR) and breathing during recovery (compared with your rest state).

Your liver uses a small part of the oxygen repayment to convert some of the lactic acid produced at the onset of work into glucose.

If you were to reach your steady-state oxygen requirement earlier during the first minutes of work, a smaller oxygen deficit is incurred. Your body depletes less PC and produces less lactic acid.

Performing Endurance training speeds up your kinetics of oxygen transport, which means that it decreases the time needed for you to reach a steady state of oxygen uptake.

All of your cells NEED Oxygen and by increasing your Oxygen uptake through exercise, you create a condition that your body can allows your body to Heal and become Healthy at your Cellular level.

People in poor condition, as well as people with cardiovascular or pulmonary disease, take longer to reach their steady-state oxygen requirement.

They incur a **larger** oxygen deficit and must produce more ATP from their immediate and short-term sources of energy when beginning work or transitioning from one intensity to the next.

This is goes into the importance and foundation of Moving YourSelf … incurring a larger oxygen deficit is at the root cause of cellular oxidation and cellular death.

Lack of exercise goes hand-in-hand with poor diet as the #2 Actual Cause of Death… you can successfully eliminate both by applying the Science of Eating To Live and Moving SomeThing!

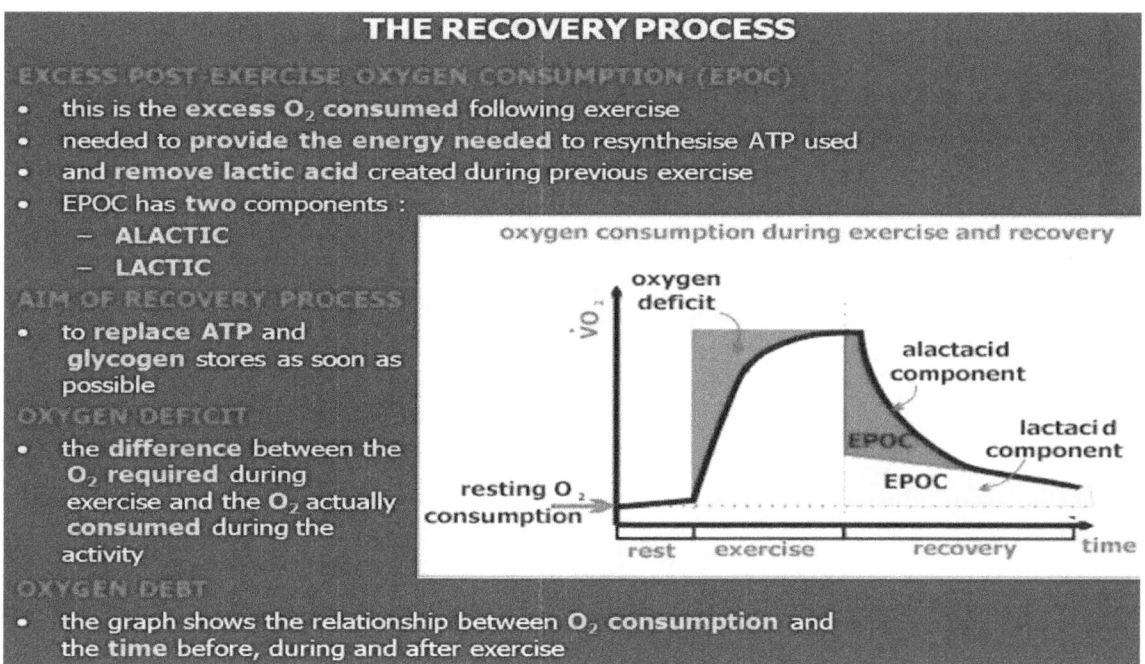

THE RECOVERY PROCESS

EXCESS POST-EXERCISE OXYGEN CONSUMPTION (EPOC)
- this is the **excess O$_2$ consumed** following exercise
- needed to **provide the energy needed** to resynthesise ATP used
- and **remove lactic acid** created during previous exercise
- EPOC has **two** components:
  - **ALACTIC**
  - **LACTIC**

AIM OF RECOVERY PROCESS
- to **replace ATP** and **glycogen** stores as soon as possible

OXYGEN DEFICIT
- the **difference** between the **O$_2$ required** during exercise and the **O$_2$ actually consumed** during the activity

OXYGEN DEBT
- the graph shows the relationship between **O$_2$ consumption** and the **time** before, during and after exercise

Your Heart Rate and Pulmonary Ventilation

The link between your cardiorespiratory responses to work and the time it takes to reach the steady-state oxygen requirement should be no surprise.

In addition, your muscles contribute to the lag in oxygen uptake at the onset of work.

An **untrained** muscle has relatively few mitochondria available to produce ATP aerobically and relatively few capillaries per muscle fiber to bring the oxygen-enriched arterial blood to those mitochondria.

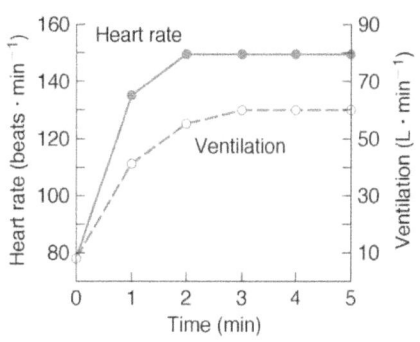

Heart Rate and Pulmonary Ventilation Responses to Submaximal Work

Following endurance training, both of these factors increase so that your muscle can produce more ATP aerobically at the onset of you beginning to work. In addition, less lactic acid is produced at the onset of work and your blood lactic acid concentration is lower for a fixed submaximal work rate.

This means that you can Move Longer, Faster and Stronger!

This is WHY we need to exercise from our childhood all the way to the grave. Life s based on MOTION!

A Body IN Motion will STAY IN MOTION …. The MORE Motion builds MORE Mitochondria in your Muscles that create MORE Power = Constant MOTION OF LIFE = Enjoying Your Abundant Life!

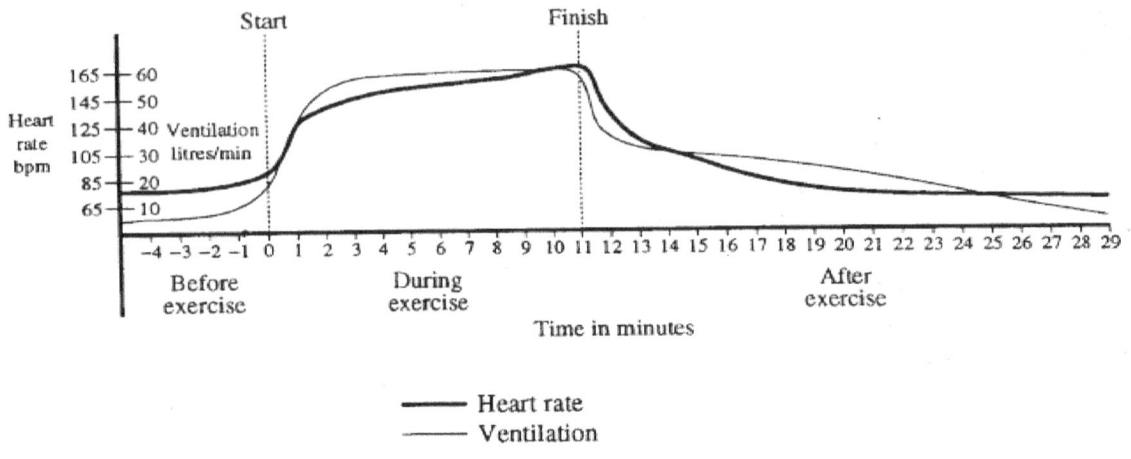

Your Oxygen Uptake and Maximal Aerobic Power

Maximal aerobic power describes the greatest rate at which your body (primarily muscle) can produce ATP aerobically during dynamic exercise involving a large muscle mass (e.g., running, cycling). It is also the upper limit at which your cardiovascular system can deliver oxygen-enriched blood to your muscles.

Therefore, your maximal aerobic power is not only a good index of your Cardio Respiratory Fitness (CRF), it is also a good predictor of your performance capability in aerobic events such as distance running, cycling, cross-country skiing, and swimming.

In the apparently healthy person, maximal aerobic power is the quantitative limit at which their cardiovascular system can deliver oxygen to their tissues.

This usual interpretation must be tempered by the mode of exercise (test type) used to impose the work rate on the subject.

Importance of the Aerobic System

The aerobic system is by far the most important source for energy. The reason why the anaerobic system was introduced first is because it is important to understand the dual role of lactate: an *output of the anaerobic system* and the *most important fuel for the aerobic system*.

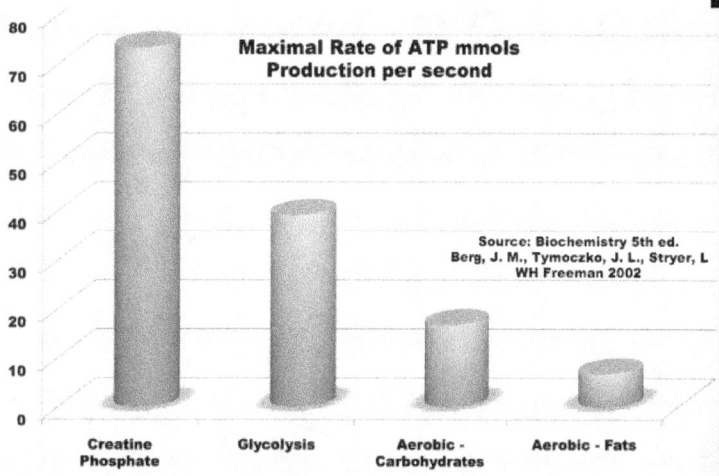

For a long race, the pyruvate/lactate for fuel is limited and your muscles will use a large amount of fats for fuel. The more carbohydrates available, the faster you will race. Without your anaerobic system providing the carbohydrates and some high energy molecules in addition to the small amounts of ATP, your aerobic metabolism would be much slower.

Carbohydrates (in the form of lactate) are the most desirable fuel for endurance sports because they lead to a faster rebuild of ATP and enable faster contraction and a speedier race for the athlete. But the supply is limited. There are only enough carbohydrates stored in your muscles to enable intense aerobic exercise for about 90-100 minutes.

On the other hand, there is enough fat stored in your body to fuel slower speed aerobic exercise for several days. The proportion of fats and carbohydrates used during an activity/exercise depends upon your conditioning level and the speed required.

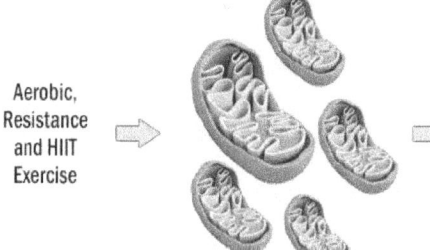

There are no negative byproducts of your aerobic system: only **water** and **carbon dioxide** which an you **sweat** and **exhale**.

The one negative is **heat**, and this has to be carefully considered during training.

As you use your aerobic system at high levels a lot of heat is generated in your cells and this heat accelerates the breakdown of your cells. Too much breakdown and you will lose your aerobic capacity.

That is why training at or above threshold must be limited in a sensible training program.

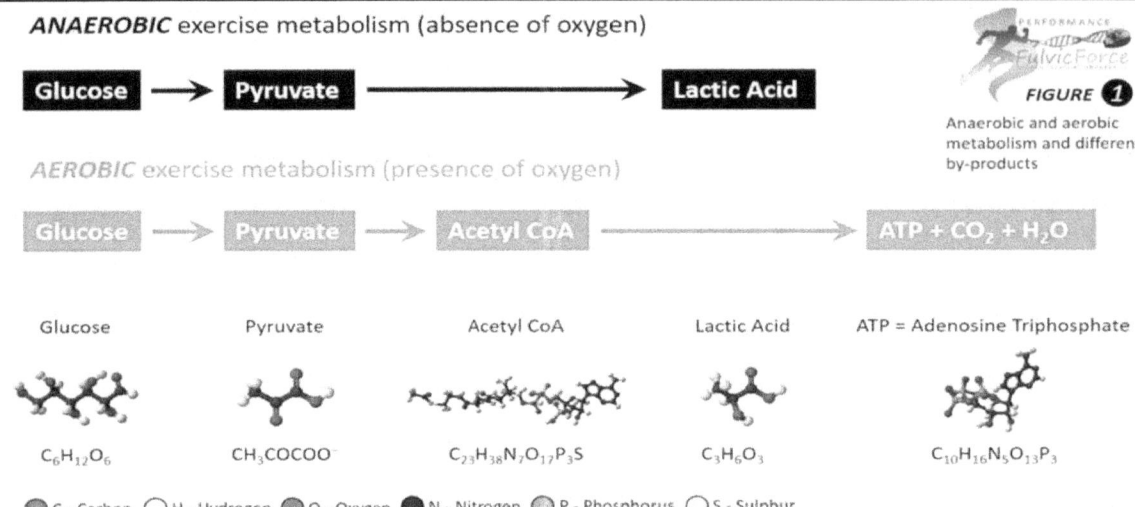

FIGURE 1. Anaerobic and aerobic metabolism and different by-products

The aerobic system is the most important of your energy systems and provides most of your energy for any race over 2 minutes. It is extremely important for the triathlon, both for training and for the race itself. A **strong aerobic system** not only provides energy for the race but enables the athlete to raise the intensity and volume of training.

Also, a **strong anaerobic system during the training period** enables the athlete to complete more intense and longer workouts than would a low anaerobic capacity. However, during a race a high anaerobic capacity will inhibit performance.

Your aerobic system is more trainable than your anaerobic system and improvements or declines in your aerobic system are more easily measured. This is another reason why more attention is paid to your aerobic system.

Aerobic energy is produced in small subsections of the cell called mitochondria. These are complicated little biological entities and the normal muscle cell has about 2% of its volume in mitochondria.

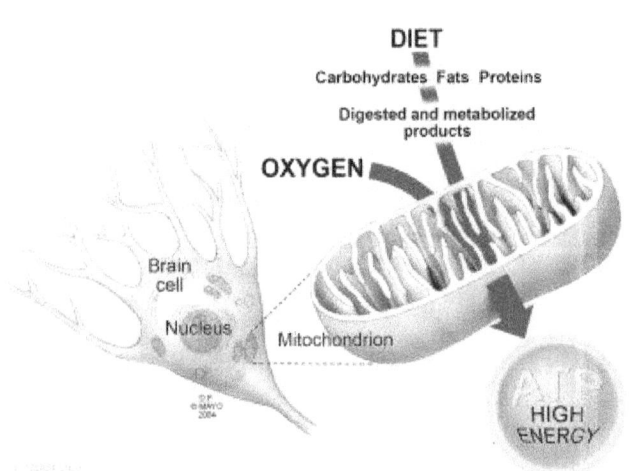

Endurance athletes might have up to 10% of their cells composed of mitochondria.

So, essentially, those that complete at least 60 minutes a day of cardiovascular aerobics, have five times as many little energy factories (mitochondria) as the average person and this is why they can run so fast for so long.

This means that the more that you Move YourSelf = The More Energy your body can produce and the longer it can maintain and sustain your Energy production!

This is why exercise is so vital to your Health and Wellness and is included along with your dietary choices as in the category of being the 2nd ACTUAL CAUSE OF DEATH!

You can Eat To Live, but without Moving YourSelf – You will not significantly Expand your Life to Successfully Enjoy Your Abundant Life!

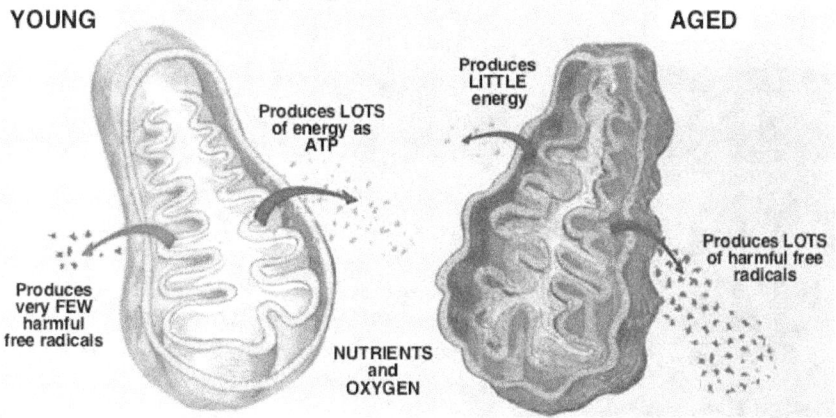

Move Something!

AGE	BEGINNER 60% - 70%		INTERMEDIATE 70% - 80%		ADVANCED 80% - 90%	
	Beats/min	Beats/10 sec *	Beats/min	Beats/10 sec *	Beats/min	Beats/10 sec *
to 19	121 - 141	20 - 24	141 - 161	24 - 27	161 - 181	27 - 30
20 - 24	119 - 139	20 - 23	139 - 158	23 - 26	158 - 178	26 - 30
25 - 29	116 - 135	19 - 23	135 - 154	23 - 26	154 - 174	26 - 29
30 - 34	113 - 132	19 - 22	132 - 150	22 - 25	150 - 169	25 - 28
35 - 39	110 - 128	18 - 21	128 - 146	21 - 24	146 - 165	24 - 28
40 - 44	107 - 125	18 - 21	125 - 142	21 - 24	142 - 160	24 - 27
45 - 49	104 - 121	17 - 20	121 - 138	20 - 23	138 - 156	23 - 26
50 - 54	101 - 118	17 - 20	118 - 134	20 - 22	134 - 151	22 - 25
55 - 59	98 - 114	16 - 19	114 - 130	19 - 22	130 - 147	22 - 25
60 - 64	95 - 111	16 - 19	111 - 126	19 - 21	126 - 142	21 - 24
65 - 69	92 - 107	15 - 18	107 - 122	18 - 20	122 - 138	20 - 23
70 - 74	89 - 104	15 - 17	104 - 118	17 - 20	118 - 133	20 - 22
75 - 79	86 - 100	14 - 17	100 - 114	17 - 19	114 - 129	19 - 22
80 - 84	83 - 97	14 - 16	97 - 110	16 - 18	110 - 124	18 - 21
85 +	81 - 95	14 - 16	95 - 108	16 - 18	108 - 122	18 - 20

Anaerobic
- 85-100%
- Maximum intensity: short sprints or bursts of activity (2-5 minutes)
- Good for athletic conditioning, competitive training

Aerobic
- 75% - 80%
- Moderate intensity: power walking, running, cycling
- Good for building endurance, cardiovascular fitness

Weight Loss
- 60% - 75%
- Light/Moderate intensity: brisk walking, jogging, cycling
- Good for burning fat, increasing endurance, heart health

Light
- 50% - 60%
- Light intensity: warming up, cooling down, new exercisers
- Good for beginners, getting in shape, overall health

Resting Heart Rate

Trained athletes have a lower resting heart rate due to increased efficiency of the cardiovascular system and higher stroke volume

This is most evident in the recovery phases

The trained athlete can recover faster (HR ↓'s faster) due to a more efficient cardiovascular system.

Recovery Heart Rate

What did we say the purpose of a cool-down is at the end of a workout?

Recovery Heart Rate – Existing heart rate just after exercise

Normal Recovery Heart Rate Range	
5 minutes after exercise	120 bpm
10 minutes after exercise	100 bpm

If your heart rate does not drop to this range after exercise, you need to reduce the intensity of your workout

If your heart rate drops quicker, you may want to increase the intensity of your workout

Resting Heart Rate for MEN

Age	18-25	26-35	36-45	46-55	56-65	65+
Athlete	49-55	49-54	50-56	50-57	51-56	50-55
Excellent	56-61	55-61	57-62	58-63	57-61	56-61
Good	62-65	62-65	63-66	64-67	62-67	62-65
Above Average	66-69	66-70	67-70	68-71	68-71	66-69
Average	70-73	71-74	71-75	72-76	72-75	70-73
Below Average	74-81	75-81	76-82	77-83	76-81	74-79
Poor	82+	82+	83+	84+	82+	80+

Resting Heart Rate for WOMEN

Age	18-25	26-35	36-45	46-55	56-65	65+
Athlete	54-60	54-59	54-59	54-60	54-59	54-59
Excellent	61-65	60-64	60-64	61-65	60-64	60-64
Good	66-69	65-68	65-69	66-69	65-68	65-68
Above Average	70-73	69-72	70-73	70-73	69-73	69-72
Average	74-78	73-76	74-78	74-77	74-77	73-76
Below Average	79-84	77-82	79-84	78-83	78-83	77-84
Poor	85+	83+	85+	84+	84+	84+

Supreme Health & Fitness!   *Health & Wellness Series ... Vol 3!*

Daily Energy Expenditure = Resting Metabolic Rate + Physical Activity
DEE = RMR + PA (All units are expressed in Cal/day)

- Given: **RMR** = 1 Cal × hr × kg (Divide weight in lb by 2.2 to get kg)

  Two examples:

  121-lb. person: **RMR** = 1 × 24 × (121 / 2.2) = **1,320 Cal/day**
  154-lb. person: **RMR** = 1 × 24 × (154 / 2.2) = **1,680 Cal/day**

- To estimate your **Resting Metabolic Rate**, enter your weight and calculate:

  RMR = 1 × 24 × (_____ / 2.2) = _____ Cal/day

- Next, select your average **Physical Activity (PA)** level:

  - **Sedentary** (no regular physical activity): **PA** = 25% of **DEE**
  - **Moderately active** (30 mins/day moderate activity): **PA** = 33% of **DEE**
  - **Very active** (60 mins/day moderate/vigorous exercise): **PA** = 40% of **DEE**

- To estimate **DEE**, divide **RMR** by 1.00 minus **PA** level expressed as a decimal (.25, .33, or .40). See examples below.

  Estimate of **Daily Energy Expenditure** for **121-lb.** person who is

  - **Sedentary:** **DEE** = 1320 / .75 = **1,760 Cal/day**
  - **Moderately active:** **DEE** = 1320 / .67 = **1,970 Cal/day***
  - **Very active:** **DEE** = 1320 / .60 = **2,200 Cal/day**

  Estimate of **Daily Energy Expenditure** for **154-lb.** person who is

  - **Sedentary:** **DEE** = 1680 / .75 = **2,240 Cal/day**
  - **Moderately active:** **DEE** = 1680 / .67 = **2,507 Cal/day***
  - **Very active:** **DEE** = 1680 / .60 = **2,800 Cal/day**

- To estimate your **Daily Energy Expenditure**, enter your **RMR** and divide by the appropriate decimal (.75 for Sedentary, .67 for Moderately active, or .60 for Very active):

  DEE = (_____ / _____) = _____ Cal/day

*The daily energy expenditures of 2,000 and 2,500 Cal printed on food labels are based on a moderately active 121-lb. woman and a moderately active 154-lb. man.

Move Something!

Chapter Ten

Exercise & Your Heart Beat, Target Rate & Output

*****

The main purpose of exercise is to improve the quality of your physical body. You should exercise according to your most important system, organ and/or tissue – 1st!

If your most important tissue is unhealthy, then the rest of your body is soon to follow. There is no Health, Energy or LIFE without your Cardio-Respiratory System – your Heart and Lungs.

By performing Cardio-Vascular exercise – you exercise both of your Life determining Systems at the same time!

Exercise is a science and if you don't know and understand HOW your body operates, then you increase the chances of you causing a bodily injury instead of improving your health. With this chapter, you will learn how your heart functions, but more importantly, you will learn how to use your heart to get the maximum Oxygen and Energy intake, without causing exhaustion or injury.

You need your heart to Successfully beat you into the Enjoyment of your Abundant Life!

Your Heart Rate

Your Heart rate (HR) often is used as a fitness indicator for both, at-rest and during a standard submaximal-work task. The Maximal HR is useful for determining your Target Heart Rate (THR) for fitness workouts, but it is not a good fitness indicator because it changes very little with training.

Once the HR reaches about **110 beats min^{-1}**, it increases linearly with work rate during an exercise until near-maximal efforts.

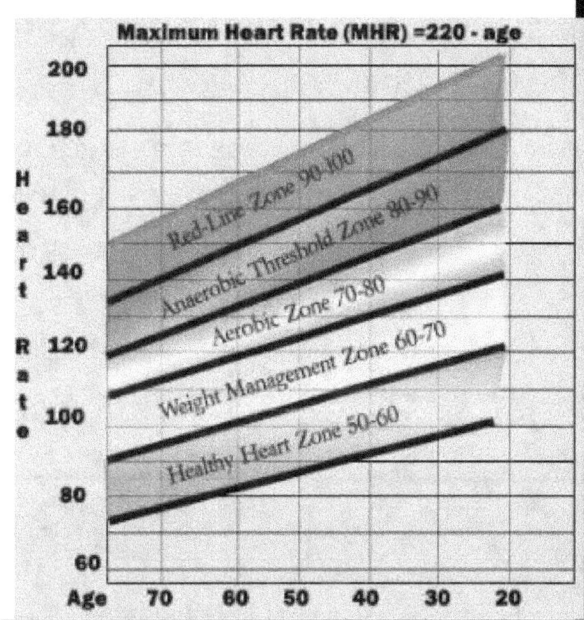

Heart rates

Your Resting Heart Rate (RHR) is your pulse at rest

Your Recovery Heart Rate is your pulse after and activity when your body goes back to normal. It should be at 120 BPM 5-6 minutes after your activity. It should be 100 BPM 10 minutes after the activity

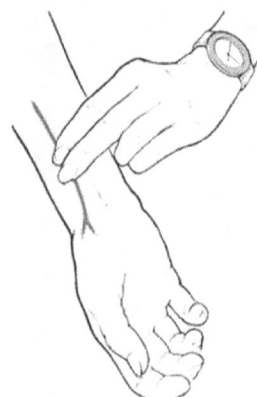

Radial Pulse

1. Extend one hand and locate your radial pulse in the groove in your wrist above your thumb joint.
2. Use the index and middle fingers of your other hand to press firmly but lightly on the pulse point.
3. Count the number of beats in exactly six seconds and multiply by 10 to find the number of beats per minute.

Taking your pulse is rather simple. Use the index and middle finger of one hand to palpate (feel) the arterial pulse in your radial artery on your wrist.

Count for 15 seconds and multiply by 4 to determine the number of times your heart beats in one minute.

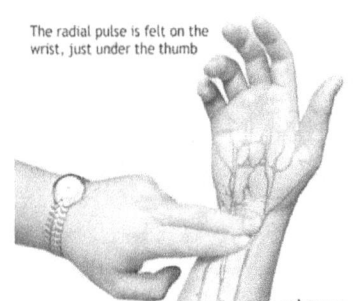

The radial pulse is felt on the wrist, just under the thumb

Pulse Rate

Trial #1 ____ X 4 = ____ bpm

Trial #1 ____ X 4 = ____ bpm

Trial #1 ____ X 4 = ____ bpm

Note: The NYSED "Making Connections" Lab measures for 20 seconds and multiplies by 3, but any calculation that leads to a count of 60 seconds is acceptable.

The lower your HR is at submaximal work rates, it increases in its beneficial effect because it decreases the oxygen needed by your heart muscle – allowing the parts of your body that need oxygen to receive and have available as much oxygen required for Success completion.

When an ECG is recorded, the HR can be taken from the ECG strip. Without an ECG, HR can be taken with an HR watch, a stethoscope, or manual palpation of an artery at the wrist or neck. HR watches are accurate and are the easiest way to measure HR.

When palpating, fingers (not the thumb) should be used, preferably at the **wrist** (radial artery). Taking the HR at the **neck** (carotid artery) requires caution because applying too much pressure can trigger a reflex that slows the HR.

Your HR for at-rest or during steady-state exercise should be taken for **30 seconds** for higher reliability.

When your HR is taken after exercise, measurement should begin soon after exercise ends (within 5 sec) and should be taken for **10 or 15 seconds** because your HR changes so rapidly.

The **10 or 15 seconds** rate is multiplied by **6 or 4**, respectively, to calculate your **beats per minute**.

For an example, if you have a **10 second** post-exercise HR **is 20 beats · min^{-1}**, then your **HR is 120 beats · min^{-1}** (6 · 20).

Understanding and knowing your Heart Rate is not just vital to exercise, your Heart Rate is also the foundation of your LIFE!

Heart Rate	Effort	Effect
171 - 190	Very hard 90-100%	**Performance Redline Zone** Develops maximum preformance and speed
152 - 171	Hard 80-90%	**Threshold Zone** Increases maximum preformance capacity
133 - 152	Moderate 70-80%	**Aerobic Zone** Improves aerobic fitness
114 - 133	Light 60-70%	**Temperate Zone** Improves basic endurance and fat burning
95 - 114	Very light 50-60%	**Healthy Heart Zone** Improves overall health and helps recovery

Understanding Your Target Heart Rate

Your Target Heart Rate is your optimal beat speed that you would want your heart to beat or perform at. At this beat, your heart is operating efficiently, and you have a steady, consistent and constant flow and supply of Oxygen to successfully complete any exercise or activity.

This is the heart rate that will beat you into the Enjoyment of your Abundant Life!

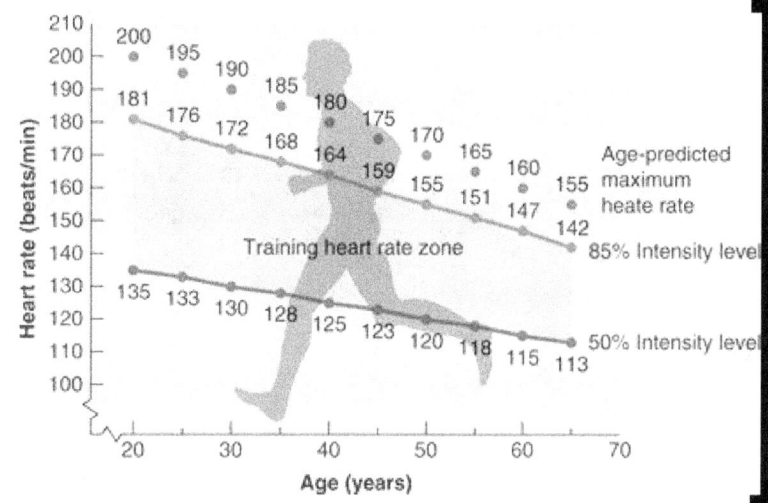

Your ability to complete a workout depends on your physiological responses and your perception of effort rather than your metabolic cost of the activity itself.

Fortunately, by using specific HR values that are approximately equal to **60% to 80% VO2 Max** is possible to formulate an exercise prescription that takes these and many other beneficial and health factors into consideration.

These HR values form the **target heart rate (THR)** range.

Determine Your THR range

Direct Method - Determining Your Target Heart Rate

Heart Rate increases linearly with your metabolic load, so you would test yourself (or be tested) in an exercise where you would gradually increase your intensity.

Finding Target Heart Rate Zone

- **A simple way to determine your maximum heart rate is to use the following formula:**
  220 - age = Maximum Heart Rate

- **Maximum Heart Rate** An example for a 15 year old person would be as follows: 220 – 15 = 205

- 205 x .60 = 123
- 205 x .85 = 174

- **Target Heart Rate Zone** 123 – 174
- This range is what a 15 year old should work at in order to improve cardiorespiratory endurance.

To determine your THR, you would monitor and record your HR at each stage of a maximal exertion. Your HR is then plotted on a graph against your VO_2 (or MET) equivalents of each stage of the exercise.

Work rates of **60% to 80%** of maximal METs demanded HR responses of **132 to 156 beats · min^{-1}**. The HR values become the intensity guide for you and represent your THR range.

Target Heart Rate: Indirect Methods

In contrast to the direct method, which requires the participant to complete a maximal GXT, two indirect methods have been developed to estimate an appropriate THR. These are the HRR method and the %HRmax method.

*Heart Rate Reserve Method

Heart Rate Reserve

Subtract your Resting Heart Rate (RHR) from your Maximum Heart Rate (MHR). This gives your Heart Rate Reserve (HR$_{max}$ Reserve).

$$MHR - RHR = HRmax\ Reserve$$

Using the 20 year-old with a resting heart rate of 60 beats per minute (BMP) for our example:

$$200 - 60 = 140$$

HRR is the difference between **resting** and **maximal** HR. For a **maximal HR** of **200 beats · min^{-1}** and a **resting HR** of **60 beats · min^{-1}**, the **HRR** is **140 beats · min^{-1}**.

The HRR method of determining the THR range, requires a few simple calculations:

1. Subtract the **resting HR** from the **maximal HR** to obtain the **HRR**.

2. Calculate **60%** and **80%** of the **HRR**.

3. Add each value to the resting **HR** to obtain the **THR** range.

*Percentage of Maximal Heart Rate Method

Another method of determining THR range is to use a fixed percentage of the maximal HR (%HRmax). The advantage of this method is its simplicity and the fact that it has been validated across many populations.

Rate of Perceived Exertion (RPE)

2-3	Easy	Can talk with no problem, feels easy
4-5	Moderately Easy	Talking is still fairly easy – feeling bit of exertion
6-7	Moderately Hard	Talking takes more effort – feeling like some work
8	Very Difficult	Can't keep up a conversation – feeling like hard work
9-10	Extremely Difficult	Can't really talk at all

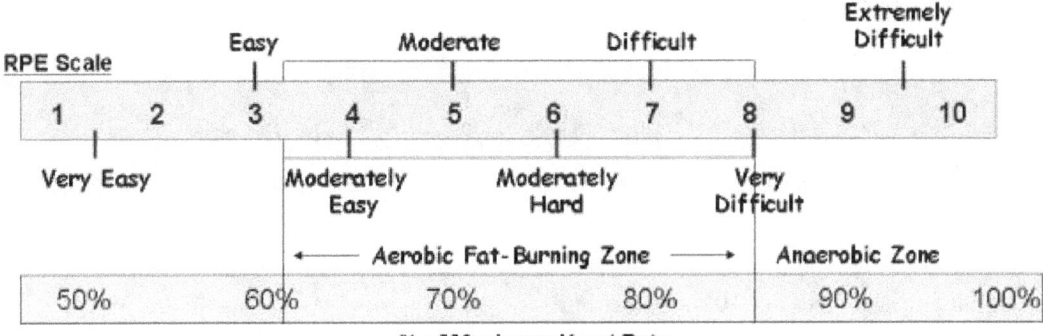

Finding Your Threshold

As mentioned earlier, the intensity of exercise that provides an adequate stimulus for cardiorespiratory improvement varies with activity level and age and spans the range of 40% to 84% VO2R and VO_2max. For a majority of the population, the optimal intensity threshold is in the following ranges:

- 60% to 80% of VO2max, HRR, and VO2R

- 75% to 90% of HRmax

As we discussed at the beginning of this section, the threshold is toward the lower part of the range (50%-60% HRR) for older, sedentary populations and toward the upper part of the range (>80% HRR) for younger, more fit populations.

The middle of the range (70% HRR, 70% VO2max, or 80% HRmax) is an *average* training intensity and is appropriate for the typical apparently healthy person who wishes to be involved in a regular fitness program.

Determining Your Maximal Heart Rate

If your HRmax cannot be measured, then any estimation must consider the effect of your age on it. Previously, HRmax had been estimated by subtracting your age from 220.

Age-predicted maximum heart rate (APMHR)

$$HRmax = 220 - age$$

Karvonen formula

$$\% HRR = ([HRmax - RHR] \times \% \text{ intensity}) + RHR$$

Use of Your Target Heart Rate

Your THR can be divided by 6 to provide the desired 10 second THR. If your HRmax is unknown, the estimated THR for 10 seconds is found by age and activity level. You can learn to exercise at your THRs by walking or jogging for several minutes and then stopping and immediately taking a 10 second HR. If your HR is not within the target range, you should adjust the intensity by going slower or faster for a few minutes and then taking another 10 second count.

Determining Intensity

1. Estimate Maximal Heart Rate (MHR)
   - MHR= 220 - age
2. Check Resting Heart Rate (RHR)
3. Determine HRR
   - HRR= MHR - RHR
4. Calculate training intensities (TI) at 40-85% using *Karvonen Formula*.

The concept of an intensity threshold provides the basis for regular fitness workouts. Low-intensity activity around the house, yard, and office should be encouraged, but specific workouts above the intensity threshold are necessary to achieve optimum CRF results.

At the other extreme, people who push themselves near their maximum do not have a fitness advantage because similar results can be obtained at a lower intensity that is above the threshold.

Your THR can be used as an intensity guide for large-muscle-group, continuous, whole-body activities such as walking, running, swimming, rowing, cycling, skiing, and dancing. However, the same training results may not occur from activities using small muscle groups or resistance exercises, because these exercises elevate your HR much higher for the same metabolic load.

Your THR range that is associated with improvements in CRF and health-related outcomes is between **50 to 84 %HRR**, however, for those people who are less active and have more risk factors, then they should use the **lower** end of their THR range.

For an example, moderate-intensity activity, equal to only **40 to 59 %HHR**, is well within the capabilities of most people and carries a low-risk of injury or complications. That is why it is the best starting place for most sedentary deconditioned people.

You may wish to continue doing moderate-intensity activity and not move to vigorous-intensity activity, because it suits you and offers you the best way to include exercise it into your schedule.

More active people with fewer risk factors can use the upper end of the THR range.

Using your THR to set exercise intensity has many advantages:

- It has a built-in individualized progression (i.e., as you increase your fitness, you have to work harder to achieve your THR).

- It accounts for environmental conditions (e.g., you decrease your intensity while working in very hot temperatures).

- It is easily determined, learned, and monitored.

These recommendations are appropriate for most people, but individuals differ in terms of the threshold needed for a training effect, the rate of adaptation to the training, and how exercise feels to them. If the work is so easy that you experience little or no increase in ventilation and is able to work without effort, then the intensity should be increased.

At the other extreme, if you shows signs of working very hard and is still unable to reach your THR, then a lower intensity should be chosen. In this case, the top part of the THR range might be above the person's true HRmax because the 220 − age formula only roughly estimates the true value.

WHAT'S YOUR TARGET HEART RATE?

220 Always start with 220
-40 Subtract your age
180 Maximum heart rate

Multiply your maximum heart rate by .65 and .80 to find your target heart range.

180 x .65 = 117
180 x .80 = 144

CONCLUSION: The target heart range for a 40 year old is between 117—144 beats per minute.

	Target zone	% of max HR bpm range	Example duration	Training benefit
Maximize Performance	5 MAXIMUM	90–100% 171–190 bpm	Less than 5 minutes	**Benefits:** Increases maximum sprint race speed **Feels like:** Very exhausting for breathing and muscles **Recommended for:** Very fit persons with athletic training background
	4 HARD	80–90% 152–171 bpm	2–10 minutes	**Benefits:** Increases maximum performance capacity **Feels like:** Muscular fatigue and heavy breathing **Recommended for:** Fit users and for short exercises
Improve Fitness	3 MODERATE	70–80% 133–152 bpm	10–40 minutes	**Benefits:** Improves aerobic fitness **Feels like:** Light muscular fatigue, easy breathing, moderate sweating **Recommended for:** Everybody for typical, moderately long exercises
Lose Weight	2 LIGHT	60–70% 114–133 bpm	40–80 minutes	**Benefits:** Improves basic endurance and helps recovery **Feels like:** Comfortable, easy breathing, low muscle load, light sweating **Recommended for:** Everybody for longer and frequently repeated shorter exercises
	1 VERY LIGHT	50–60% 104–114 bpm	20–40 minutes	**Benefits:** Improves overall health and metabolism, helps recovery **Feels like:** Very easy for breathing and muscles **Recommended for:** Basic training for novice exercisers, weight management and active recovery

Your Stroke Volume

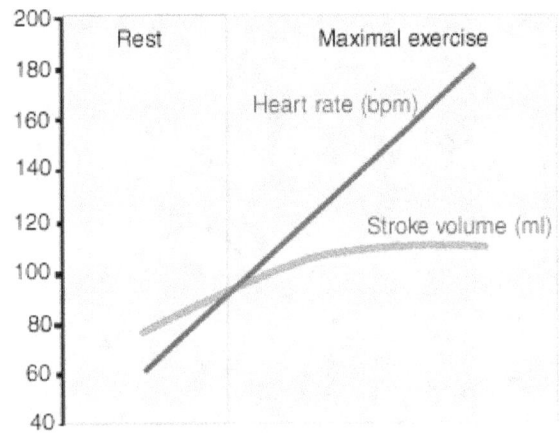

Regulation of Stroke Volume

1. Regulated by three variables:
   a. **End diastolic volume (EDV)**: volume of blood in the ventricles at the end of diastole
      1) Sometimes called **preload**
      2) *Stroke volume increases with increased EDV.*
   b. **Total peripheral resistance**: Frictional resistance in the arteries
      1) *Inversely related to stroke volume*
      2) Called **afterload**

The volume of blood pumped by your heart per beat (ml · beat^{-1}) is called your ***stroke volume (SV)***. If you were doing work in the upright position (cycling, walking), your SV increases in the early stages of your activity until about 40% VO$_2$max is reached and then it levels off.

Consequently, when your VO$_2$ is greater than 40% VO$_2$max, your HR is the sole factor responsible for the increased flow of blood from your heart to your working muscles. ***This causes detrimental STRESS on your Heart – causing it to over-work and a potential injury. The immediate effect is a lack of Energy and Power to complete your activity.***

This is what makes HR a good indicator of the metabolic rate during exercise — it is linearly related to exercise intensity from light exercise to heavy exercise.

Exercise is a Science and when you aren't aware of how your body functions then you can cause damage to yourself while you are pursuing Health and Fitness. In fact, this is HOW most exercise injuries occur … from lack of knowledge which causes a person to injure themselves. Especially a Cardio or Respiratory injury.

You need you heart to beat you into your Abundant Life …. And Life is Measured by and is Orchestrated by the Beat of your Heart!

The main point of exercise is to Strengthen and Condition your Heart so that it can Successfully Beat You into the Enjoyment of Your Abundant Life!

One of the primary effects of endurance training is an increase in your SV, both at-rest and during work; this increase is due to a larger volume of your ventricle that is linked, in part, to a larger blood volume. This allows a greater **end-diastolic volume**, the volume of blood in your heart just before contraction.

In the general population, **SV** is the major variable influencing maximal cardiac output.

Differences in **maximal cardiac output** and **maximal aerobic power** that exist between females and males, between trained and untrained individuals, and between world-class endurance athletes and average fit individuals can be explained largely by differences in maximal **SV**.

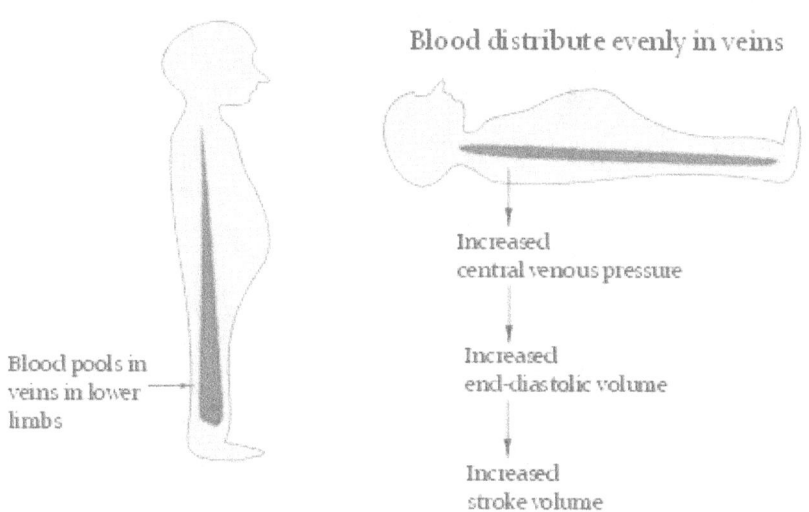

Effect of posture on stroke volume

www.physiologyplus.com

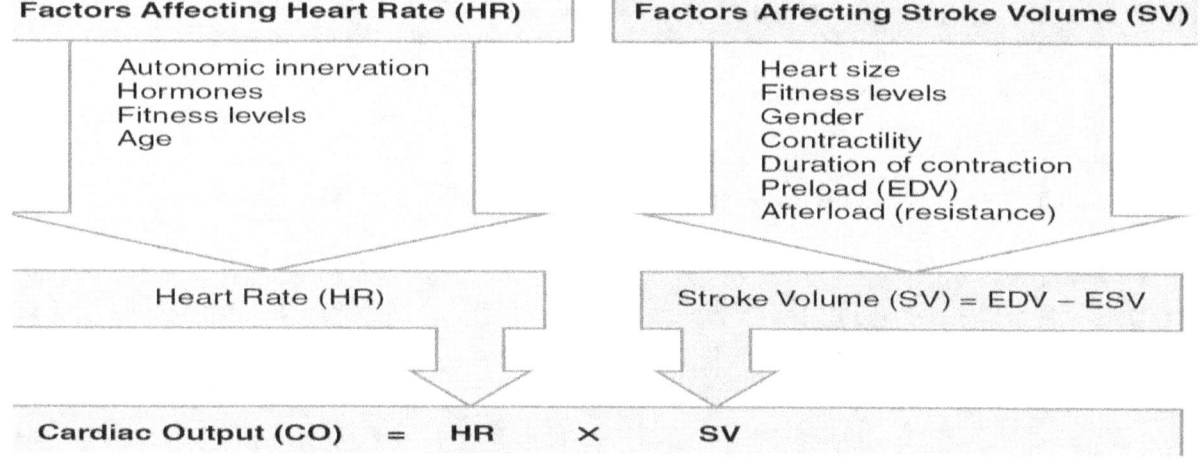

Your Cardiac Output

Your Cardiac output (Q) is the volume of blood pumped by your heart per minute and is calculated by multiplying your HR (beats · min^{-1}) by your Stroke Volume (SV) (ml · beat^{-1}).

$$\text{Cardiac Output} = HR \cdot SV$$

$$= 60 \text{ beats} \cdot \text{min}^{-1} \cdot 80 \text{ ml} \cdot \text{beat}^{-1}$$

$$= 4,800 \text{ ml} \cdot \text{min}^{-1}, \text{ or } 4.8 \text{ L} \cdot \text{min}^{-1}.$$

Your Cardiac output increases linearly with work rate. Generally, your cardiac output response to light and moderate work is not affected by endurance training.

What does change is HOW your cardiac output is achieved: with a lower Heart Rate and higher Stroke Volume.

Your Maximal cardiac output is the most important cardiovascular variable determining your **maximal aerobic power** because the oxygen-enriched blood (carrying about 0.2 L of O_2 per liter of blood) must be delivered to your muscle for your mitochondria to use.

If your maximal cardiac output is **10 L · min^{-1}**, then only **2 L of O_2** would leave your heart each minute (i.e., 0.2 L of O_2 per liter of blood times a cardiac output of 10 L · min^{-1} = 2 L of O_2 · min^{-1}).

Cardiac output – the volume of blood pumped from each ventricle per minute:

CO	=	SV	x	HR
cardiac output (ml/minute)	=	stroke volume (ml/beat)	X	heart rate (beats/min)

a. Average heart rate = 70 bpm
b. Average stroke volume = 70–80 ml/beat
c. Average cardiac output = 5,500 ml/minute

Endurance training increases your maximal cardiac output and the delivery of oxygen to your muscles.

This increase in maximal cardiac output is matched by greater capillary numbers in your muscle to allow the blood to move slowly enough through your muscle to maintain the time needed for oxygen to diffuse from your blood to your mitochondria.

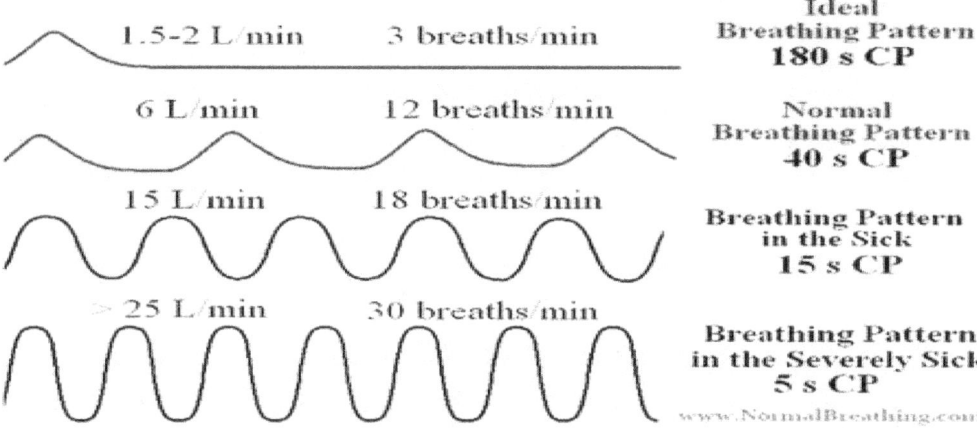

Your Oxygen Extraction

Two factors determine oxygen uptake at any time: the **volume of blood** delivered to your tissues per minute (cardiac output) and the **volume of oxygen** extracted from each liter of your blood.

Your Oxygen extraction is calculated by subtracting the oxygen content of mixed venous blood (as it returns to your heart) from the oxygen content of your arterial blood. This is your **arteriovenous oxygen difference**, or the *(a – V) O_2 difference*.

Your (a – V) O_2 difference reflects the ability of your muscle to extract oxygen and it increases with the intensity level of your exercise. The ability of your tissue to extract oxygen is a function of the capillary-to-muscle-fiber ratio and the number of mitochondria in your muscle fiber.

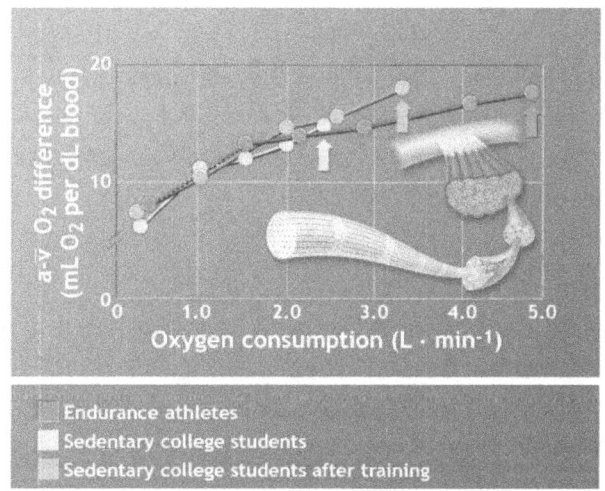

Endurance training increases both of these factors, thus increasing the maximal capacity to extract oxygen. This increase in the (a – V)O_2 difference accounts for about 50% of the increase in VO_2max that occurs with endurance training in previously sedentary individuals.

Your Blood Pressure

Your **blood pressure** (BP) is dependent on the balance between your cardiac output and the resistance your blood vessels offer to your blood flow (total peripheral resistance). The resistance to blood flow is altered by the constriction or dilation of your **arterioles**, which are blood vessels located between your artery and the capillary.

$$BP = Cardiac\ Output \cdot Total\ Peripheral\ Resistance.$$

Blood Pressure Categories

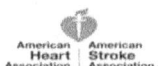

BLOOD PRESSURE CATEGORY	SYSTOLIC mm Hg (upper number)		DIASTOLIC mm Hg (lower number)
NORMAL	LESS THAN 120	and	LESS THAN 80
ELEVATED	120 – 129	and	LESS THAN 80
HIGH BLOOD PRESSURE (HYPERTENSION) STAGE 1	130 – 139	or	80 – 89
HIGH BLOOD PRESSURE (HYPERTENSION) STAGE 2	140 OR HIGHER	or	90 OR HIGHER
HYPERTENSIVE CRISIS (consult your doctor immediately)	HIGHER THAN 180	and/or	HIGHER THAN 120

Your BP is sensed by **baroreceptors** in the arch of your aorta and in your carotid arteries. When your BP changes, the baroreceptors send signals to the cardiovascular control center in your brain, which in turn alters cardiac output or the diameter of your arterioles.

For an example, if you have been lying supine and suddenly stand, blood pools in your lower extremities, your SV decreases and your BP drops.

If your BP is not restored, less blood flows to your brain and you might experience a faint. The baroreceptors monitor this decrease in your BP and your cardiovascular control center simultaneously increases your HR and reduces the diameter of your arterioles (to increase total peripheral resistance) to try to return your BP to normal.

During exercise, your arterioles dilate in the active muscle to increase blood flow and meet your metabolic demands. This dilation is matched with a constriction of the arterioles in your liver, kidneys, and gastrointestinal tract and an increase in your HR and SV, as already mentioned. These coordinated changes maintain your BP and direct most of the cardiac output to your working muscles.

These steps are in-place to ensure your Success of completing any activity or exercise.

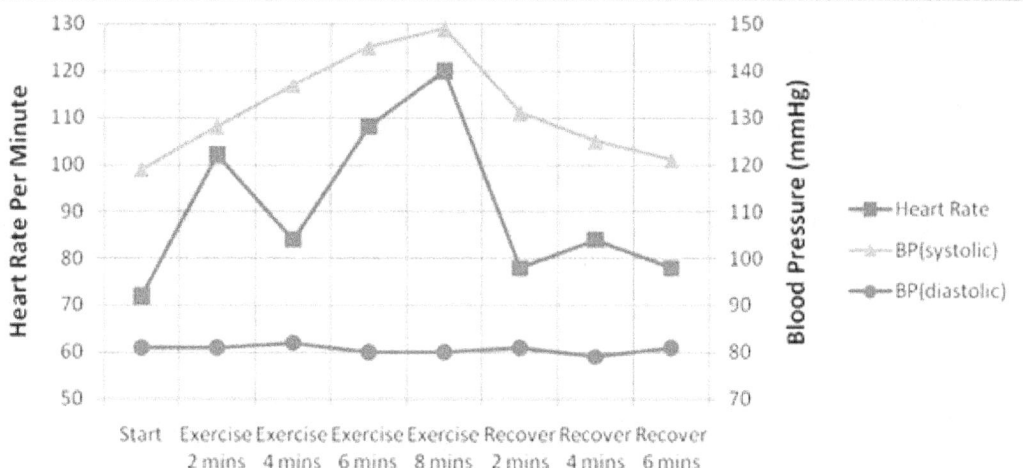

Your **Systolic blood pressure (SBP)** increases with each stage until your **maximum work tolerance** is reached. At that point, your SBP might **decrease**. A fall in your SBP with an increase in work rate is used as an indicator of **maximal cardiovascular function** and can aid in determining the **end point** for an exercise or activity.

Your Diastolic blood pressure (DBP) tends to remain the same or decrease during n activity. An increase in your DBP toward the end of an activity is another indicator that you may have reached the limits of your **functional capacity**.

Endurance training reduces your BP responses at fixed submaximal work rates.

Two factors that determine the oxygen demand (work) of your heart during aerobic exercise are your HR and your SBP. The product of these two variables is called your **rate–pressure product,** or your **double product,** and is proportional to your myocardial oxygen demand (i.e., the volume of oxygen the heart muscle needs each minute to function properly).

Factors that decrease your HR and BP responses to work increase the chance that the coronary blood supply to your heart muscle will adequately meet the oxygen demands of your heart.

This means you will create the circumstance for your Success of completing your activity or exercise!

You need your Heart to beat you into your Abundant Life ... Knowing how to improve and increase the Strength and Health of your Heart increases your ability to Heal, become Healthy and make manifest your Power!

Endurance training decreases your HR and BP responses to fixed submaximal work and protects against any diminished blood supply (ischemia) to your myocardium.

Your SBP increases with each stage of an activity or exercise, whereas your DBP remains the same or decreases. The work of your heart is proportional to the product of your HR and your SBP.

Blood Pressure During Exercise

Systolic blood pressure has a much higher increase during exercise than diastolic blood pressure due to:

- Increased contractility of the heart
- Increased stroke volume
- The muscular need for greater force and pressure to deliver blood to the exercising muscles
- Vasodilation within the exercising muscle, which results in more blood draining from the arteries, through the arterioles, and into muscle capillaries, minimizing the change in diastolic pressure

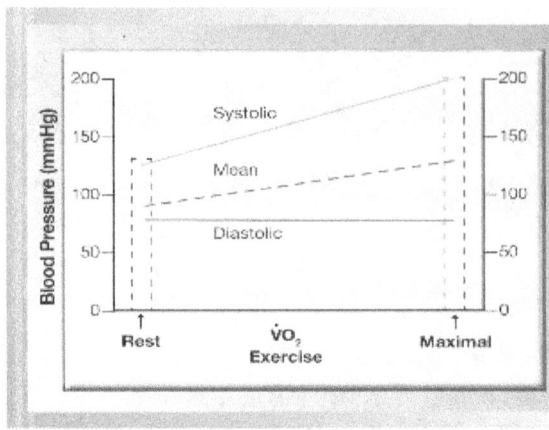

Normal responses to blood pressure during exercise

Training lowers both, making it easier for your coronary arteries to meet the oxygen demand of your heart.

Your HR and BP are higher during arm work compared with leg work at the same work rate. If you perform the same rate of work with your arms as with your legs, then your HR and BP responses are considerably higher during your arm work.

Given that the load on your heart and the potential for fatigue are greater for arm work, you should choose activities that use the large muscle groups of your legs.

Such activities ultimately result in lowering your Heart Rate, Blood Pressure and perception of fatigue at the same work rate.

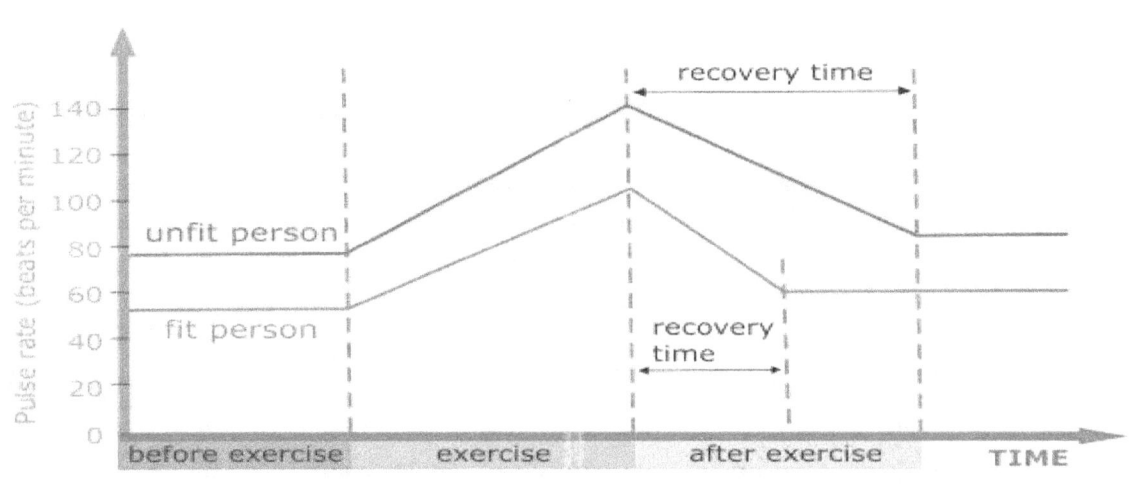

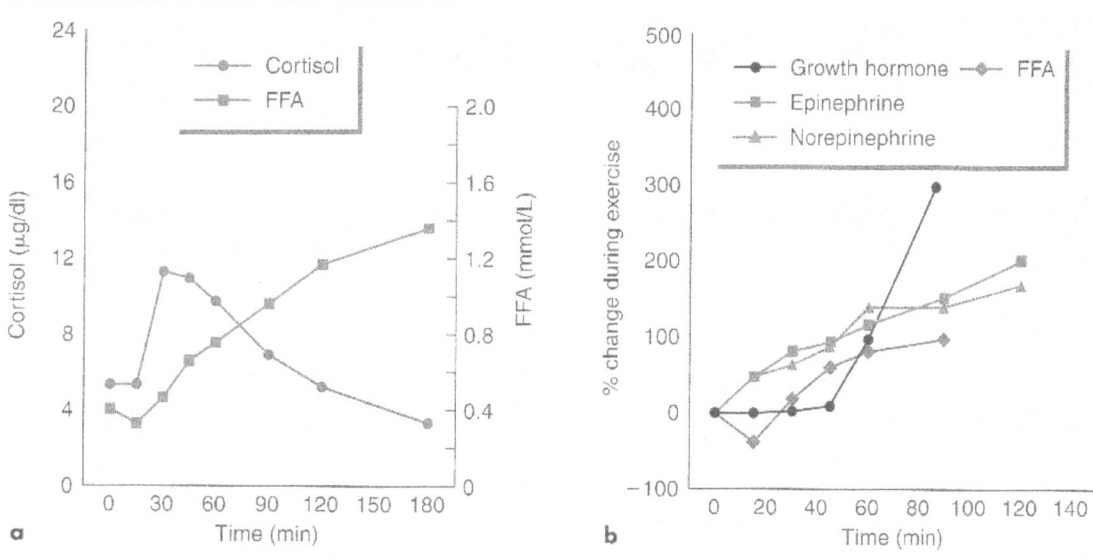

▲ **Figure 5.11** Changes in plasma levels of (a) free fatty acid (FFA) and cortisol and (b) epinephrine, norepinephrine, growth hormone, and FFA during prolonged exercise.

Effects of Endurance Training and Detraining on Your Physiological Responses

Many observations have been made about the effects of endurance training on various physiological responses to exercise.

• Endurance training increases the number of mitochondria and capillaries in your muscle, causing all active fibers to become more oxidative. This effect is manifested by the increase in type IIa fibers and decrease in type IIx fibers. These changes boost the endurance capacity of your muscle by allowing fat to be used for a greater percentage of energy production, sparing your muscle glycogen store and reducing lactate production. The lactate threshold shifts to the right, and performance times in endurance events improve.

You 'BURN' your fat, while conserving your energy and increasing your ability to produce energy. By using your fat first, you keep your natural energy stores in your muscles HIGH – ensuring that you always have the energy you need to Move YourSelf and maintain your Motion!

• Endurance training decreases the time it takes to achieve a steady state in submaximal exercise. This reduces your oxygen deficit and reliance on PC and anaerobic glycolysis for energy.

You are an Aerobic Life form, and operating under an anaerobic condition is for emergency efforts only. Endurance training helps you to maintain your energy production under aerobics conditions = Stronger, Longer and Constant Motion!

- Endurance training enlarges the volume of your ventricle. This accommodates an increase in your end-diastolic volume such that more blood is pumped out per beat. The increase in your Stroke Volume is accompanied by a decrease in your Heart Rate during submaximal work, so your cardiac output remains the same.

Your heart works less to meet the oxygen needs of your tissues at the same work rate.

You can Move Faster, Stronger and Longer WITHOUT wearing out your Heart!

You need your Heart to beat you into your Abundant Life. With endurance training you can condition your body to move at a Faster speed WITHOUT Stressing your Heart and Energy levels – your perpetual Motion of Life!

Endurance training increases the ability of your muscle to use your fat as a fuel and to spare your carbohydrate level while decreasing the time it takes for your body to achieve a steady state during your submaximal work.

Endurance training effects (lower HR, lower blood lactate) do not transfer when untrained muscles are used to perform the work.

Maximal oxygen uptake decreases when training stops.

The initial decrease is caused by a decrease in SV and, later, in oxygen extraction.

To maintain your Maximal oxygen uptake, *This means that you have to constantly and consistently Exercise and keep YourSelf in the Motion of Life!*

Move Something!

WHAT Are YOU Moving?

YourSelf!

WHERE Are YOU Going?

Abundant LIFE!

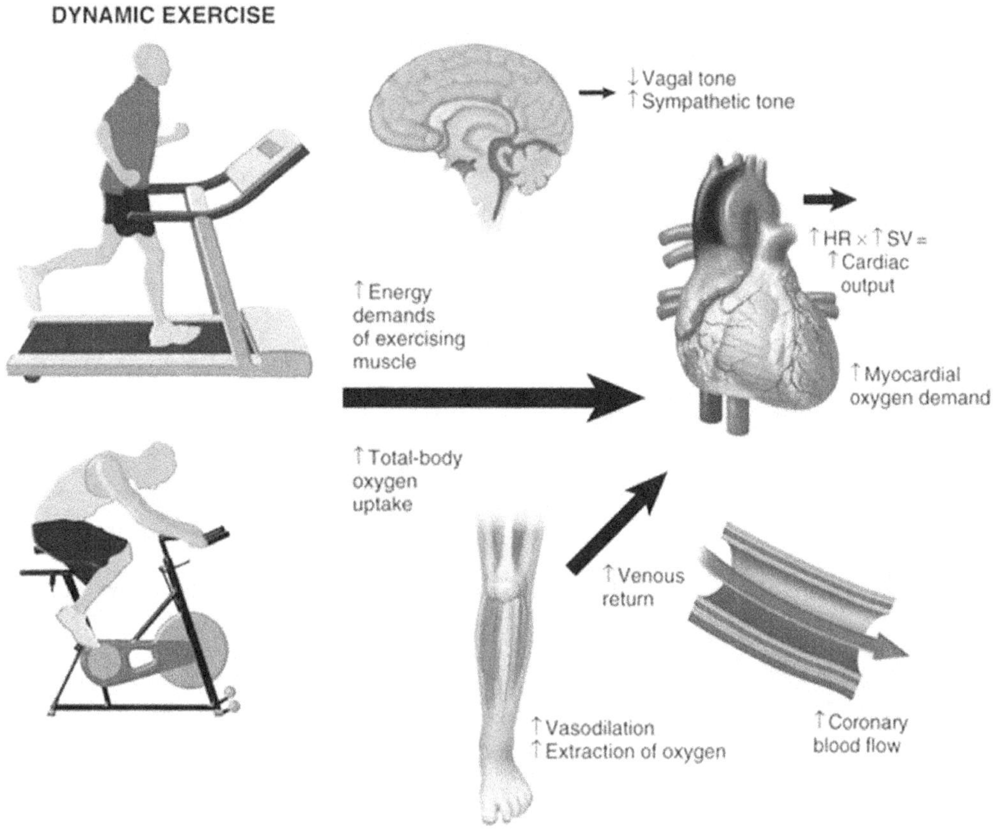

Move Something!

DYNAMIC EXERCISE

↓ Vagal tone
↑ Sympathetic tone

↑ Energy demands of exercising muscle

↑ Total-body oxygen uptake

↑ Venous return

↑ Vasodilation
↑ Extraction of oxygen

↑ HR × ↑ SV = ↑ Cardiac output

↑ Myocardial oxygen demand

↑ Coronary blood flow

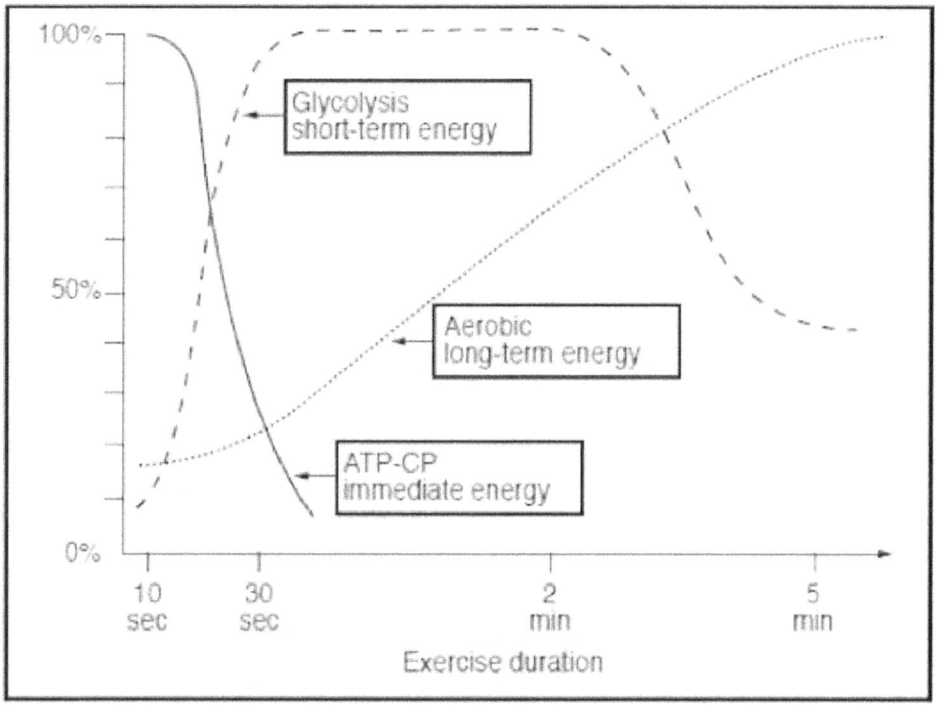

- Glycolysis — short-term energy
- Aerobic — long-term energy
- ATP-CP — immediate energy

Exercise duration: 10 sec, 30 sec, 2 min, 5 min

Supreme Health & Fitness!   Health & Wellness Series ... Vol 3!

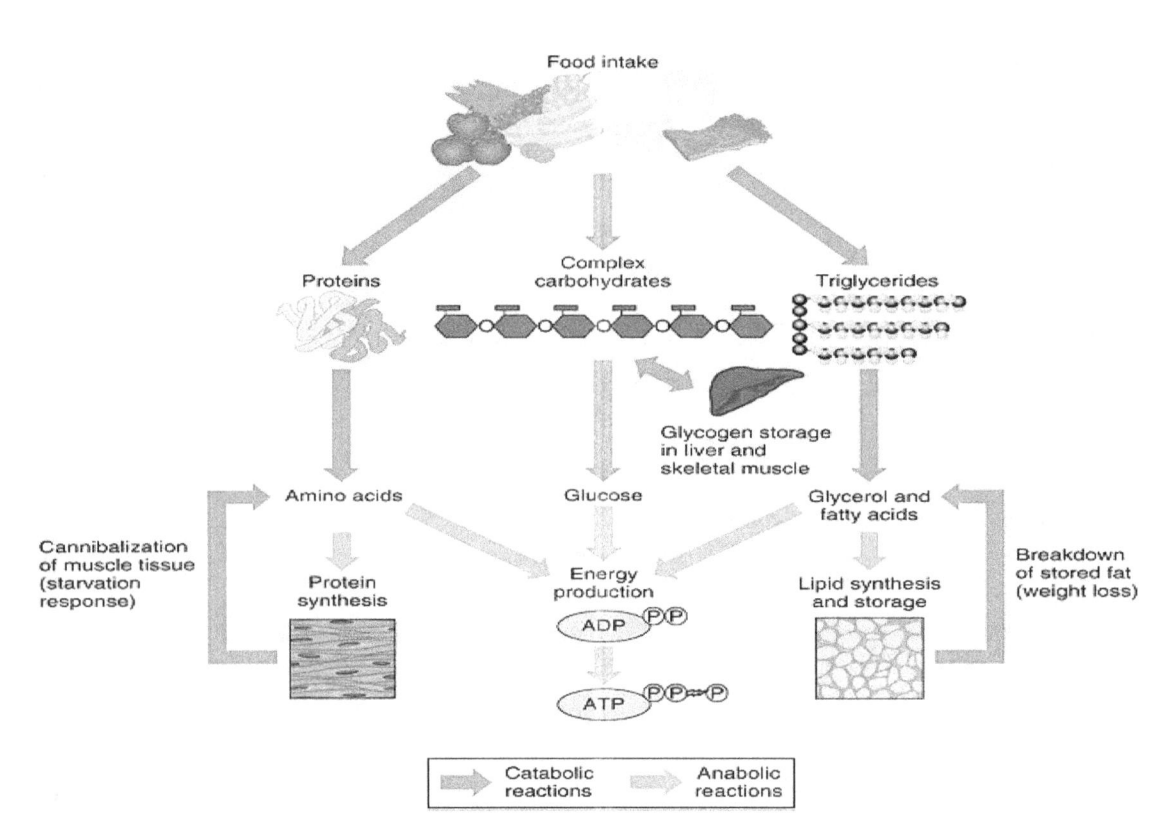

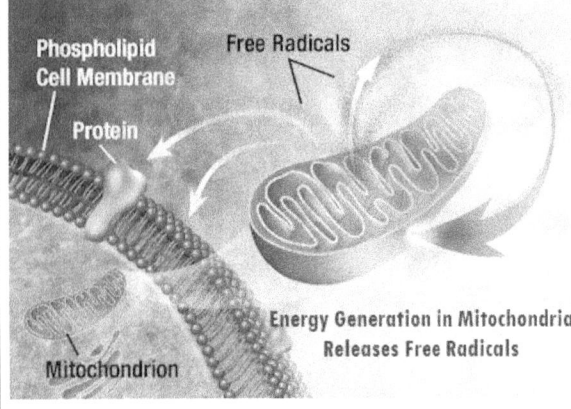

Energy Generation in Mitochondria Releases Free Radicals

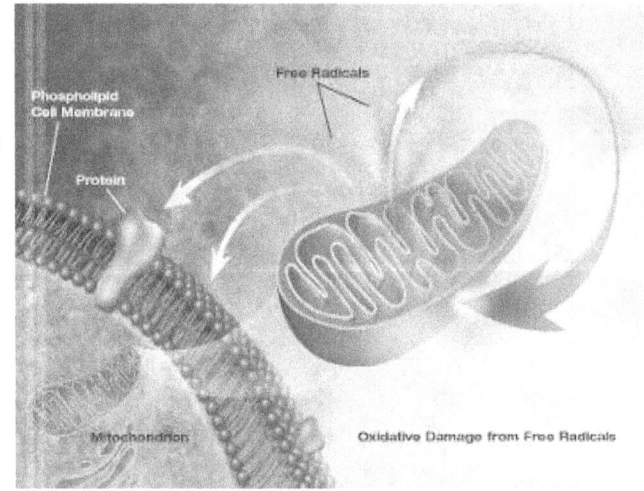

Oxidative Damage from Free Radicals

Table 1. Etiologic Factors of Sarcopenia

Reduced level or lack of physical activity

Loss of neuromuscular function: denervation; loss of alpha motor-neuron axons

Altered endocrine function
- Insulin: increased risk of insulin resistance
- Estrogens: declining levels in women
- GH and IGF-1: waning levels
- Testosterone: declining levels in men
- Vitamin D: declining levels in women
- PTH: high levels

Increased levels of cytokines: IL-6, particularly in older women; TNF-alpha, particularly in men

Mitochondrial dysfunction: cumulative age-related damage to muscle mitochondrial DNA (mtDNA)

Apoptosis: pattern of cell death

Genetic influence

Increased dietary protein needs, low nutritional intake, and low protein intake

Table 2. Benefits of Strength-Training Exercise in Older Adults

Aerobic activities when supplemented with strength-training exercises at least twice weekly help to:
- Build strength
- Maintain bone density
- Improve balance, coordination, and mobility
- Reduce risk of falling
- Maintain independence in performing activities of daily living

Table 3. Strength Training Reduces Signs and Symptoms of Diseases and Chronic Conditions

Arthritis: Decreases pain and stiffness; increases strength and flexibility

Diabetes: Improves glycemic control

Osteoporosis: Increases bone density; reduces risk of falls

Heart disease: Improves lipid profile and overall fitness, reducing cardiovascular risk

Obesity: Increases calorie burning through increase in metabolism; assists with long-term weight control

Back pain: Strengthens back and abdominal muscles, which reduces stress on the spine

Regular Physical Activity Health Benefits for Seniors

➤ Helps to reduces symptoms of anxiety and depression and fosters improvements in mood and feelings of well-being.

➤ Reduces risk of developing neurodegenerative diseases, high blood pressure, colon cancer, and diabetes.

➤ Helps maintain the ability to live independently and reduces the risk of falling and fracturing bones.

➤ Can help reduce blood pressure in some people with hypertension.

➤ Helps people with chronic, disabling conditions improve their stamina and muscle strength.

➤ Helps maintain healthy bones, muscles, and joints.

➤ Helps control joint swelling and pain associated with arthritis.

Protective Effects of Exercise

- Being physically fit reduces the risk of cardiovascular disease, with people who do not exercise being TWICE as likely to develop heart disease

- Exercise is thought to decrease the many of the risk factors for CHD by:
    - *strengthens the heart muscle (myocardium) so that it can pump more blood with each beat therefore improving efficiency of the heart*
    - *lowering resting heart rate*
    - *improves blood lipid profile by decreasing LDL and increasing HDL levels*
    - *lowers blood pressure by maintaining the elasticity of the arteries*
    - *helps weight loss by decreasing % body fat*
    - *decreasing development of atheroma*
    - *controlling stress*

- Even a small amount of moderate exercise, such as walking, can improve the quality of life and increase life expectancy

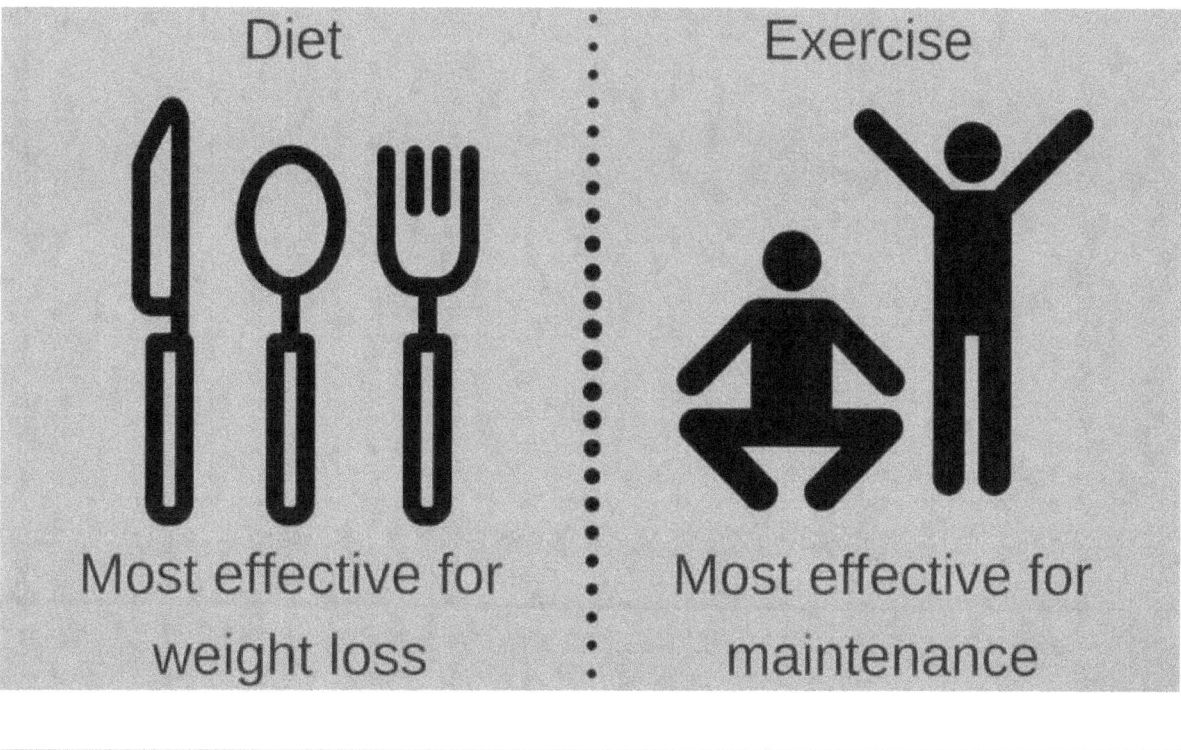

Diet	Exercise
Most effective for weight loss	Most effective for maintenance

"More Something!"

Chapter Eleven

Exercise & Weight Management

*****

- Obese individuals who lost just 5% of their body weight gained significant health benefits that would lower their risk of stroke, diabetes and heart disease

- Losing 5% body weight lowered glucose, triglyceride, insulin levels and systolic blood pressure along with liver fat and intra-abdominal fat volume

- These beneficial changes continued with progressive weight loss up to 16% of body weight, which suggests that more weight loss may lead to even greater health benefits

Working up the motivation to lose weight is half the battle, especially if you're obese and feeling overwhelmed by the number of pounds you need to lose to get healthy.

New research brings welcome news, which is that even a small amount of weight loss can yield significant health benefits.

A common treatment recommendation for obese and overweight patients is to lose between 5% and 10% of body weight to get healthier.

But as study author Dr. Samuel Klein, a professor of medicine and nutrition science chief at Washington University School of Medicine, told The New York Times:

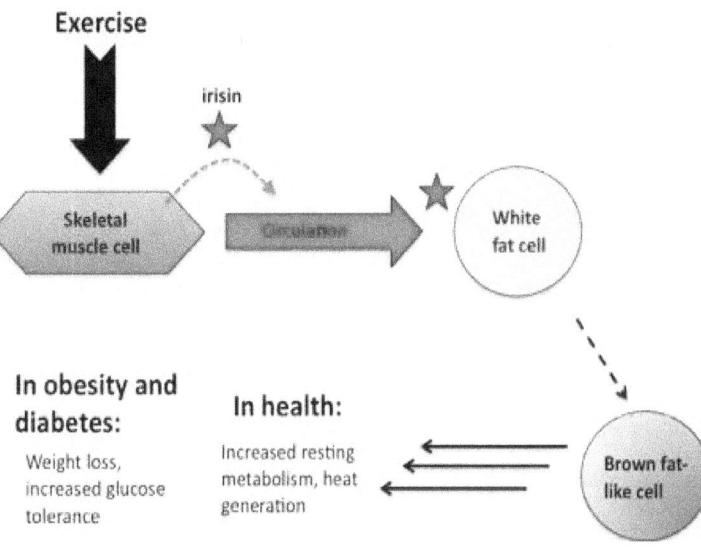

"Losing 5% is much easier than losing 10%, so it was important to understand what the differences might be ... You get a big bang for your buck with 5%."

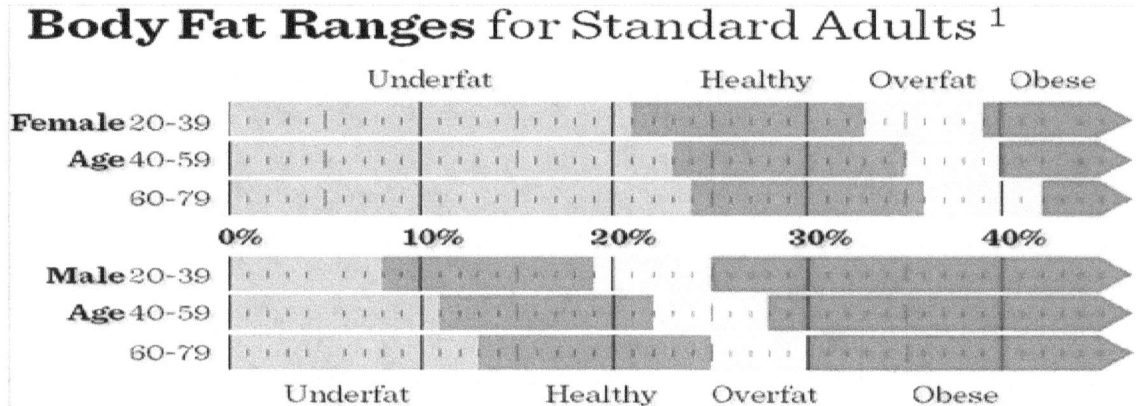

Fat Cells and Toxins

Did you know that our bodies protect us from toxins by storing them in our fat cells, and in order to **allow our body to lose weight**, we must reduce the intake of toxins (such as pesticides, chemicals, drugs, artificial sweeteners, high fructose corn syrup, partially hydrogenated oil and substances found in processed food).

These toxic chemicals are also affecting our hormones and liver functions in charge of metabolism.

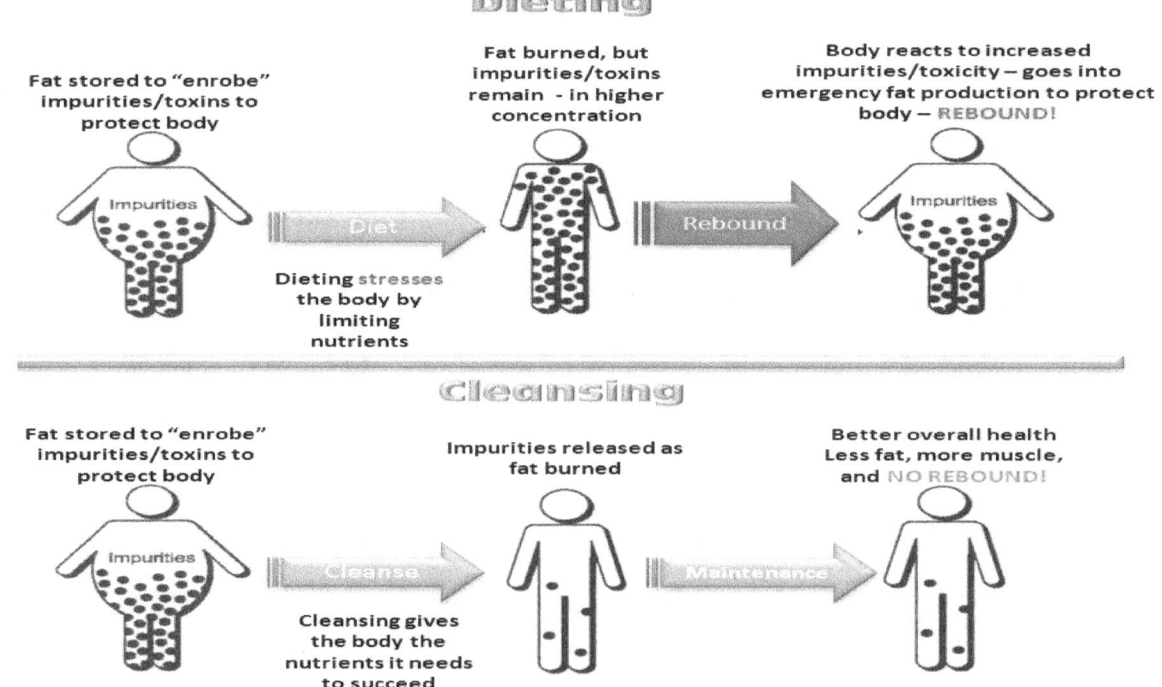

Losing Just 5 Percent of Your Body Weight Triggers Significant Health Benefits

There is a Harvard study that involved 40 obese individuals who either maintained their body weight or lost weight via a low-calorie diet. Those in the weight loss group had goals of losing 5%, 10% or 15% of their body weight.

It turned out that even the modest 5% weight loss led to significant benefits, including changes that would lower the risk of stroke, diabetes and heart disease. Specifically, the main changes were:

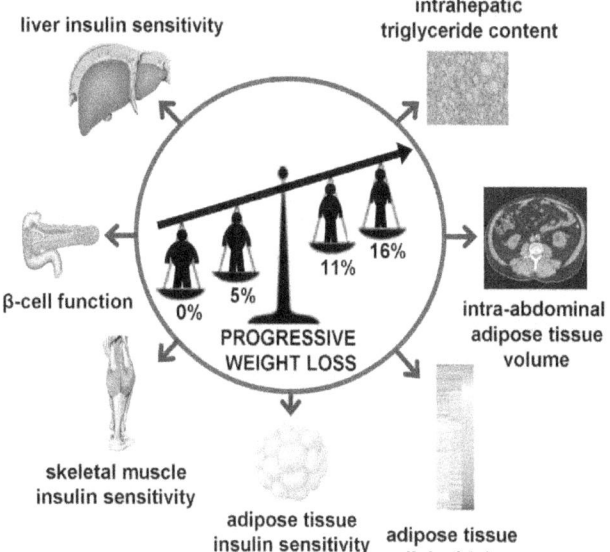

- **8% lower body fat mass**
- **7% lower intra-abdominal fat volume**
- **40% lower liver fat**
- **Lower glucose, triglyceride and insulin levels**
- **Lower systolic blood pressure and heart rates**

These beneficial changes continued with progressive weight loss up to 16% of body weight, which suggests that more weight loss will lead to even greater health benefits. Further, the 5% weight loss did not lead to improvements in markers of inflammation.

That being said, the small 5% weight loss led to noteworthy beneficial changes.

Klein told Tech Times that even if you can lose only 5% of your body weight, you should view it as a success, not a failure:

"You're much healthier on the inside, and it's a really reasonable and legitimate target for people with obesity."

This isn't the first time modest weight loss has been found to beneficial. Back in 1995, a review published in Obesity Research concluded, ***"Weight loss as low as 5% has been shown to reduce or eliminate disorders associated with obesity … "***

Obesity Rates Are Skyrocketing

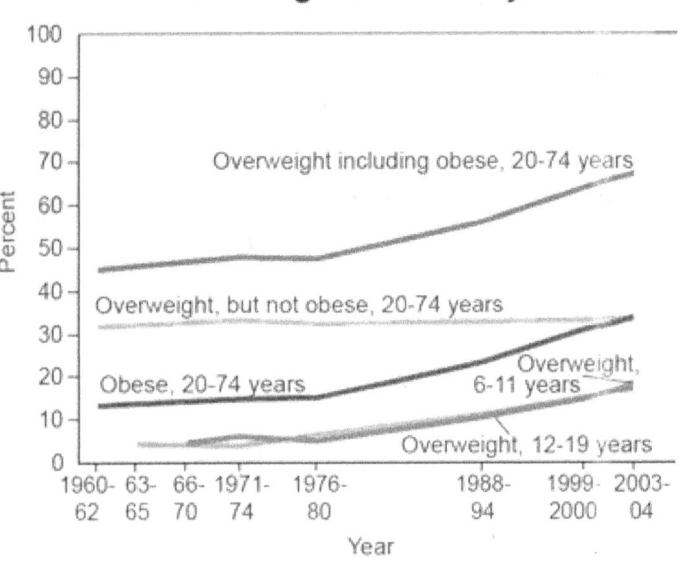

More than 2.1 billion people, or close to 30% of the global population, are overweight or obese, and obesity is responsible for about 5 percent of all deaths each year, worldwide.

Today, about 75% of U.S. men and 67 percent of U.S. women are either overweight or obese, and the trend is getting worse, not better.

In the U.S., nearly 1 in 5 deaths is now associated with obesity. The statistics for children are equally disturbing.

Over 17% of American children between the ages of 2 and 19 fall into the obese category, which can set them up for a lifetime of very serious health problems.

There has been some provocative research that suggests being overweight may be linked to a *longer* life, leading some to question whether "healthy obesity" is a potential reality. However, for the vast majority of those who carry around extra pounds, health problems will often result.

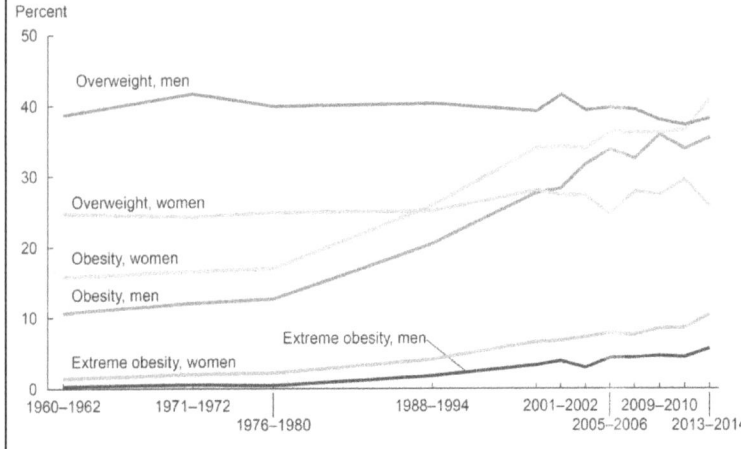

Figure. Trends in adult overweight, obesity, and extreme obesity among men and women aged 20–74: United States, 1960–1962 through 2013–2014

Why It's Important to Lose Weight If You're Obese

In a 2014 study that analyzed data from more than 5 million people over the age of 16, every 11-pound increase in body weight was associated with an increased risk for 10 types of cancer, including leukemia, uterine, gallbladder, kidney, cervix, and thyroid cancer.

Further, people who are obese have been found to be 18% *more* likely to die of any cause. A 2013 systematic review and meta-analysis also found that obese individuals were more likely to die sooner or have heart-related problems than people of normal weight — even if they were otherwise healthy.

According to the U.S. Surgeon General, obesity increases your risk for asthma, sleep disorders (including sleep apnea), depression, pregnancy complications, and poor surgical outcomes.

Further, in the U.S., eight obesity-related diseases account for a staggering 75% of health care costs.

These diseases include:

Type 2 diabetes	Non-alcoholic fatty liver disease (NAFLD)
Hypertension	Polycystic ovarian syndrome
Lipid problems	Cancer (especially breast, endometrial, colon, gallbladder, prostate and kidney)
Heart disease	Dementia

Why Are Obesity Rates Rising?

Highly processed genetically engineered (GE) foods are a primary culprit, as they're chockfull of ingredients that both individually and in combination contribute to metabolic dysfunction and hard-to-control weight gain.

GE corn syrup, trans fats, and GE sugar — along with heavily processed refined grains — these ingredients are now foundational in the U.S. diet and are increasingly found worldwide. There is virtually no doubt that they are the *primary* contributors to Americans' failing health and rising rates of obesity.

Non-starchy, carb-rich, and highly processed (and typically genetically-engineered) foods, along with being in continuous feast mode, are primary drivers of these statistics. Wherever a highly processed food diet becomes the norm, obesity inevitably follows.

Adding to the problem is extremely aggressive marketing of junk food that's laboratory-created to be addictive and to encourage you to eat more. Then there's the overuse of antibiotics in food production and medicine. Mice given antibiotics for the first four weeks of life grew up to be 25% heavier and had 60 percent more body fat than the controls in one study.

And it's become quite clear that changes to your microbiome (such as antibiotics use) can have a serious and long-term impact on your body's metabolism, especially when they occur early in life.

Endocrine-disrupting chemicals, including pesticides and plastics chemicals, also likely play a role in rising weights, as do inactivity and lack of sleep.

Easy Four-Step Plan to Lose Weight

If you're overweight or obese and want to lose some weight, you may be wondering where to start. It helps to look at the foundational reasons why you may be struggling with your weight.

Generally, in order for you to significantly gain weight, you must first become leptin resistant. Leptin is a hormone that helps you regulate your appetite. When your leptin levels rise, it signals your body that you're full, so you'll stop eating. However, as you become increasingly resistant to the effects of leptin, you end up eating more. Many people who are overweight also have an impairment in their body's ability to oxidize fat, which leads to a low-energy state.

Dr. Richard Johnson's research clearly shows that refined sugar (in particular fructose) is exceptionally effective at causing leptin resistance in animals, and it's very effective at blocking the burning of fat.

If you are insulin or leptin resistant, as long as you keep eating fructose and grains, you're literally programming your body to Create and Store FAT!

This is one of the key reasons why, if you are overweight (which means you are also likely insulin or leptin resistant), it would be prudent for you to restrict your fructose consumption to about 15 to 25 grams of fructose per day from all sources. Not only will this help you to avoid additional weight gain, it will also help you to avoid further metabolic dysfunction. You may find this fructose chart helpful in estimating how many grams of fructose you are consuming each day.

Dietary sugar, especially fructose, is a significant "tripper of your fat switch." However, if you are serious about losing weight, you'll need a c*omprehensive* plan that includes the following. This plan will help most people lose weight but, also, it will help you to gain metabolic health. So even if your weight is normal, you can follow this plan to ensure that you're metabolically healthy as well.

1. Apply the Science of Eating To Live! Eliminate or strictly limit fructose in your diet, and follow the healthy eating program in my comprehensive nutrition plan. Replace processed foods with real food.

2. Fasting is our BEST Solution ... Prescribed by GOD! You can also use intermittent fasting strategically with this program to greatly boost your body's fat-burning potential. Intermittent fasting helps reset your body to use fat as its primary fuel, and mounting evidence confirms that when your body becomes adapted to burning FAT instead of sugar as its primary fuel, you dramatically reduce your risk of chronic disease.

Exercising in a fasted state (such as first thing in the morning) will bring it up yet another notch.

3. Move YourSelf and Engage in high-intensity exercise to burn fat and increase muscle mass (a natural fat burner). Also, strive to sit less (much less, such as only three hours a day) and walk 7,000 to 10,000 steps a day in addition to your regular exercise program.

4. Eliminate Your STRESS. Address the emotional component of eating. For this I highly recommend the Emotional Freedom Techniques (EFT), which helps eliminate your food cravings naturally.

What Emotional Freedom Technique (EFT) Does

Another name for Emotional Freedom Technique (EFT) is Meridian Tapping. This is because EFT utilizes **the same energy-meridian system that traditional Chinese acupuncture uses – minus the needles**.

EFT is done by lightly tapping on specific points on your body (usually eight or nine) between your chest and the top of your head.

While tapping, you vocalize first the negative issue at hand (and your feelings about it) and then vocalize a more positive perception of the issue (even if it is just to accept it).

This combination works on an energetic, emotional, and physiological level to clear emotional blocks and bring your mind and body back into balance.

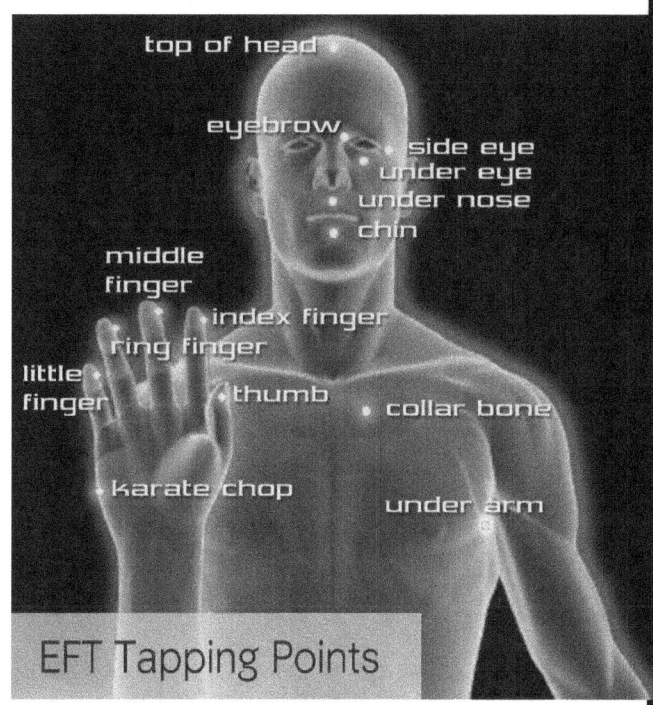

On an anatomic level, regularly practicing Tapping and utilizing it in times of stress helps stabilize your hormone levels. It will also calm your amygdalae, the part of your limbic system that responds to emotional stimuli and is responsible for your "fight or flight" response.

EFT Tapping has been shown to significantly decrease (and in some cases eliminate) conditions such as:

- **Anxiety**
- **Depression**
- **PTSD /Trauma**

- **Food Cravings**
- **Addictions**
- **Phobias**
- **Test and Public Speaking Anxiety**
- **Physical Pain**

How to Determine Your Healthy Weight

Body Mass Index (BMI) is a flawed measurement tool, so branding yourself as overweight or obese simply based on your BMI is not recommended. Your waist-to-hip ratio is a more reliable indicator of your future disease risk because a higher ratio suggests you have more visceral fat.

Excess visceral fat — the fat that accumulates around your internal organs — is extremely more hazardous to your health than subcutaneous fat (which is the more noticeable fat found just under your skin). A measure that BMI tells you nothing about.

The danger of visceral fat is related to the release of proteins and hormones that can cause inflammation, which in turn can damage arteries and enter your liver, affecting how your body breaks down sugars and fats.

To determine your waist-to-hip ratio, get a tape measure and record your waist and hip circumference. Then divide your waist circumference by your hip circumference.

Waist-to-Hip Ratio	Men	Women
Ideal	0.8	0.7
Low Risk	<0.95	<0.8
Moderate Risk	0.96 to 0.99	0.81 to 0.84
High Risk	>1.0	>0.85

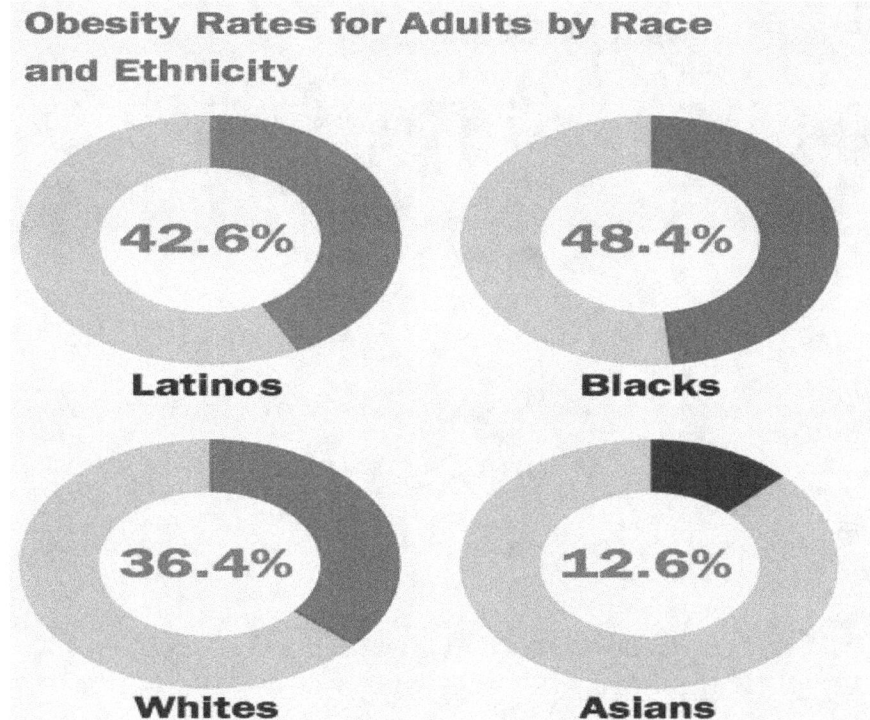
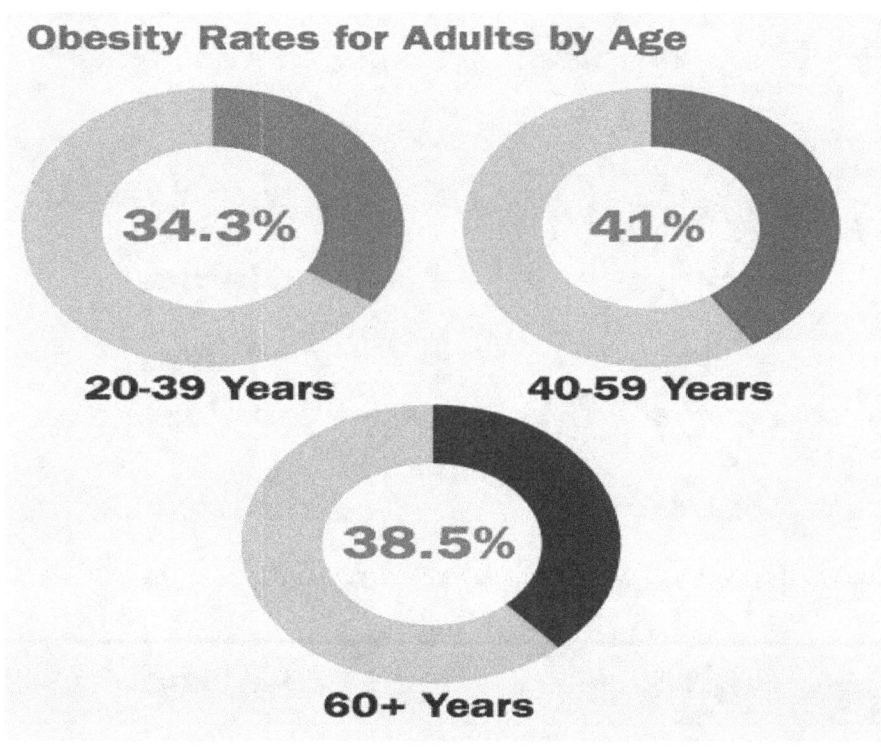

African American Obesity or Overweight

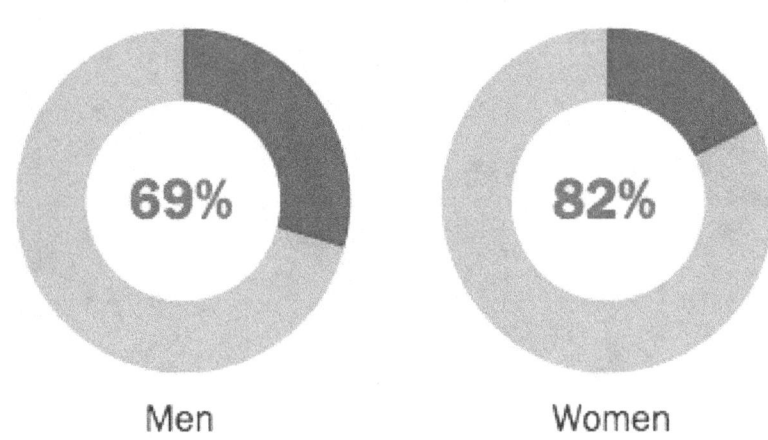

Men — 69%
Women — 82%

Obesity Rate for Children Ages 2 to 19 by Race and Ethnicity

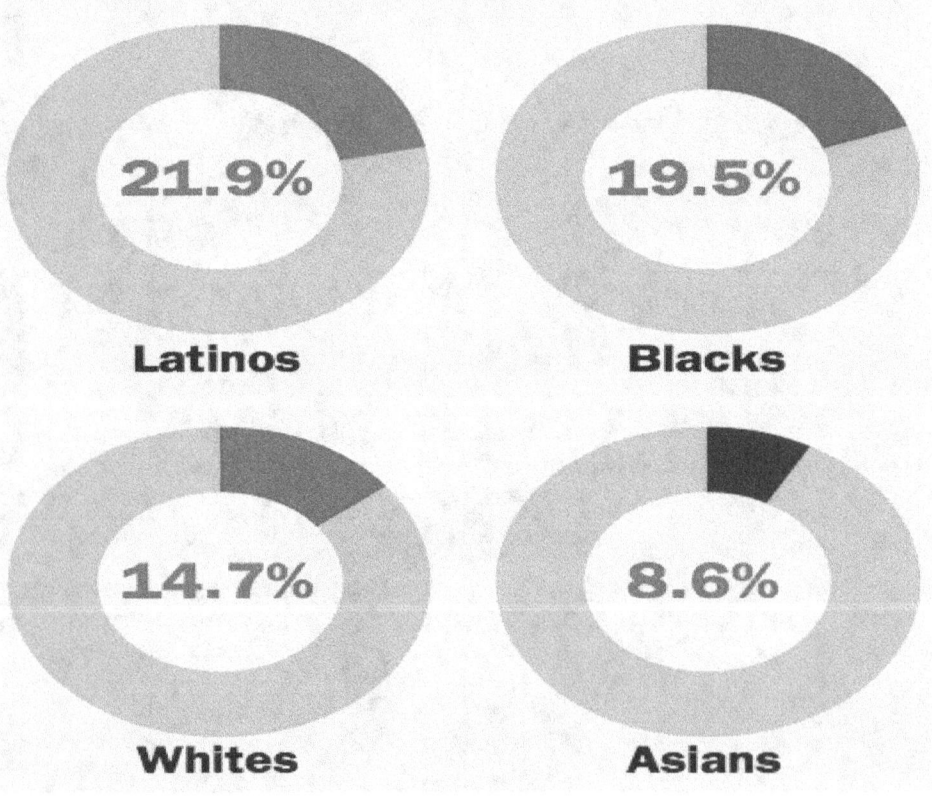

Latinos — 21.9%
Blacks — 19.5%
Whites — 14.7%
Asians — 8.6%

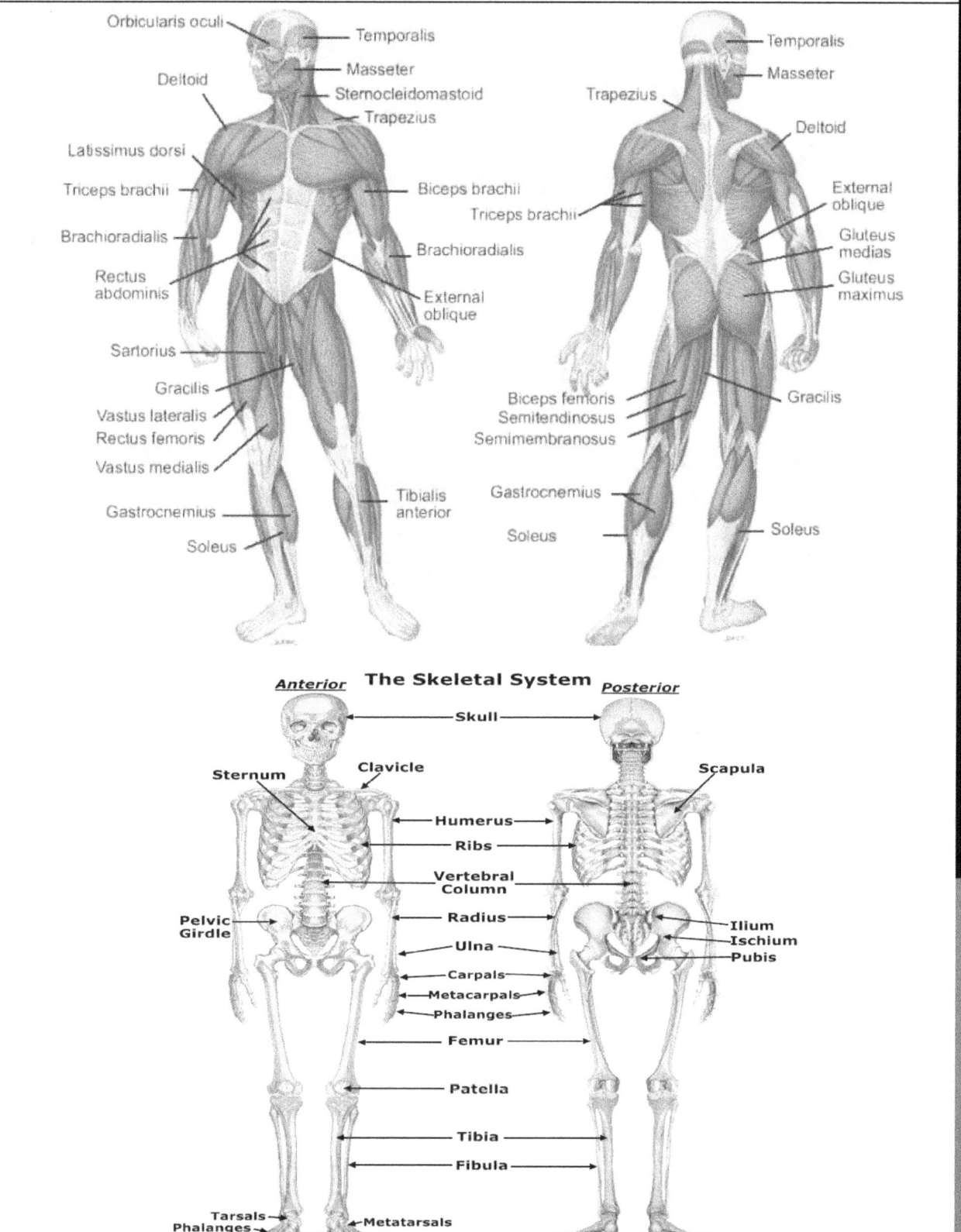

Move Something!

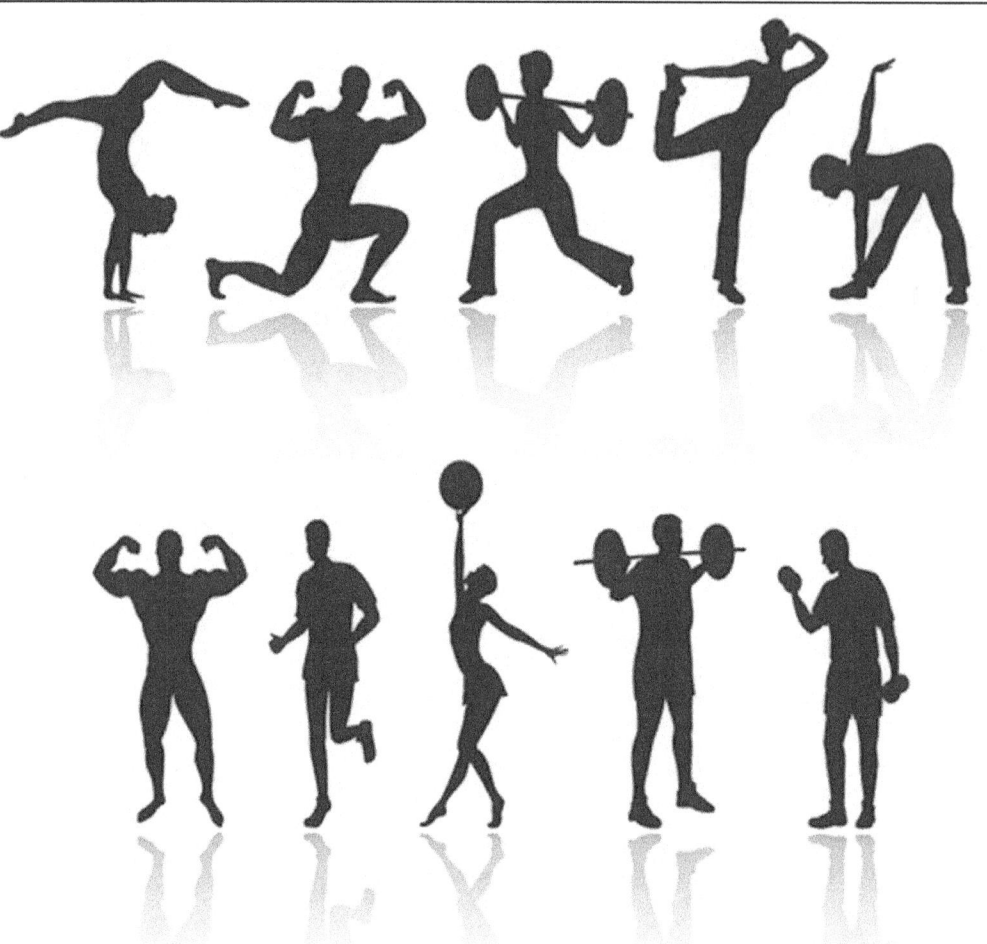

Supreme Health & Fitness! Health & Wellness Series...Vol 3!

Chapter Twelve

Your Musculoskeletal Health

*****

Your musculoskeletal is combined of 2 of your systems – Muscle and Skeletal - systems that you need to carry you into the Successful Enjoyment of Your Abundant Life!

These are the system that form the physical Foundation of your God-Body!

The most common health complaints involve your musculoskeletal system, from back pain to arthritis, to osteoporosis and joint pain. Musculoskeletal problems can stem from chronic diseases and syndromes such as fibromyalgia and rheumatoid arthritis to acute injuries like a pulled muscle or sprained ankle.

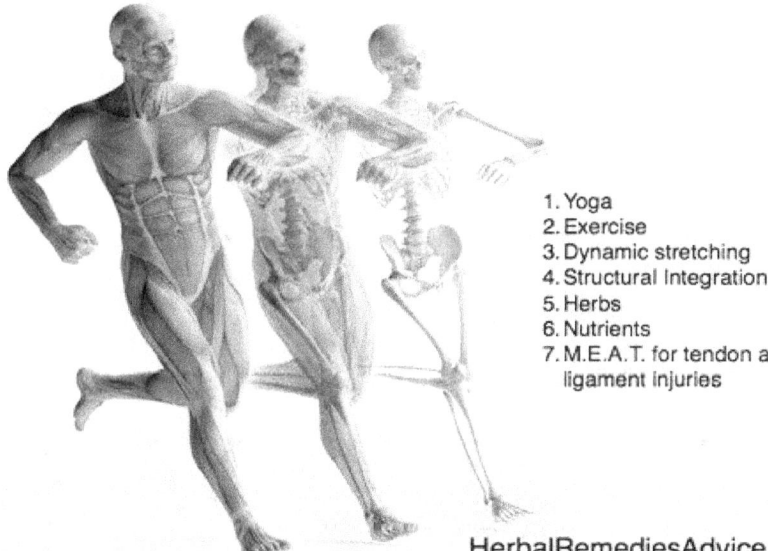

Keeping this system healthy will improve your quality of life for the rest of your life! Healthy muscles and bones keep you moving and vibrant.

And now, here are 7 tips to keep you moving with ease.

1. Yoga

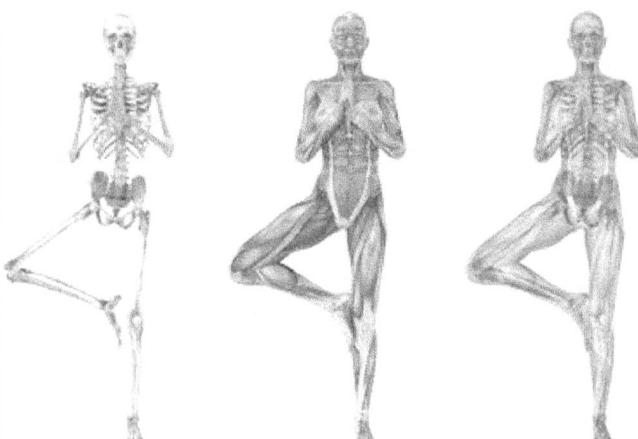

Yoga is phenomenal for supporting the health of muscles, bones and connective tissues. Through different asanas or poses, yoga helps to gently stretch muscles and connective tissue, resulting in more flexibility.

It helps to build your bones and promote bone flexibility through weight-bearing exercises.

It increases your ability to balance and of course it builds muscles.

Yoga is a lifelong practice that not only benefits the physical body but also supports your mental and emotional body. Yoga relieves stress, induces relaxation and strongly supports the nervous system.

There are many types and styles of yoga out there. If you are starting yoga look for a beginning yoga class but also shop around to find a teacher and style that suits you. I especially like and recommend yoga instructions that integrate your core strength and breath into your yoga practice.

2. Move YourSelf!

Muscular System Response to Long Term Exercise

- Increased number of **Mitochondria** and **Myoglobin** stores
  - Myoglobin is a site for oxygen storage in the muscle
  - Mitochondria produce energy as glucose combines with O_2 to produce ATP
- Increased **Muscle Strength**
  - This is a response to muscles being used more than they are used to – they are overloaded. Overloading can be done by increasing resistance (weight).

Exercise, when done properly, can offer many of the same benefits as yoga.

I believe exercise is a key aspect of health and there is no substitute for it!

I work with many people to get them started on an exercise program.

It's amazing to me how many people think they hate exercise because it doesn't feel good or because they don't have enough time. If you've had these same excuses I've got great news for you.

Moving YourSelf should feel good … It's The MOTION OF LIFE!

And long gone are the days when we think that proper exercise is an hour of time spent on the elliptical machine at the gym.

Functional exercise is an emerging field of exercise that promotes strength training using functional movement and body weight. Workouts are often 20 minutes or less. High intensity interval training is a type of exercise that has been proven to be incredibly more effective at building cardiovascular endurance than regular low intensity aerobic exercise.

Long Term Effects of Exercise on the Energy Systems

- At cellular level muscles need what to contract? **ATP**
- What adaptations may occur at cellular level ?
  Increase in level of enzymes for aerobic and anaerobic systems.
  Increase in size of mitochondria.
- Increased use of fat as an energy source
- Fat combustion powers almost all exercise at 25% of aerobic power.
- Fat oxidation increases if exercise extends to long periods as glycogen depletes
- Trained athletes burn more fat as fuel than non-trained athletes.

3. Warm up, cool down, and stretch correctly

Never stretch "cold muscles". I see this all the time in people preparing to engage in exercise. The first thing they do is stretch their muscles by holding a pose for 20 - 30 second. *This is a great way to get an injury!*

Instead, learn the principles of dynamic stretching. Your body is first warmed up aerobically, then stretching is done while moving at the same time. Studies repeatedly show that dynamic stretching better prepares the body for exercise and increases both strength and flexibility.

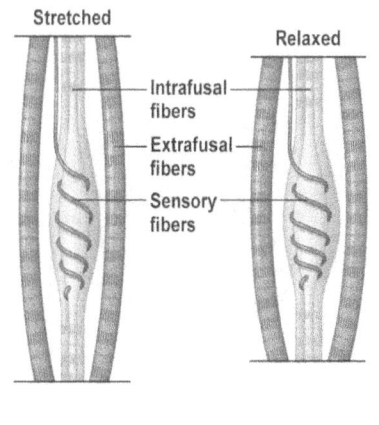
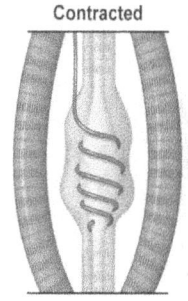

Static stretching, when you stretch and hold the pose for 20 - 30 seconds can prevent injuries and support the health of the muscles, if it is done *after* your exercise, not before!

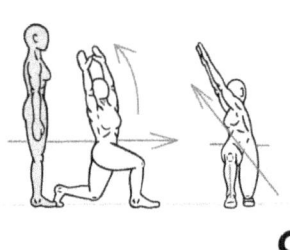

Examples of DYNAMIC STRETCHES

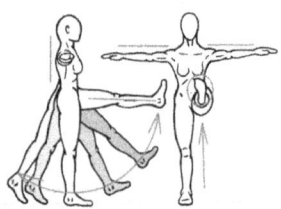
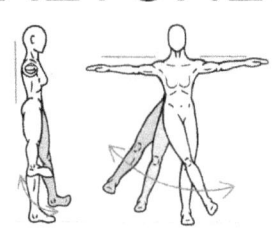
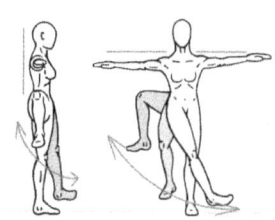

What Exactly Happens When a Muscle Stretch Is Performed?

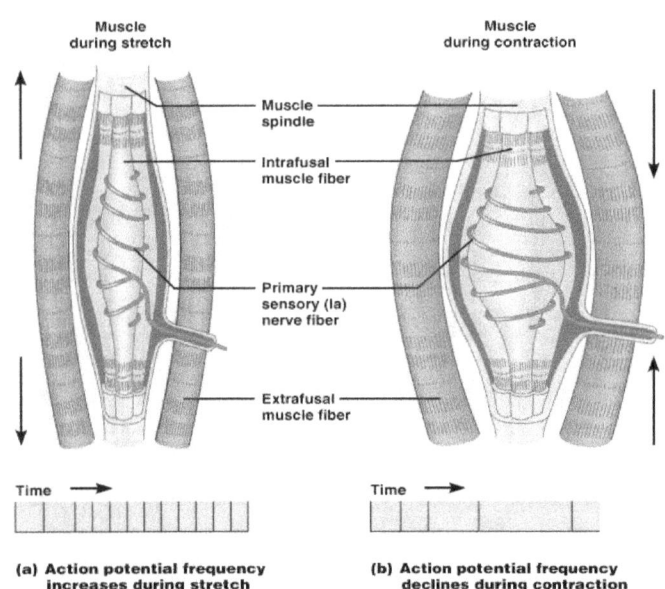

When a muscle is contracted, the thick filaments start pulling the thin ones to the center of the sarcomeres, which is actually the basic unit of contraction.

An overlap between the thick and thin myofilaments is initiated, becoming bigger as the stretch is developing; when the sarcomeres stretch, the overlap area diminishes and the muscle fibers elongate.

When every sarcomere is completely extended, the muscle fibers have reached the largest degree of their resting length as well, so extra tension is all directed on the adjoining connective tissue.

Maximizing the tension forces the collagen fibers in the connective tissue to be lined up with the tension. At the same moment the disarranged muscle fibers straighten up in the line of the tension, and that is absolutely vital for your tissue's restoration (especially after a strenuous work-out).

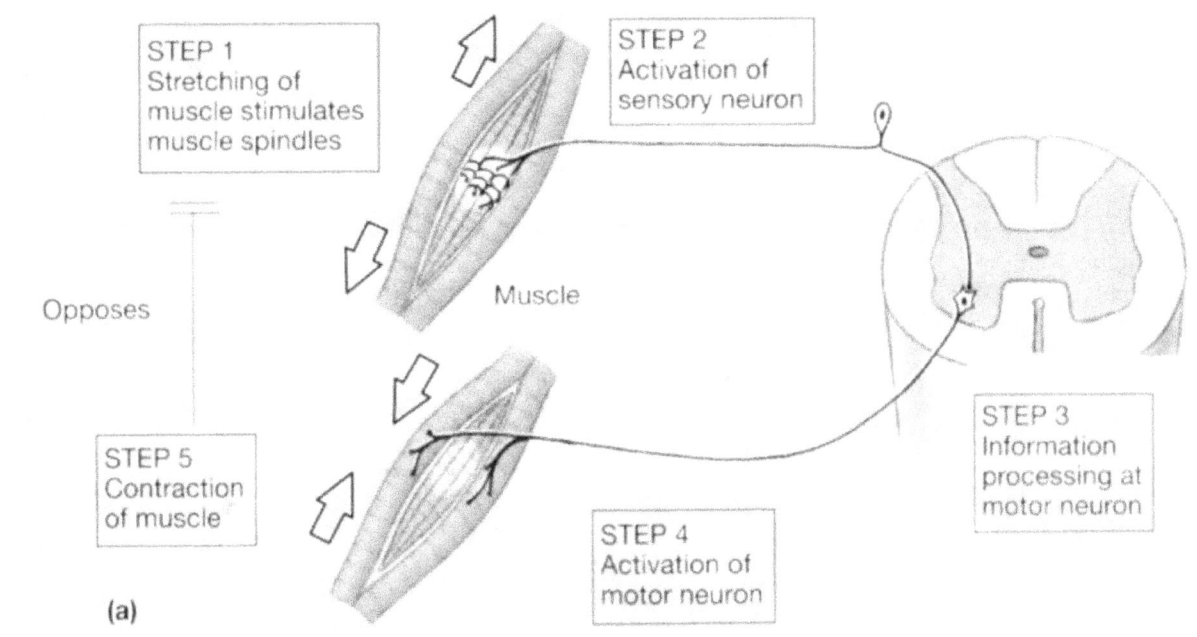

4. Structural Integration

Structural integration is a specialized type of massage. It is very effective at addressing both chronic and acute pain. Practitioners use body posture and sometimes muscle length testing to determine the root cause of problems for individuals.

Sessions are generally focused on one area (rather than the standard whole-body massage of a spa massage) and practitioners often have advanced training in how to address particular pain patterns in the body.

If you have any type of chronic pain then I highly recommend finding a practitioner of Structural Integration that can adequately help you to realign your Body..

5. Herbs for a Healthy Musculoskeletal System

Many different herbs can be used to support the musculoskeletal system.

Turmeric has long been called the herbs of the yogis and is used to increase flexibility. It is strongly anti-inflammatory and can be used to reduce overall inflammation in the body, thus relieving both chronic and acute pain.

Gotu kola is an herb that has a special affinity for the connective tissue. Bones and cartilage can benefit from mineral-rich herbs and decoctions such as nettle leaf, bone broth soup, seaweeds, burdock root and dandelion root.

Three Powerful Herbs for a Healthy Musculoskeletal System

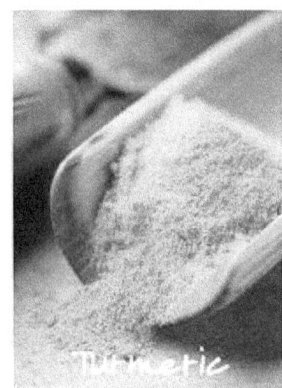
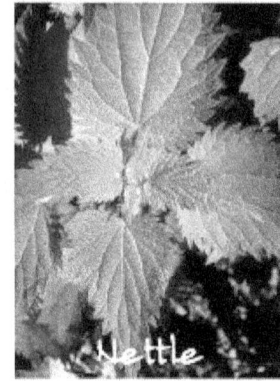
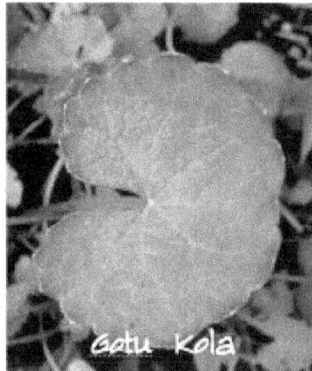

Turmeric   Nettle   Gotu Kola

6. Nutrients for a Healthy Musculoskeletal System

Many nutrients are needed to keep the musculoskeletal system healthy. Here are 3 especially beneficial nutrients for your musculoskeletal system that many people are found to be deficient in.

Vitamin D3 …. Vitamin D3 is essential for the health of your bones. Low vitamin D3 levels puts women at an increased risk for osteoporosis. Also research has shown that women with osteoporosis need higher levels of vitamin D3 than is currently recommended.

Magnesium …. Magnesium performs over 300 different actions in the body, including supporting your nervous system, bone health and muscle health. An estimated 80 - 90% of people in the United States are deficient in magnesium. In a perfect world magnesium can be found in green leafy vegetables; however, much of our soil has become deficient in magnesium and if it isn't in the soil it's not in the food! B y Growing your Own Food you can create magnesium DENSE soil that creates a Harvest of Magnesium DENSE foods. Unfortunately, many people find that supplementation is necessary.

Calcium (found in foods, not pills!) …. Calcium is undoubtedly important for musculoskeletal health. The best way to get calcium is through food such as dairy products, leafy green veggies or even stinging nettle infusions. Calcium, taken in supplement form has been repeatedly linked to cardiovascular disease so I never recommend calcium supplements. Food is definitely best in this case!

RICE VERSUS MEAT

The RICE treatment leads to incomplete healing of soft tissue whereas MEAT encourages complete healing.

Modality	Result	Modality	Result
Rest	Decreased joint nutrition	**M**ovement	Increased joint nutrition
Ice	Decreased blood flow	**E**xercise	Increased blood flow
Compression	Decreased pain control	**A**nalgesic	Increased pain control
Elevation	Incomplete healing	**T**reatment	Complete healing

7. Warmth and Blood-Moving Herbs for Injuries (DO NOT USE ICE!)

When an injury happens such as a sprain or strain many people's first reaction is to put ice on the injury. This is an antiquated practice that does more harm than good in the long term.

Move over, R.I.C.E. and make way for M.E.A.T.
Rest, Ice, Compression and Elevate used to be the gold standard in all musculoskeletal injury treatment. The main goal of this method is to reduce the rate of swelling. However, these actions have been shown to actually slow down the rate of overall healing, especially for injuries to the ligaments and tendons.

RICE VS MEAT

	RICE	MEAT
Immune System Response	Decreased	Increased
Blood Flow to Injured Area	Decreased	Increased
Collagen Formation	Hindered	Encouraged
Speed of Recovery	Delayed (lengthened)	Hastened (shortened)
Range of Motion of Joint	Decreased	Increased
Complete Healing	Decreased	Increased

RICE Versus MEAT
The RICE protocol hampers soft tissue healing, whereas MEAT encourages healing.

Healing after an acute injury is dependent on blood supply to the area. Ice stops the flow of blood to the area, thus impeding healing. You can read all about why icing a tendon or ligament injury is detrimental to the healing process here.

Movement, Exercise, Analgesics and Treatments (M.E.A.T.)

Moving the area, using gentle exercises, using pain relief besides anti-inflammatories, and treatments such as massage, myofascial release and physical therapy are far more beneficial to tendon and ligament injuries.

With their long traditions of martial arts, Traditional Chinese Medicine has very advanced methods of treating acute injuries. This generally includes applying heat to the area as well as herbs that "move the blood". Instead of congealing the fluids around the injury, the fluids which contain the ability to heal and repair tissues are encourage to move in and out of the place of injury.

MEAT method is better

- Movement
- Exercise
- Analgesics medication NOT Brufen but Enzymes like Papaya (Chymoral)
- Treatment is the best way to heal torn ligaments and tendons.(Surgical / rehabilitation / brace)

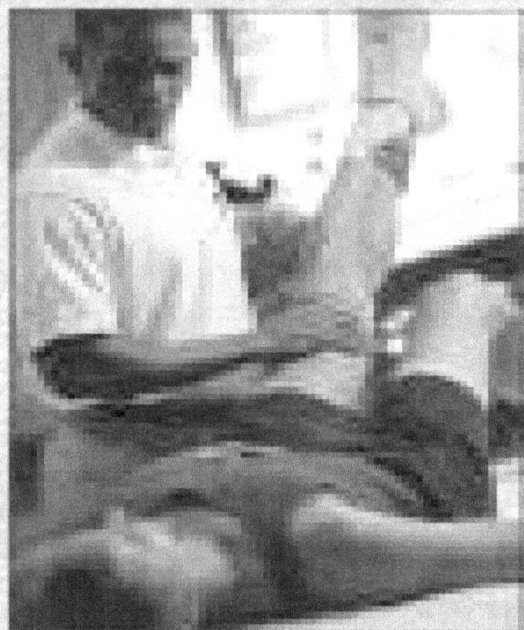

You can maintain and improve your musculoskeletal health by moving appropriately and by getting the right nutrients and supportive herbs in your body.

A lot has changed in the world of fitness in the past decade or so. Many practices like static stretching and icing all injuries have been shown to have long term negative effects.

New principles such as dynamic stretching, M.E.A.T. and traditional food-based nutrition are pointing the way for you to have a healthier and stronger musculoskeletal system.

Remember, you need your Musculoskeletal system to Successfully Move You into Your Abundant Life!

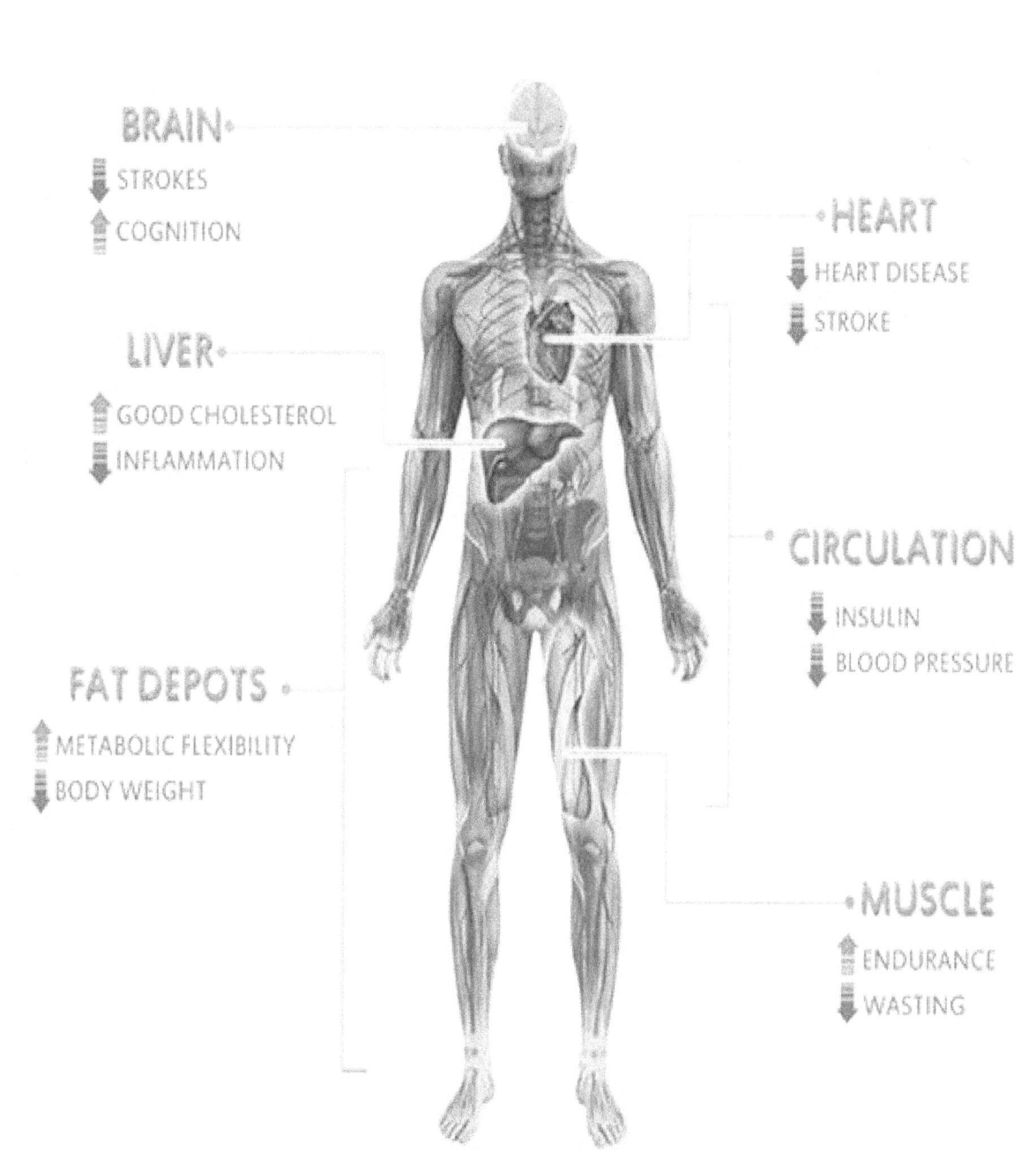

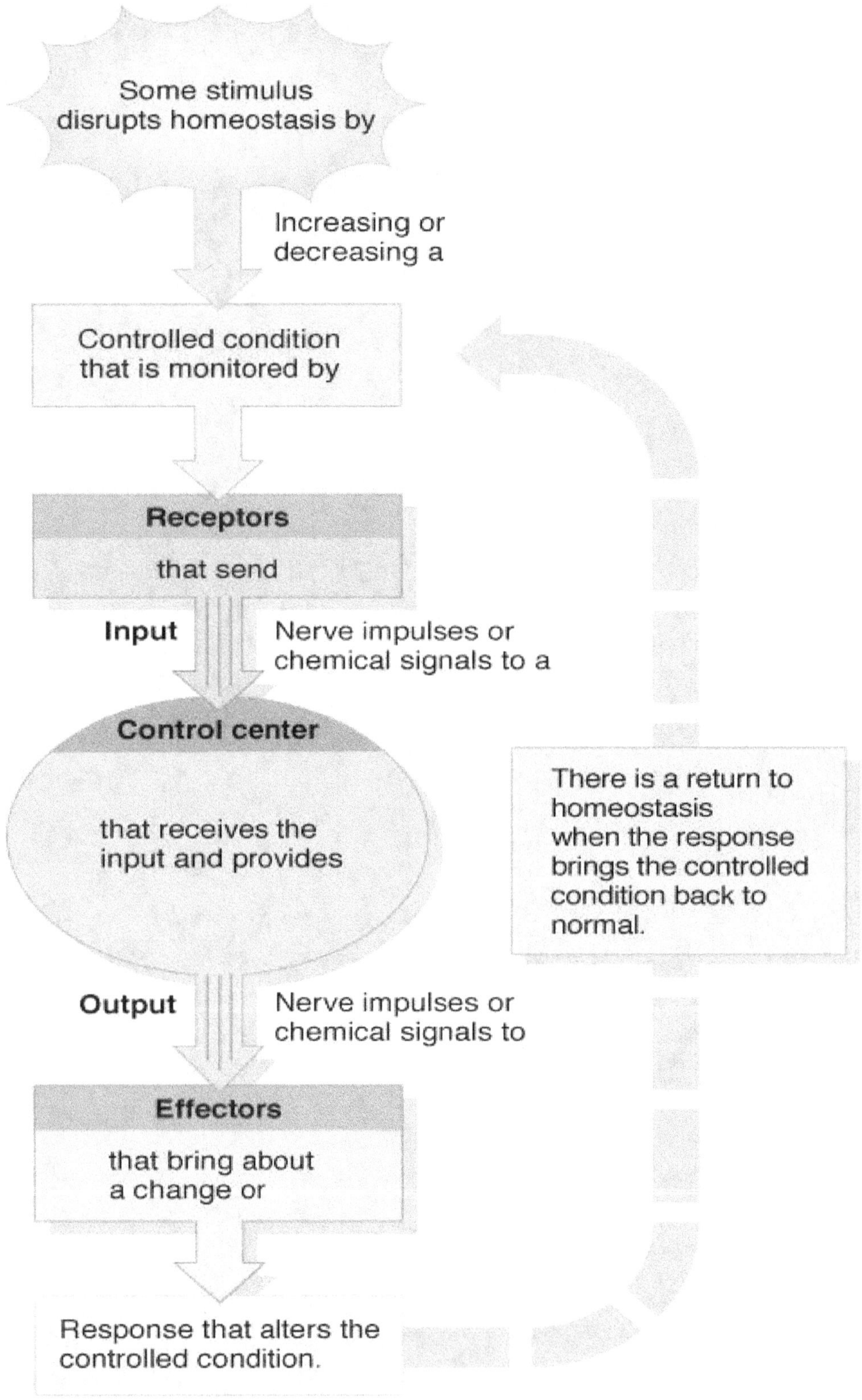

Some stimulus disrupts homeostasis by

Increasing or decreasing a

Controlled condition that is monitored by

Receptors that send

Input — Nerve impulses or chemical signals to a

Control center that receives the input and provides

Output — Nerve impulses or chemical signals to

Effectors that bring about a change or

Response that alters the controlled condition.

There is a return to homeostasis when the response brings the controlled condition back to normal.

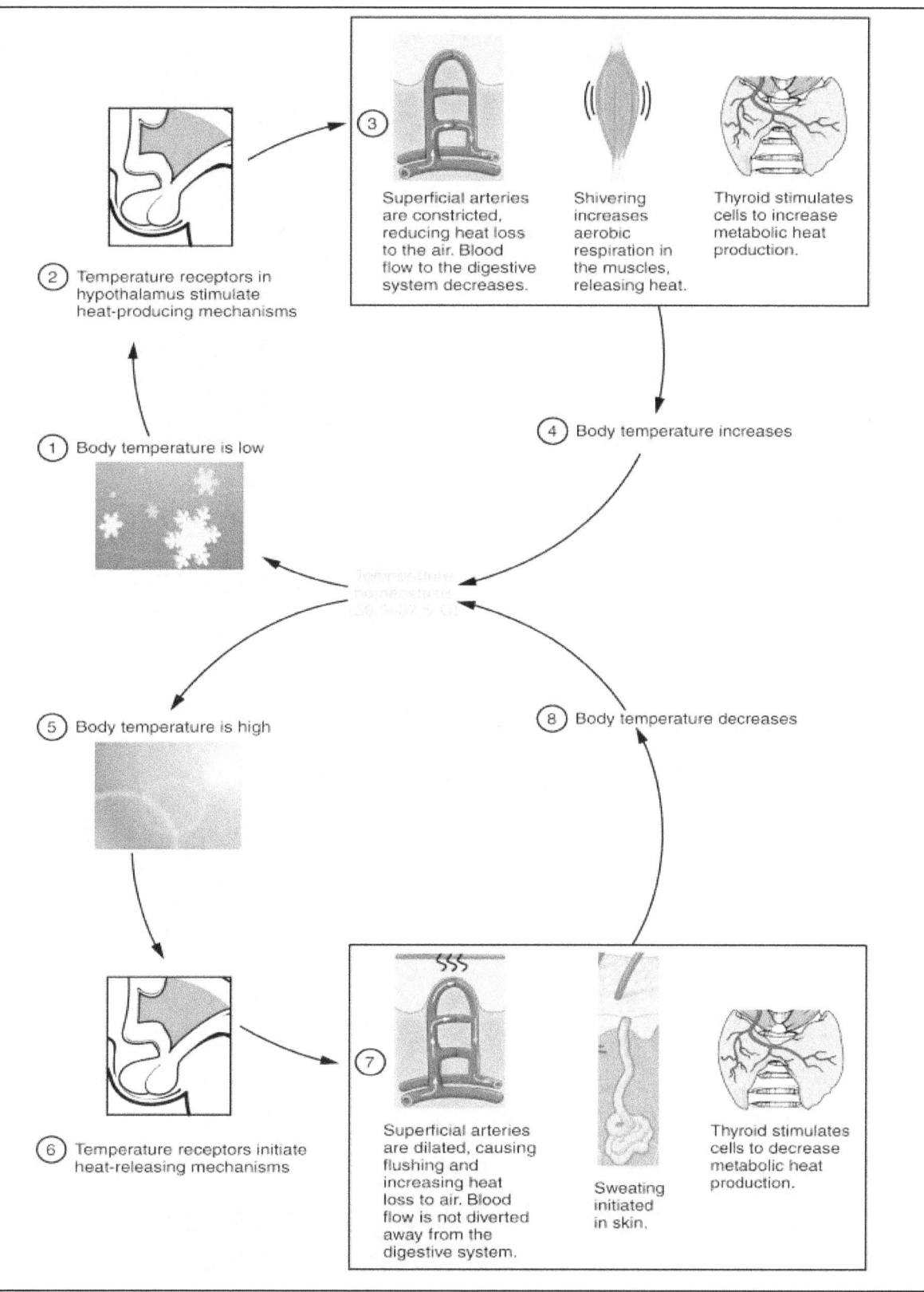

Move Something!

Chapter Thirteen

Regulating Your Body Temperature

*****

Under resting conditions, your body's core temperature is **98.6 *F / 37 °C**, and your heat production and heat loss are balanced. Mechanisms of your heat production include your basal metabolic rate, shivering, work and exercise.

During exercise, your mechanical efficiency is about **20% or less**, which means that **80% or more** of your energy production (VO$_2$) is converted to body **heat**.

For an example, if you are working on a cycle ergometer at a rate requiring a VO$_2$ of **2.0 L · min^{-1}**, your energy production is about **10 kcal · min^{-1}**.

At **20%** efficiency there is **2 kcal · min^{-1}** that is used to do work and **8 kcal · min^{-1}** are converted to heat.

If most of this added heat is not lost, core temperature might quickly rise to dangerous levels.

Now let's explore HOW your body loses excess heat.

Heat-Loss Mechanisms

Your body loses heat by four processes.

In **radiation,** heat is transferred from the surface of one object to the surface of another, with no physical contact between the different objects. Heat loss depends on the temperature gradient, which represents the temperature difference between the surfaces of the different objects.

Four mechanisms of heat transfer are relevant to biological systems
- **Radiation** = By electromagnetic radiation
- **Conduction** = Directly between two objects
- **Convection** = By the movement of a gas or liquid
- **Evaporation** = Conversion of water to gas

Physics of Heat Loss from the Body

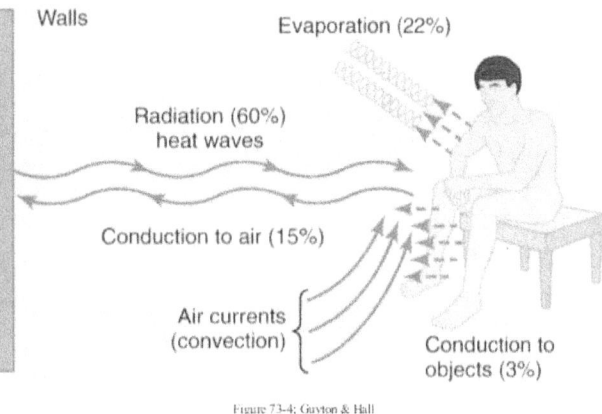

Mechanisms of heat loss from the body

For an example, if you are in a seated position, at-rest and in a comfortable environment (21-22 °C), approximately **60%** of your body heat is lost through radiation to cooler objects around you.

Conduction is the transfer of heat from one object to another by direct contact, and similar to radiation, it depends on a temperature gradient.

For an example, if you are sitting on a cold marble bench, you lose body heat by conduction.

Convection is a special case of conduction in which heat is transferred to air (or water) molecules, which become lighter and rise away from the body to be replaced by cold air (or water).

Heat loss can be enhanced by increasing the movement of the air (or water) over the surface of your body.

For an example, a fan stimulates heat loss by placing more cold air molecules into contact with the skin.

Similarly, if a fan were to place more hot air (warmer than your skin temperature) into contact with your skin, then you would gain heat. Heat gained from your environment adds to that generated by exercise and puts an additional strain on your heat-loss mechanisms.

The fourth heat-loss mechanism is the **Evaporation** of your sweat.

Sweating is the process of producing a watery solution over the surface of your body and **Evaporation** is a process in which liquid water converts to a gas.

This conversion requires about **580 kcal** of heat per liter of sweat to be evaporated. The heat for this comes from your body and this action cools your body.

In the state of At-rest, about **25%** of your heat loss is caused by **evaporation**, but during exercise evaporation becomes the primary mechanism for your heat loss.

Evaporation depends on the **water vapor pressure gradient** between your skin and the air and does not directly depend on temperature.

The water vapor pressure of the air relates to the **relative humidity** and the **saturation pressure** at that air temperature.

For an example, the relative humidity can be 90% in winter, but because the saturation pressure of cold air is low, the water vapor pressure of the air is also low, and you can see water vapor rising from your body following exercise.

Now in warm temperatures, the relative humidity is a good indicator of the water vapor pressure of the air.

If the water vapor pressure of the air is too high, your sweat will not evaporate, and sweat that does not evaporate does not allow your body to be cooled.

All of these heat-loss mechanisms can be **heat-gain mechanisms** as well.

You **gain** heat from the Sun by **radiation** across 93 million miles of space and you also gain heat by conduction if you sit on hot sand at the beach.

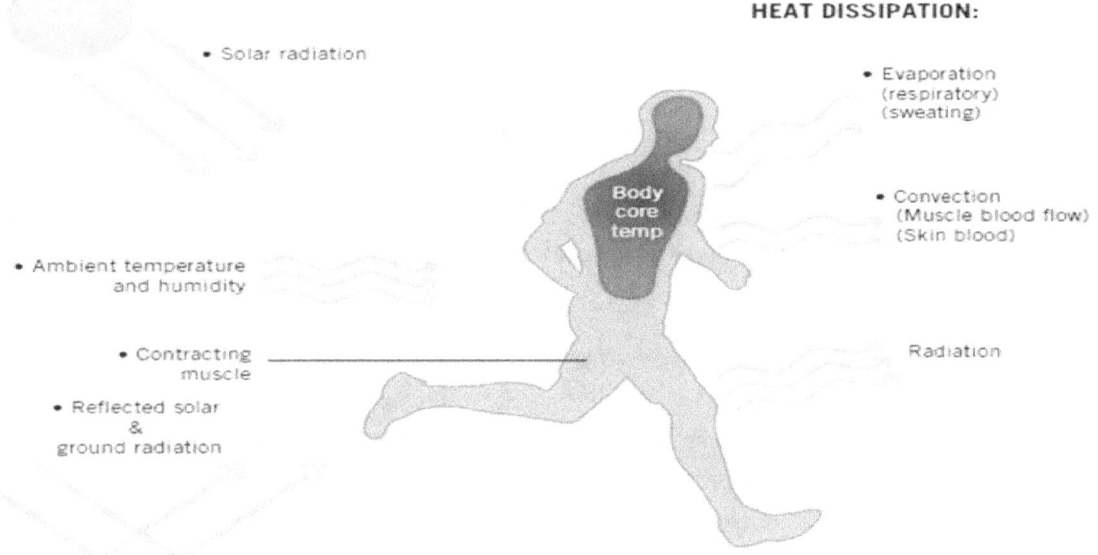

Your Body Temperature Response to Exercise

During exercise in a comfortable environment, your core temperature increases proportionally to the relative intensity (%VO_2max) of the exercise and then levels off.

The gain in your body heat that occurs early in exercise triggers the heat-loss mechanisms discussed in the preceding section. After **10 to 20 minutes**, your heat loss equals heat production and your core temperature remains steady.

Now let's look at your most important heat-loss mechanisms during exercise

Heat Exchange Mechanisms During Exercise

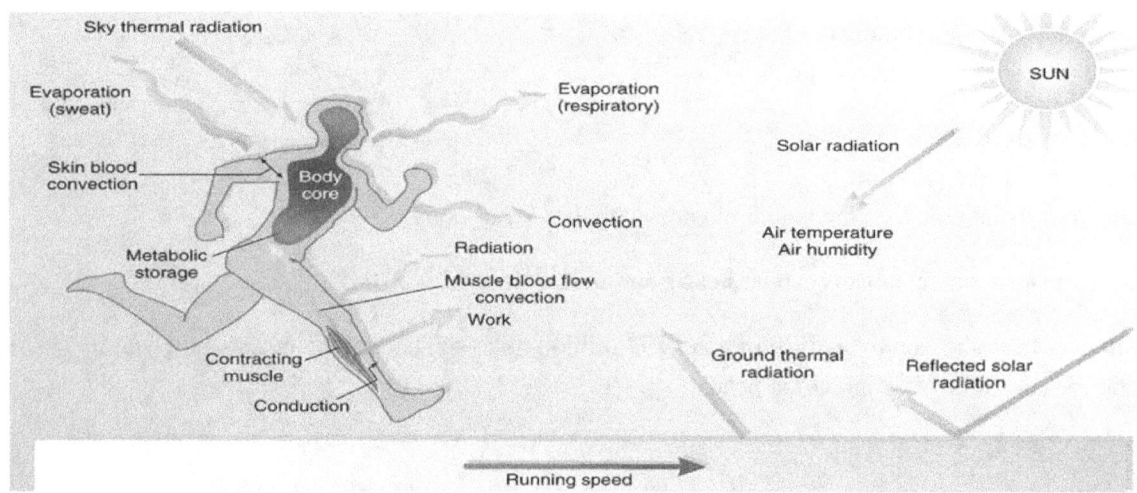

Heat Loss During Exercise

Your **Exercise intensity** and the surrounding **environmental temperature** influence which heat-loss mechanism is primarily responsible for maintaining a steady core temperature for your body during exercise.

If you participate in a progressively difficult exercise in an environment that allows heat loss by all four mechanisms, the contribution that convection and radiation make to your overall heat loss is modest. Because the temperature gradient between your skin and the room does not change much during exercise, the rate of your heat loss is relatively constant. To compensate for this, evaporation picks up when your heat losses by convection and radiation plateau, and evaporation is responsible for most of your heat loss in heavy exercise.

If you perform a steady-state exercise in a warmer environment, the role that evaporation plays now becomes even more important. The gradient for heat loss by convection and radiation decreases, and the rate of your heat loss by these processes also decreases. As a result, evaporation must compensate to maintain your core temperature.

In strenuous exercise or hot environments, evaporation is the most important process for losing heat and maintaining your body temperature in a safe range. It should be no surprise, then, that factors affecting your **sweat production** (such as dehydration) or **sweat evaporation** (such as impermeable clothing) are causes for concern.

Training in a hot and humid environment for as few as 7 to 12 days results in specific adaptations that improve your heat tolerance and, as a result, lowers your body temperature during submaximal exercise.

Adaptations that improve your heat tolerance the following:

- Increase in plasma volume

- Earlier onset of sweating

- Higher sweat rate

- Reduced salt loss through sweat

- Reduced blood flow to the skin

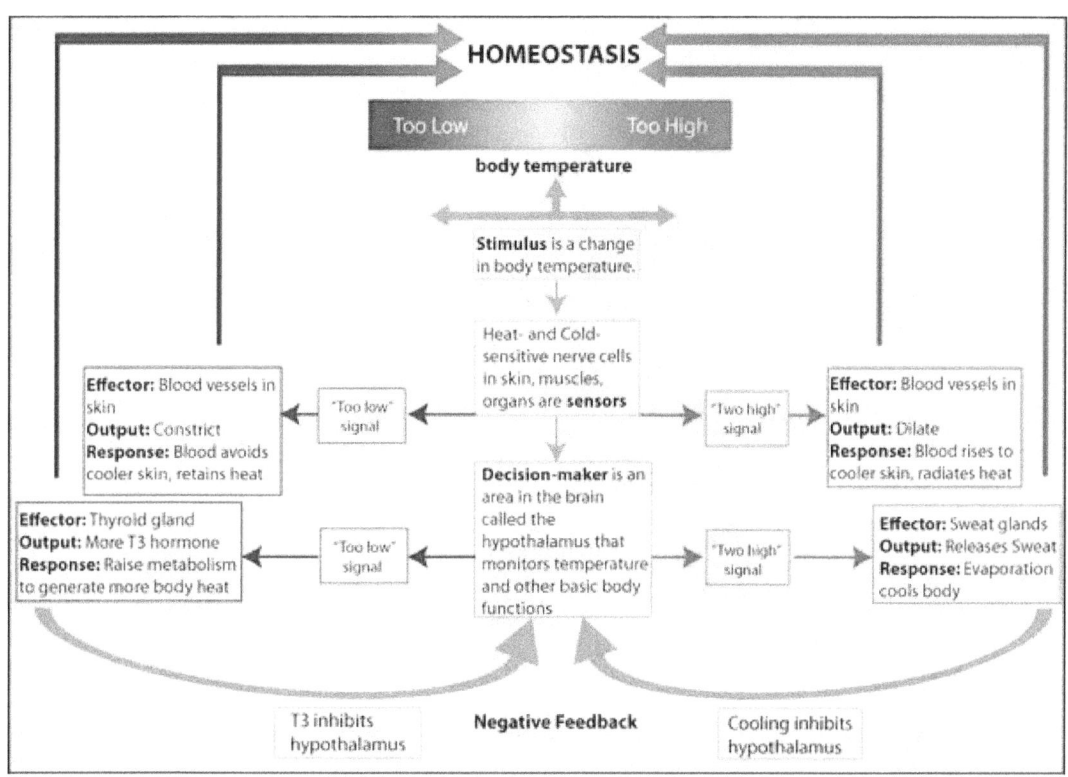

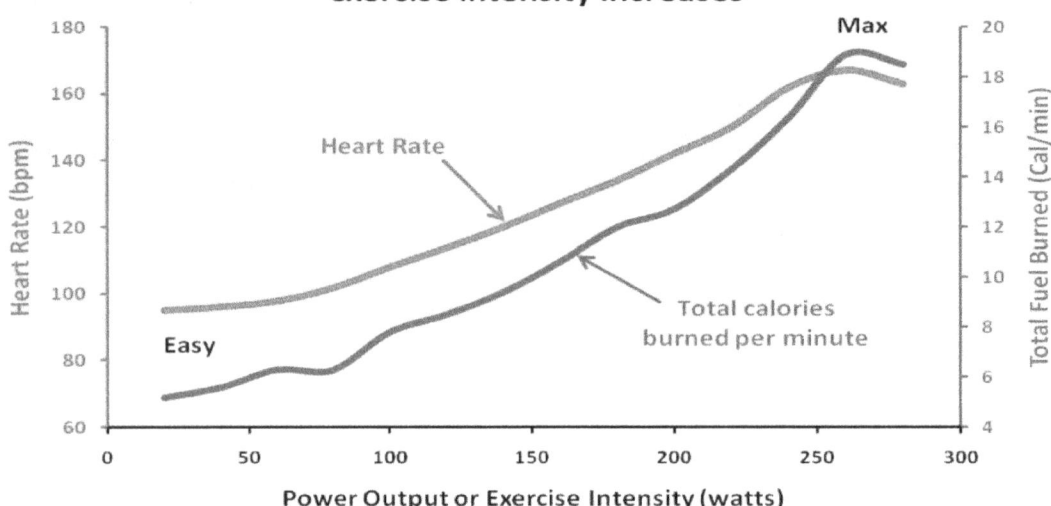

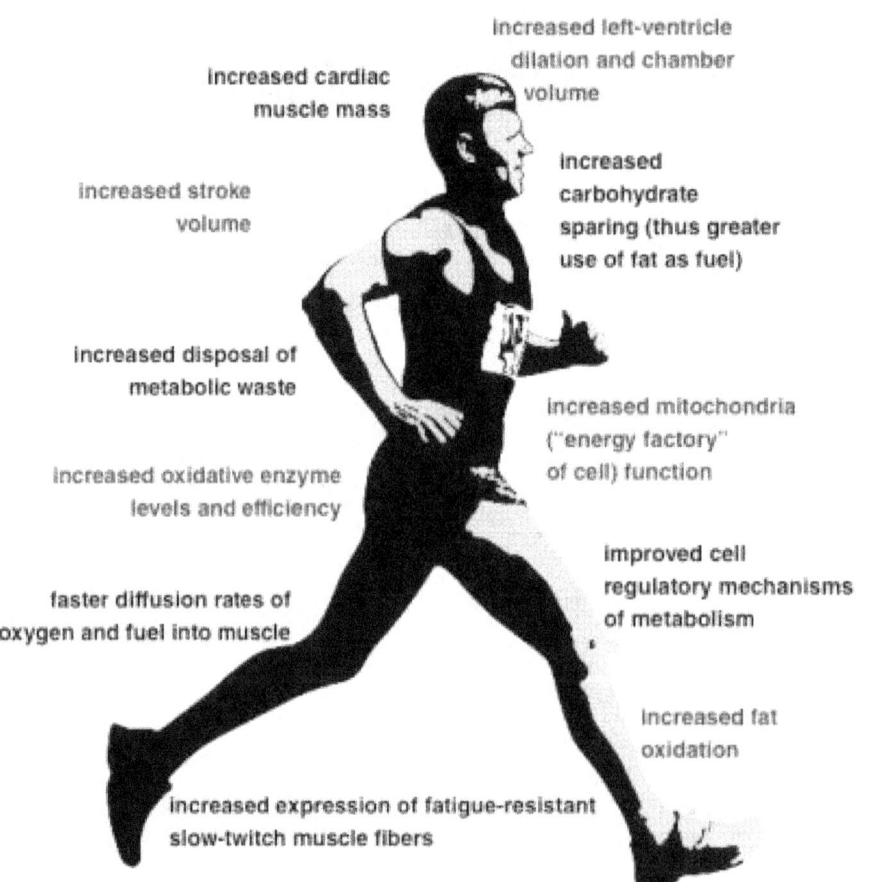

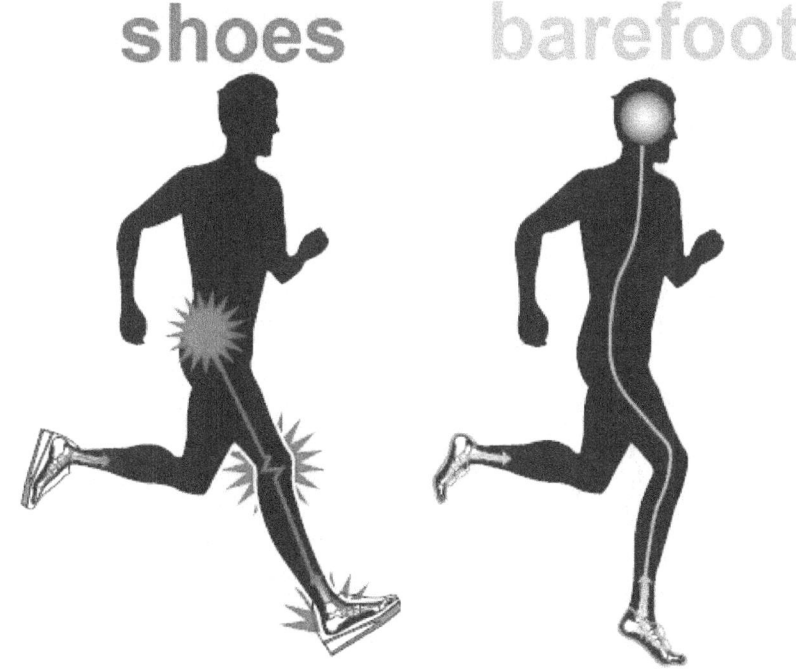

AEROBIC EXERCISE

-CARDIORESPIRATORY ENDURANCE ACTIVITIES OFTEN ARE CALLED AEROBIC EXERCISES

-ONLY AEROBIC ACTIVITIES WILL INCREASE CARDIORESPIRATORY ENDURANCE

-EXAMPLES: WALKING, JOGGING, CYCLING, ETC.

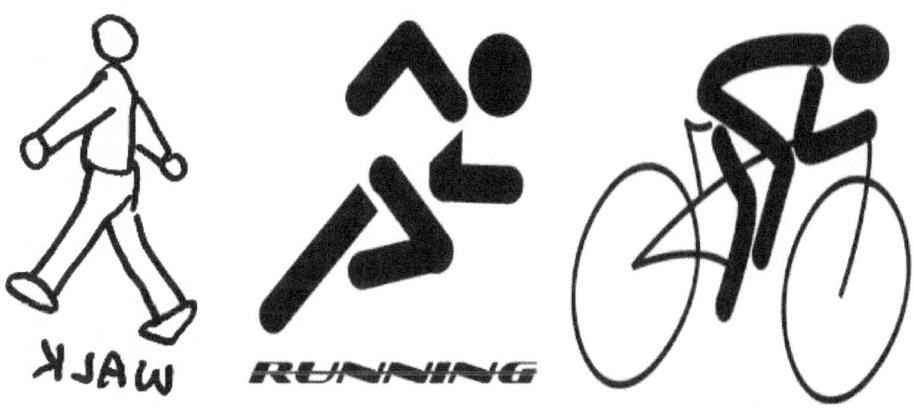

Warm Up/ Cool Downs

- Essential to every workout
- Introduce proper stretching techniques
- Targeted muscle
- Hold 10-15 seconds
- Bouncing motion is damaging to muscle

Warm Ups
- Increase heart rate and blood flow to the muscles
- Light stretching
- 10-15 minutes
- Gets body ready for exercise and reduces chances of injury

Cool Downs
- Decrease intensity in exercise gradually
- Stretch in order to minimize injuries and soreness
- Hydrate
- Lasts approx. 10 mins

WALKING → RUNNING

Fits easily in your daily routine.

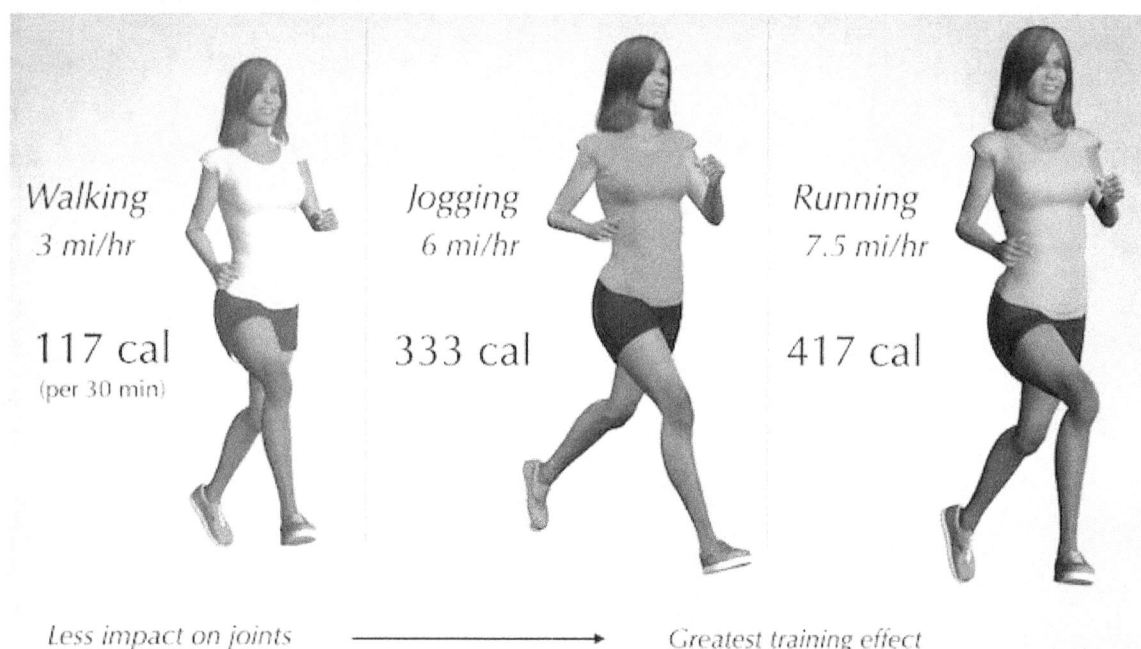

Walking
3 mi/hr
117 cal
(per 30 min)

Jogging
6 mi/hr
333 cal

Running
7.5 mi/hr
417 cal

Less impact on joints → *Greatest training effect*

Comparison of energy sources used during short-duration exercise and prolonged-duration exercise.

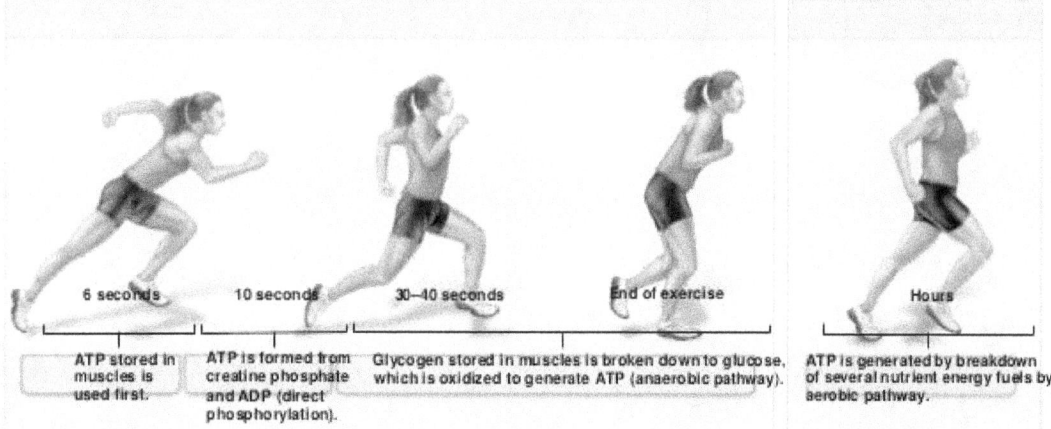

Short-duration exercise | **Prolonged-duration exercise**

- 6 seconds — ATP stored in muscles is used first.
- 10 seconds — ATP is formed from creatine phosphate and ADP (direct phosphorylation).
- 30–40 seconds — Glycogen stored in muscles is broken down to glucose, which is oxidized to generate ATP (anaerobic pathway).
- End of exercise
- Hours — ATP is generated by breakdown of several nutrient energy fuels by aerobic pathway.

Move Something! ...

Chapter Fourteen

Move Some Thing Activities

*****

Now the FUN begins as we discuss some of the best Low-Impact and High-Reward cardio to Build and maintain your Supreme Health and Fitness. The following are some of the exercises with many Benefits that range from Respiratory health, weight management/loss), energy for healing, or Building your God-Body.

Cardio exercises can simply be defined as the physical workouts that increase the rate of your heartbeat. Though it is a universal truth that our bodies are born to always move, but unfortunately, most don't give a damn to this fact and love to be in the idle mode – infected with the ***Sitting Disease***!

In lack of physical movement, we often witness decay in the strength of our muscles and the collection of extra fat accumulated around our waist.

Cardio is good to go if you just want to stay extremely fit without lifting the heavy weights in the gym.

When you apply cardio with the science of Eating To Live, it creates the environment for your Healing, the condition for you to become Healthy, as well as lays the foundation for your Fountain Of YOUTH!

Body fat is highly stubborn and if you have excess fat, you need to adopt the best methods of cardiovascular activities to get rid of it.

	Low Impact	Upper Body	Lower Body	Core	Full Range of Motion
Rowing Machine	✓✓✓	✓✓✓	✓✓✓	✓✓✓	✓✓✓
Treadmill	✓		✓✓✓	✓	✓✓
Upright Bike	✓✓✓	✓	✓✓✓	✓	✓✓✓
Recumbent Bike	✓✓✓		✓✓✓		✓
Elliptical	✓✓✓	✓	✓✓✓	✓✓	✓✓
Stair Stepper	✓✓		✓✓✓	✓	✓
Swimming	✓✓✓	✓✓	✓✓✓	✓	✓✓

Now we are going to discuss the top most cardio workouts for your Achieving and Maintaining your Supreme Health and Wellness.

Understanding Precautions, Proper Techniques and Safety

While walking, you should remember to always keep at least one foot on the ground at all times. In jogging and running, more muscular force is exerted to propel your body completely off the ground, creating a nonsupport phase.

The distinction between jogging and running is not as clearly defined. Some people view speed as being the difference, but no single criterion for speed is commonly accepted. Others have come to distinguish between the two by the intent of the participant—a jogger is simply interested in exercise, whereas a runner trains to achieve performance goals in road races.

WITH SHOES   **BAREFOOT**

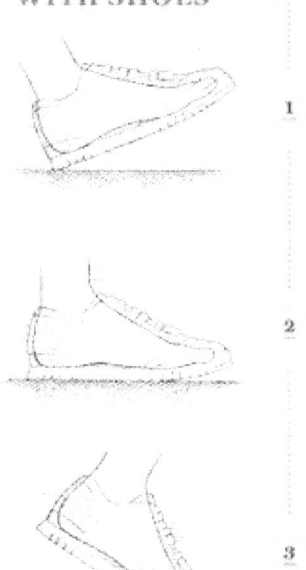
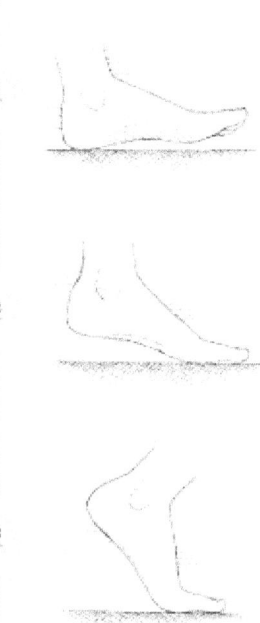

Padded heels encourage a hard landing—which New Yorkers exacerbate by walking with long, hurried strides.

A thick sole keeps your foot from rolling through the step. This flat-footed plodding is sometimes referred to as "cow-walking."

An inflexible shoe prevents your toes from fully pushing off—so your legs have to work to lift your feet up and down.

Shorter strides allow you to land softly on your heel with your knees slightly bent—i.e., how you might walk on a beach.

A natural step rolls through the outside edge of the foot, before the ball lands—and spreads slightly—on the ground.

Your toes are designed to give you a powerful push forward—sending you striding smoothly into the next step.

Your General Safety

Safety is an important consideration for all participants, independent of the activity they choose to do. In this context, there are a variety of safety factors common to both walking and jogging that we will explore before we discuss how to institute walking and jogging programs.

Your Footwear

Any comfortable pair of well-supported shoes can be worn for a beginning walking program. Serious walkers and all joggers should invest in appropriate shoes with well-padded heels that are higher than the soles and have fitted heel cups.

The shoes you wear should be flexible enough to bend easily. The same kind of socks that will be worn while exercising should be worn during the shoe fitting to ensure a proper fit.

Only the serious competitive runner needs racing shoes, which are a lighter weight and offer less cushioning.

Your Clothing

The weather conditions and your level of activity intensity determine the clothing that you should choose to wear. Warm weather dictates light, preferably cotton, loose-fitting clothing.

Nothing should be worn that prevents your perspiration from reaching the outside air. A brimmed hat should cover your head on hot, sunny days.

In cold weather, you should dress in layers so you can easily can remove or add clothing when necessary. Wool and polypropylene fabrics are good choices for extreme cold, but most joggers tend to overdress. A hat, preferably a wool stocking cap that can be pulled down over your forehead and ears, and gloves or mittens also should be worn. Cotton socks worn as mittens are useful not only to keep hands warm but also to act as wipers for the sniffling nose that often accompanies cold-weather walking and jogging.

Surface

The surface is not as crucial for walkers as it is for joggers, although some walkers (especially those with orthopedic problems) should exercise on a soft surface such as grass or a running track with a shock-absorbent surface. Many people prefer exercising off the track for visual stimulation and interest, but regular jogging on hard surfaces such as concrete or blacktop can lead to stress problems in the ankle, knee, and hip joints and in the low back. Joggers need to observe special precautions when running on the road: Jog facing traffic, assume cars at crossroads do not see joggers, and beware of cracks and curbs.

Your Safety Tips

Practice the following tips to ensure safety when walking or jogging:

- Move toward the oncoming traffic.

- Yield the right of way to cars.

- Listen to music only while exercising on a quiet street, and always listen for and be aware of traffic.

- Walk or jog with a partner if you must exercise at night.

Both walkers and joggers should wear supportive, flexible shoes, and they should wear clothing that accommodates weather conditions and exercise intensity.

They should always follow the rules of the road and walk or jog in safe areas at safe times.

Special Considerations

Participants at any fitness level can do and should perform the warm-up and cool-down activities that are associated with most games. Some additional stretching and easy movements in different directions should be included as part of the warm-up for games.

The more vigorous games, however, usually involve high-intensity bursts, stopping, starting, and quickly changing directions. They are not recommended for the **early stages** of a fitness program.

In addition to warm-up and cool-down activities, higher and lower intensities should be alternated to prevent undue fatigue.

You should always exercise at your own pace, and your THR should be checked regularly to ensure that you are within your range.

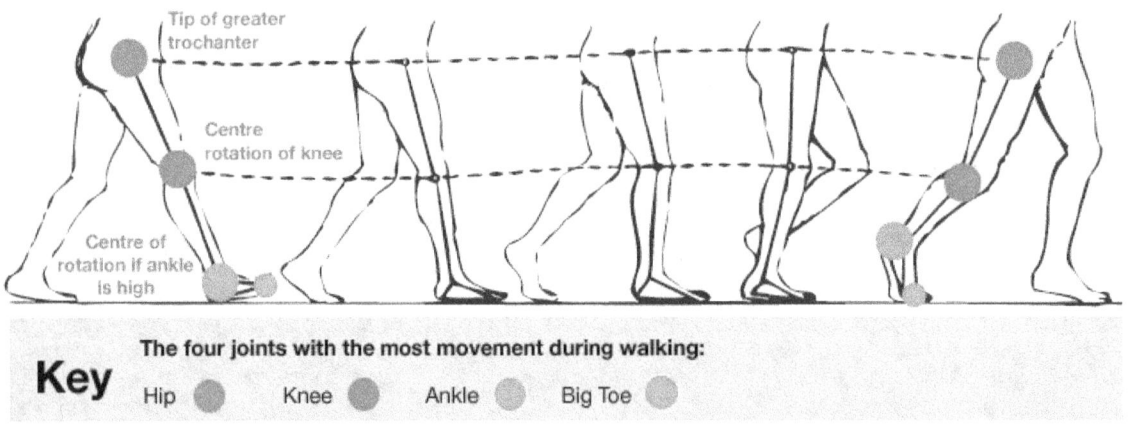

Key — The four joints with the most movement during walking: Hip, Knee, Ankle, Big Toe

Supreme Walking Program – Walk YourSelf into Healing & Your Abundant Life!

Walking is our 1st activity or exercise. The advantages of walking include its convenience, practicality, and naturalness. Walking is an excellent activity, especially for people who are overweight and poorly conditioned and whose joints cannot handle the stresses of jogging. It is the most popular physical activity for adults.

As with all exercise programs, you should begin with a warm-up. You should start your walk with a slow speed and gradually increase to a pace that feels comfortable to you. Your arms should swing freely, and your trunk should be kept erect with a slight backward pelvic tilt. Your feet should point forward at all times.

Your Walking activity can easily progress by simply increasing your distance or your speed. Your 1st Goal is to accomplish the accumulation at least **60 minutes of moderate-intensity physical activity each day.** This is an important milestone and has clear health benefits.

To help achieve this, your 60 minutes can be realized in bouts of 10 min or longer. You should gradually increase the distance you walk until you can easily walk for at least 60 minutes at a moderately brisk pace on a daily basis.

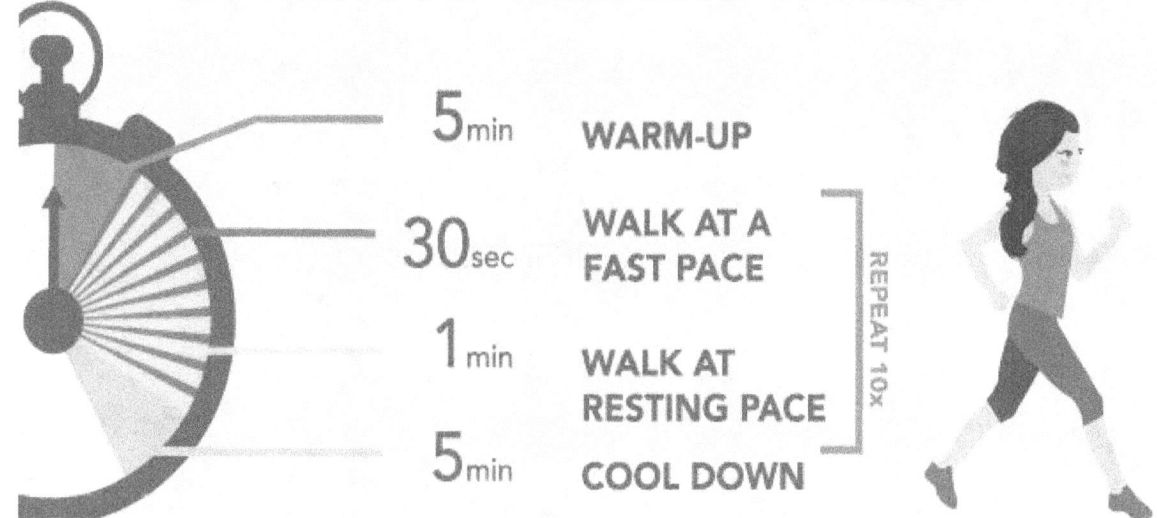

Walking Program Rules:

1. **Start at a level that feels comfortable to you.**

2. **Be aware of new aches or pains.**

3. **Don't progress to the next level if you are not comfortable.**

4. **Monitor and record your Heart Rate.**

5. **Walk at least 5 days $\cdot$ wk^{-1}**

Life is Motion and the 1st Law of the Universe is Motion. Walking is our 1st form of creating Motion.

Life is Energy. There are 2 types of Energy – Potential (Rest/Death) and Kinetic (Motion/Life).

Walking creates the Kinetic Energy of Life that your PaceMaker in your Heart needs, your Cells Need and that causes your Brain to secrete the Endorphins of Growth, Healing and Power!

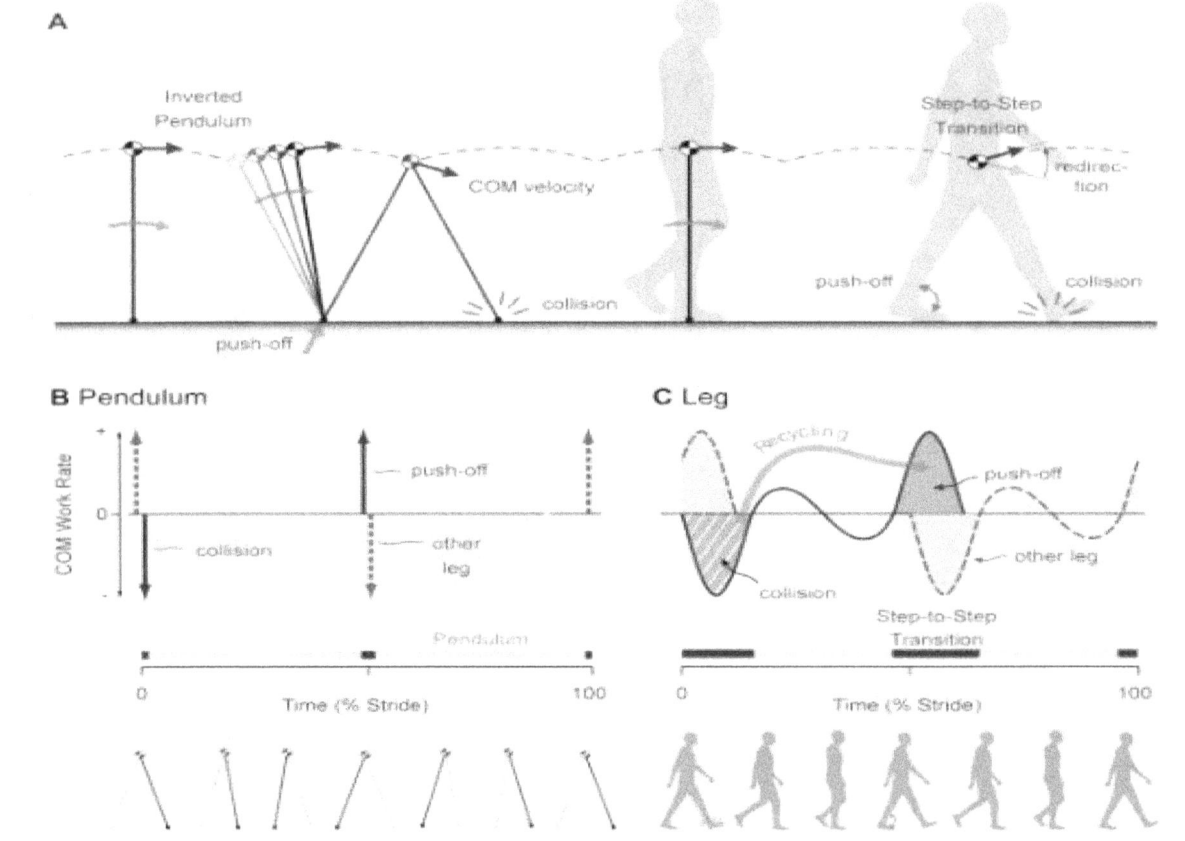

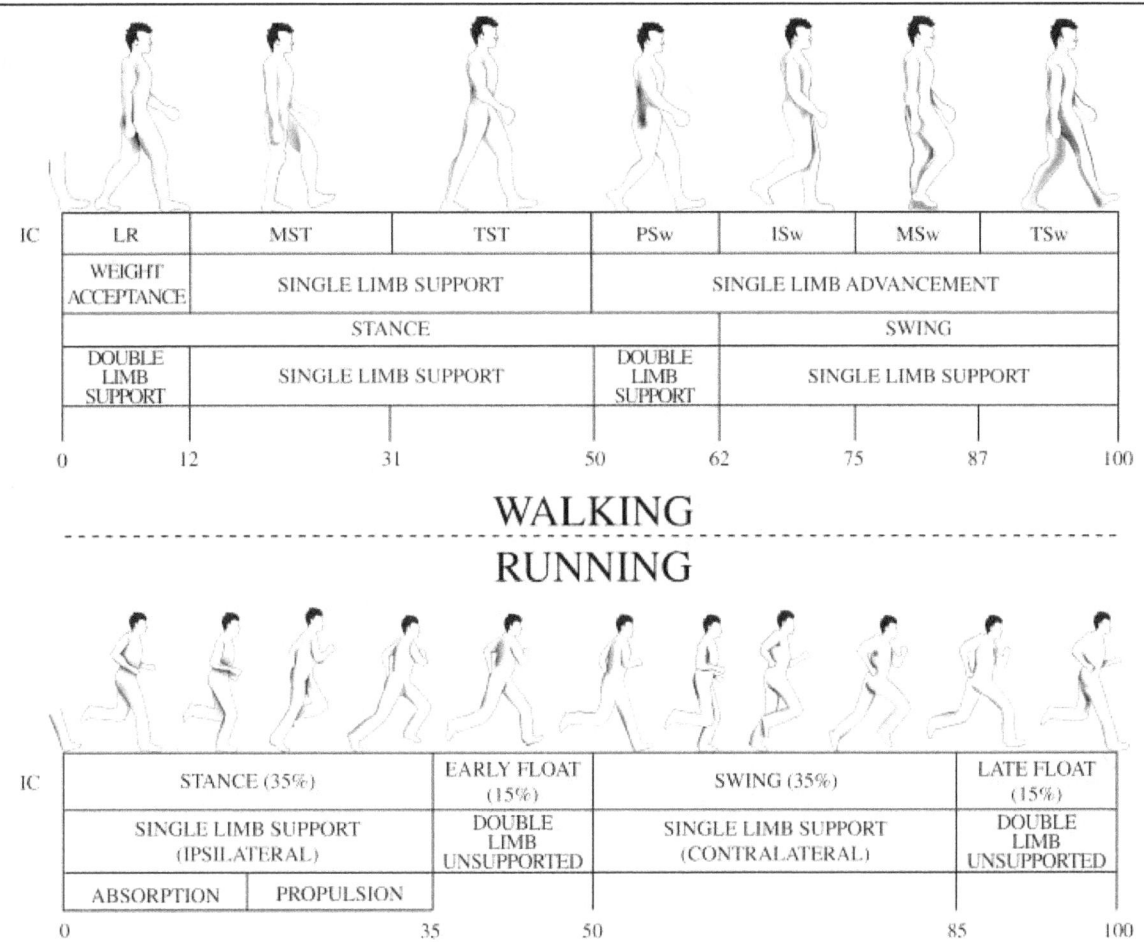

Supreme Jogging Program

No single factor determines when a person can begin jogging. If you are able to walk briskly for 30 min but are still unable to reach your **Target Heart Rate** (THR) range, then you should consider a jogging program for additional improvements in you **Cardio Respiratory Fitness** (CRF) and health. If you can perform moderate walking with a HR that is within your THR zone, then you should increase the distance or speed of walking rather than begin jogging. Also, the ability of your joints to withstand the additional stresses of jogging should be considered.

Remember, walking may be the first and only activity for many people; it is more important to stay active doing what they like than move to more intense activities just because others choose to do so.

Techniques for jogging are basically the same as those for walking. Jogging requires greater flexion of the knee of the recovery leg, and the arms are bent more at the elbows.

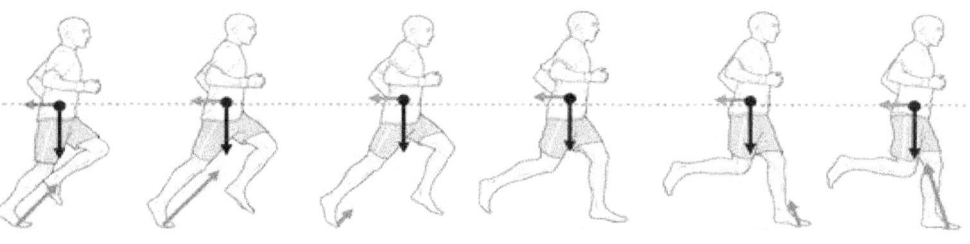

External forces* on a runner during various phases of the gait cycle

F_g — Force of gravity
F_r — Ground reaction force
F_d — Aerodynamic drag force

● Center of mass of runner

*force vectors not drawn to scale

Most people are familiar with pedometers, devices that can track the number of steps a person takes. Pedometers have been used successfully in programs aimed at increasing the amount of activity participants do, and popular books have been written about how to help people achieve a physically active lifestyle using these devices.

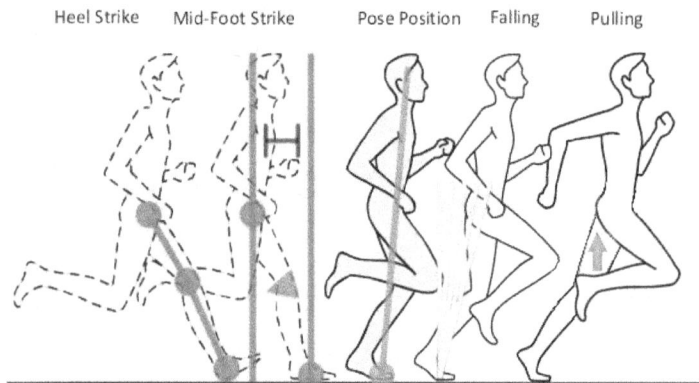

Anatomy of a Stride

Heel Strike — Joints Absorb Impact
Mid-Foot Strike — Excess Strain on Knee
Pose Position — The Running Pose
Falling — Running Faster
Pulling — Running Longer

Pedometers are simple to use, effective, and worth considering, especially with walking being the most popular activity for adults.

Your arm swing is exaggerated slightly but should still be in the forward and backward direction.

Your heel makes the first contact with the ground; then your foot immediately rolls forward to the ball of your foot and then to your toes. As your speed increases, the landing foot may contact the ground in an almost flat position.

Your Breathing should occur through your nose – with your mouth used only for an emergency.

Common faults of the beginning jogger include breathing with their mouth opened, also insufficiently bending their knee during the recovery phase, and swinging their arms across the body.

Many people begin jogging at too high a speed, which results in an inability to continue long enough to accomplish the desired amount of total work and often causes people to dislike jogging.

This problem can be prevented by jogging at a speed slow enough to allow conversation and by using work–relief intervals, which for beginners is slow jogging for a few seconds, then walking, then slow jogging, continuing in this pattern until you build your endurance and stamina.

After you can jog 20 to 40 min (about 2-3 mi, or 3.2-4.8 km) continuously within your THR zone, you can begin to increase your intensity level.

Jogging Program and Stage Progression:

1. **Complete the walking program before starting this program.**

2. **Begin each session with walking and stretching.**

3. **Be aware of new aches and pains.**

4. **Don't progress to the next level if you are not comfortable doing so.**

5. **Stay at the low end of your THR zone and record your HR for each session.**

6. **Do the program on a work-a-day, rest-a-day basis.**

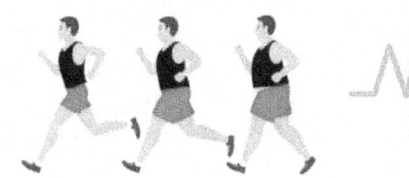

Health Benefits ♥ of Running

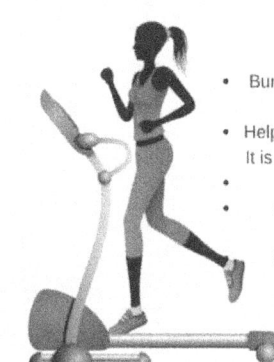

- Burn Up To 1200 Calories in 1 hrs.
- Help To Build Strong Bones, As It is a Weight Bearing Exercise.
- Strengthen Muscles.
- Improve Cardiovascular Fitness.
- Help Maintain A Healthy Weight.

Stage Progression:

* **Stage 1** - Jog 10 steps; walk 10 steps. Repeat 5 times and take your HR. Stay within THR zone by increasing or decreasing walking phase. Do 20 to 30 min of activity.

* **Stage 2** - Jog 20 steps; walk 10 steps. Repeat 5 times and take your HR. Stay within THR zone by increasing or decreasing walking phase. Do 20 to 30 min of activity.

* **Stage 3** - Jog 30 steps; walk 10 steps. Repeat 5 times and take your HR. Stay within THR zone by increasing or decreasing walking phase. Do 20 to 30 min of activity.

* **Stage 4** - Jog 1 min; walk 10 steps. Repeat 3 times and take your HR. Stay within THR zone by increasing or decreasing walking phase. Do 20 to 30 min of activity.

* **Stage 5** - Jog 2 min; walk 10 steps. Repeat 2 times and take your HR. Stay within THR zone by increasing or decreasing walking phase. Do 30 min of activity.

* **Stage 6** - Jog 1 lap (400 m, or 440 yd) and check your HR. Adjust pace to stay within the THR zone. If HR is still too high, go back to stage 5. Do 6 laps with a brief walk between each.

* **Stage 7** - Jog 2 laps and check HR. Adjust pace to stay within the THR zone. If HR is still too high, go back to stage 6. Do 6 laps with a brief walk between each.

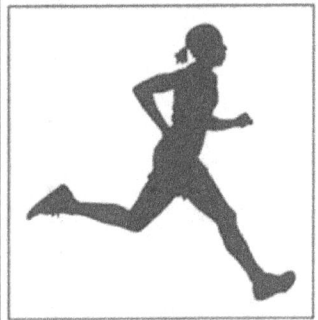
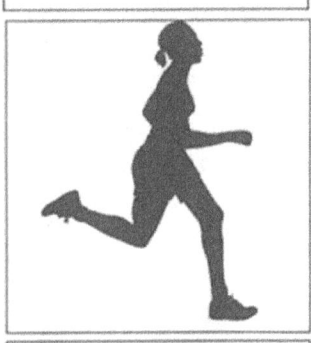
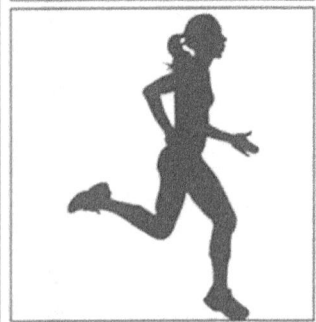
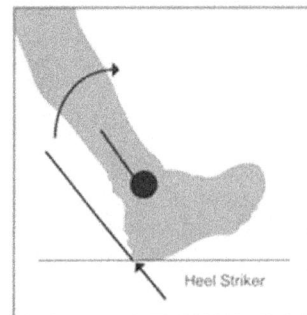
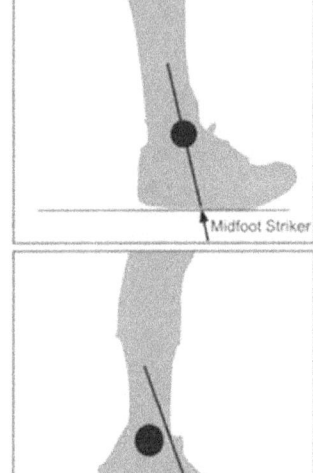

* ***Stage 8*** - Jog 1 mi (1.6 km) and check HR. Adjust pace during the run to stay within THR zone. Do 2 mi (3.2 km).

* ***Stage 9*** - Jog 20 to 40 min (2-3 mi [3.2-4.8 km]) continuously. Check HR at the end to ensure that you were within THR zone.

Stages 1 through 5 of the jogging program are appropriate intervals to use at the beginning of a jogging program. Once the program is established, variety can be introduced by jogging on a variety of surfaces, jogging over a variety of terrains, or doing paced or timed workouts leading up to a fun run.

If you are training for performance – then you will work at the top of your THR range, 3-4 days · wk^{-1} and for approximately 30 to 40 minutes at a time.

You don't want to cause an injury to yourself, so you must be careful when performing high intensity activities.

At any sign of pain or discomfort – STOP!

The purpose of exercise is to improve your Health and to create Energy and Power … So you want to avoid injuries.

You are striving to condition your body to Successfully Move YourSelf into the Enjoyment of Your Abundant Life!

Supreme Cycling – Cycle into Your Healing, Health & Abundant Life!

Riding a bicycle or stationary exercise cycle is another excellent fitness activity. Some people who have problems walking, jogging, or playing sports may be able to cycle without difficulty.

Cycling is counted amongst the best cardiovascular workouts that transform your chubby body in a great shape. An hour of cycling can burn 600 calories from your body.

Cycling not only burns the calories but also gives your leg muscles the immense strength. Blend of vigorous cycling session and sincere eating habits are sure to burn the extra belly fat and the pounds that make you chubby.

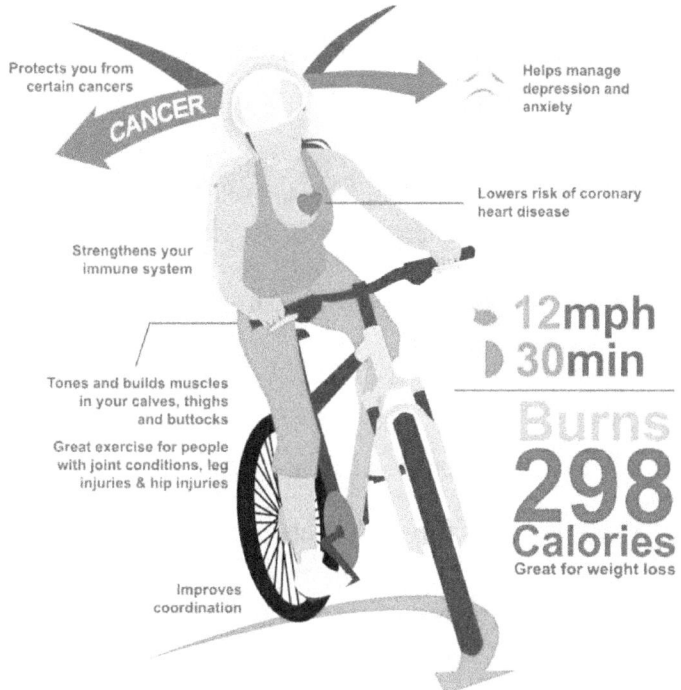

This cycling program applies and follows guidelines for improving your CRF – which is the foundation for your total Health and Wellness.

Although bicycles and terrain vary widely, checking THR allows cyclists to adjust the speed so that they work at the appropriate intensity.

Generally, cyclists cover 3 to 4 times the distance compared with jogging; a person works up to 3 miles (4.8 km) jogging or 9 to 12 miles (14.5-19.3 km) cycling in each workout.

The seat should be comfortable, and its height should be adjusted so that the knee is slightly bent at the bottom of the pedaling stroke.

For those who want a challenging indoor cycling program, spinning classes are worth investigating.

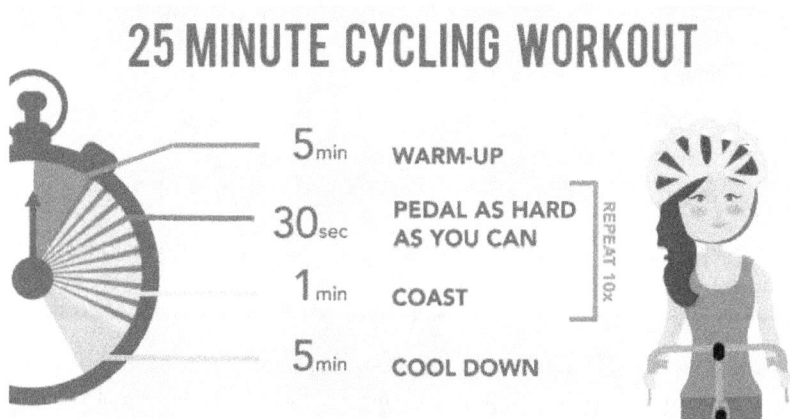

The cycles are designed to accommodate most people because the handlebars and seat height and their fore–aft positions can be adjusted.

At the beginning, you should check in with me or another instructor and get helpful pointers to avoid doing too much during the first session.

Cycling is an excellent activity, especially for those who cannot walk or jog due to joint-related problems. In general, participants should cycle 3 to 4 times the distance they would jog for an equivalent caloric expenditure and cardiorespiratory workout.

The following calculations represent rough estimates of how many calories you can potentially burn during cycling.

Calories Burn 30min:

- Recreational, 5mph: 75-155kcal
- Moderate, 10mph: 190-415kcal
- Vigorous, 15mph: 300-670kcal

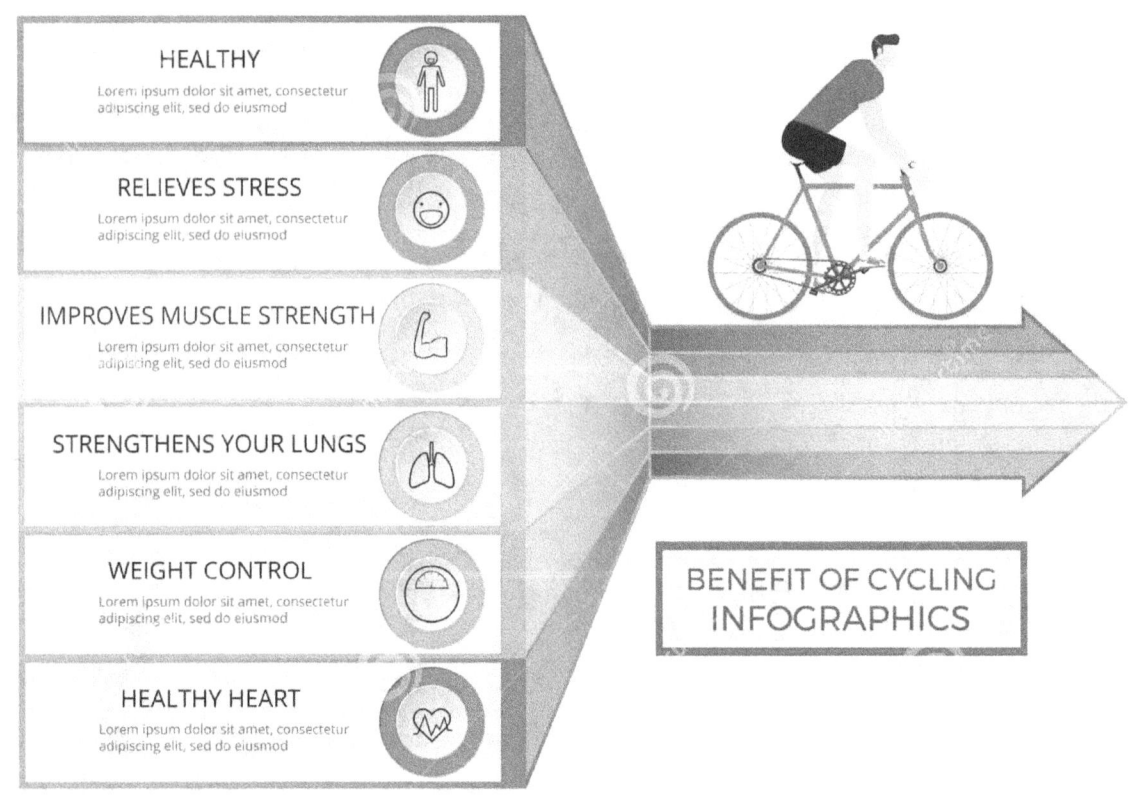

Supreme Aquatic Activities – Swim into Healing & Your Abundant Life!

Being in water or a pool is equivalent to being in the Womb. You are approximately 75% Water. The 1st Atom is Hydrogen – the foundation to Water. The most common bond of Atoms and Molecules is the Hydrogen Bond!

All Life is Created and Built on and with Water!

Aquatic activities can and should be a major part of your exercise and fitness program - especially during injury. The intensity of the activity can suit the needs of the least and the most fit, from the patient who's just survived an MI to the endurance athlete.

Your HR can be checked at regular intervals to see whether your THR has been reached as well as having your specific caloric expenditure goal can be achieved, given the high energy requirement of aquatic activities.

For those people with orthopedic problems who cannot run, dance or play games, they can successfully accomplish their fitness goals exercise in water. The water supports your body weight, minimizing problems associated with weight-bearing joints.

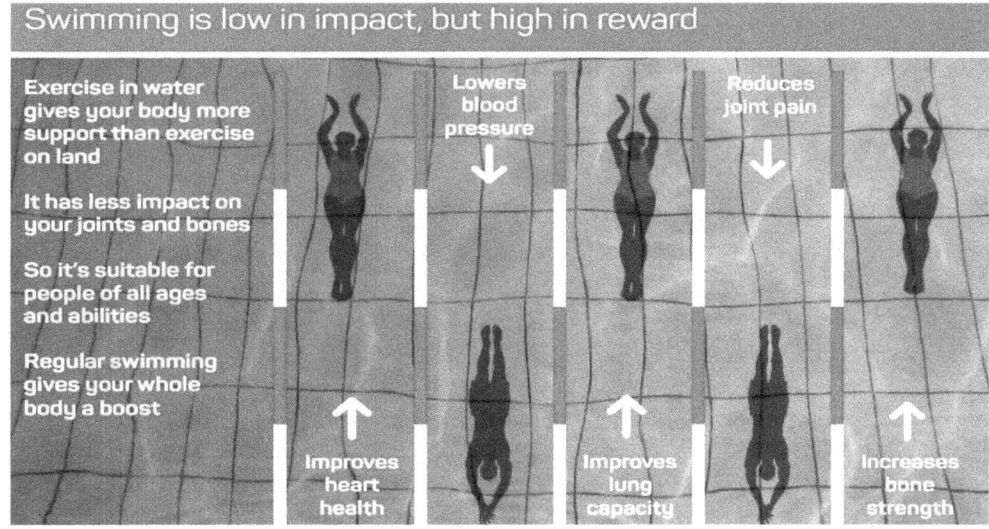

Swimming - Embrace Water and Build Your Health & Lose Fat

Swimming is an excellent cardio workout to lose weight in 2 weeks and helps to promotes blood circulation. It burns calories at an extremely high and efficient rate.

It is recommended by the cardiovascular experts the most because of the health benefits you can reap through even a half an hour swimming session becomes very significant when in comparison of the wear and tear on the body.

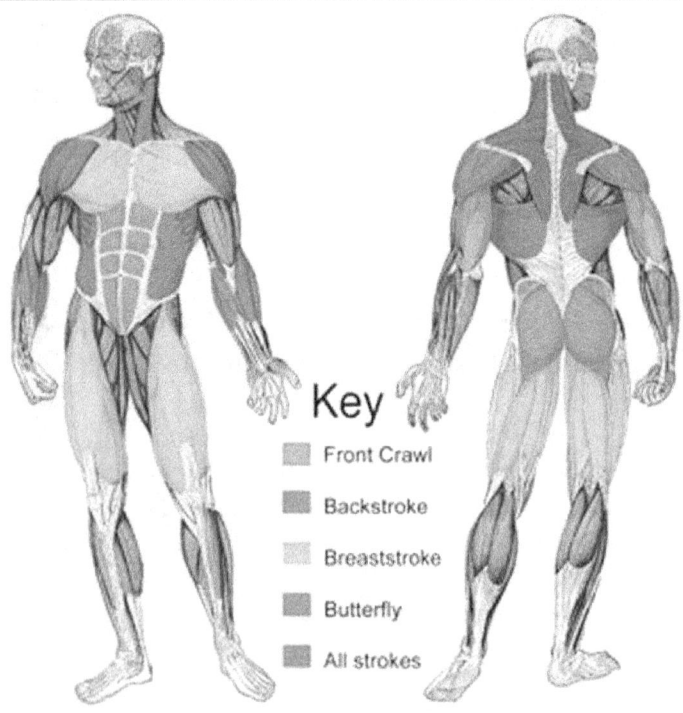

Apart from rapid weight loss, the thing what makes swimming the fastest way to lose weight. is that it burns around 500 calories just in 30 minutes.

Needless to say, it lets the capacity of your lungs reach the peak. Our research data from 1hrs of swimming estimated.

Swimming and Your Muscle Building

Swimming is a resistance exercise, similar to weight-lifting. But, unlike weight-lifting, swimming places almost no stress on your joints and bones. So not only does swimming work your muscles but it doesn't have some of the negative impacts that lifting weights has. There are many muscles that swimming can strengthen.

Swimming is a low-impact sport that incorporates a wide range of your muscle groups and most muscles in your body are worked in different ways. Because of this, risk of injury is **very low** and the benefits are numerous.

When stroke techniques are executed properly, your muscles lengthen and increase in flexibility. This is why most competitive swimmers have broader shoulders and extremely toned physiques.

<u>Although each stroke uses different muscle groups to execute different techniques, all swimming strokes will develop the following muscles:</u>

- Core abdominal and lower back muscles that keep your body steady in streamlined positions in the water to reduce drag.

- Deltoid and shoulder muscles to help your hands have proper entry in the water and to reach out far.

- Forearm muscles that are worked when pulling in the water for more propulsion.

- Upper back muscles that stabilize your shoulders throughout the swimming strokes.

- Glutes and hamstring muscles to keep your body in a balanced position and to aid in propulsion.

Freestyle and Backstroke

- Core abdominal and obliques are important in rotating your torso for a longer stroke.
- Hip flexors are used to maintain a compact and steady kick.

Butterfly

- Core abdominal and lower back muscles lift your body out of the water when breathing.
- Glutes ensure that your legs move as one like a dolphin or mermaid.

Breaststroke

- Pectoral and Latissimus dorsi muscles are used to sweep your arms inwards against the water.
- Glutes and Quadriceps muscles power the breaststroke kick.

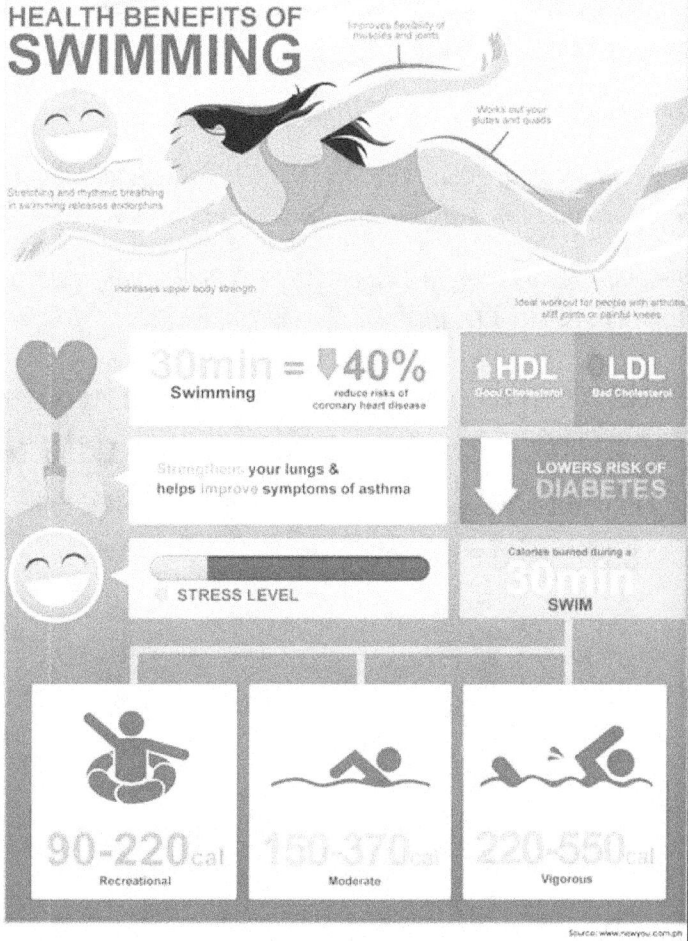

Posture

Many of us spend a lot of time in front of the computer and this causes us to have a slouched posture with hunched shoulders. As swimming strengthens the level of your core stability with regards to your back and shoulder region, a great side effect of that is helping you obtain a better and stronger posture.

A few reasons Posture is important:

- Having good posture keeps you straighter in the water in a streamline position. This means you will use less energy for the same distance.
- Better posture gives you a stronger upper body stroke which makes your technique more powerful.

Your Breathing

The nature of breathing in swimming is timed and precise movement.

Additionally, taking in air is limited in volume and frequency. This promotes greater lung capacity and a consistent intake of oxygen.

This allows you to have a Full Breath of Oxygen.

Every Cell IN Your Body NEEDS OXYGEN …. By developing the ability to fully inflate your Lungs you ensure that you are constantly at your maximum oxygen level.

When your body becomes oxygen DEFICIENT – your cells become oxidized = Cellular Oxidation = Cellular Decay and Death.

The Respiratory System is the system that helps you breathe, you would not be able to stay underwater without your respiratory system. Therefore you would not be able to swim.

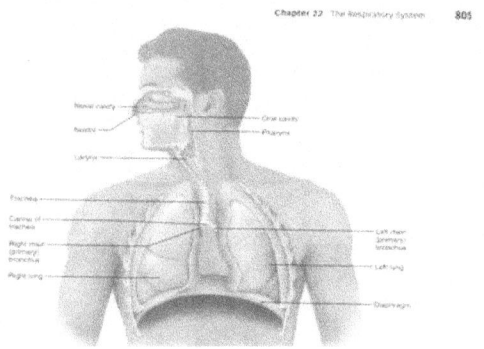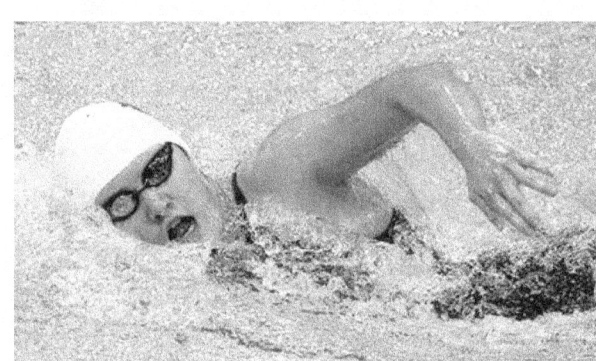

Constant repetition of strokes significantly improves your muscle endurance and because water is much denser than air, the higher resistance against the body's movements causes your muscles to be **strengthened** and **toned**. Swimming gives your body a work out that is significantly superior to training in the gym. In fact, the concept of a gym is a new concept that came with the Greeks and involved way more than exercise. Instead of having artificial weights, you are using the natural density of water for resistance training.

Your Target Heart Rate

One consistent finding is that the maximal HR response to a swimming test is about **18 beats · min^{-1}** lower than that found in a maximal treadmill test (linked to the mammalian diving reflex). This suggests that for swimming, your THR should be shifted downward (2 beats less for a 10 sec count) to achieve the goal of **60% to 80% VO$_2$max** associated with your endurance training effect.

Your Progression

Swimming activities can be graded not only by varying the speed of the swim but also by varying the activity. A patient who has just survived an MI and has an extremely low functional capacity will benefit from simply walking through the water. People who have had recent bypass surgery benefit from moving the arms as they walk across the pool.

> Swimming works your whole body including your circulatory/cardiovascular system. Your circulatory system benefits because swimming directly affects the heart. This means that it improves your body's use of oxygen without overworking your heart.

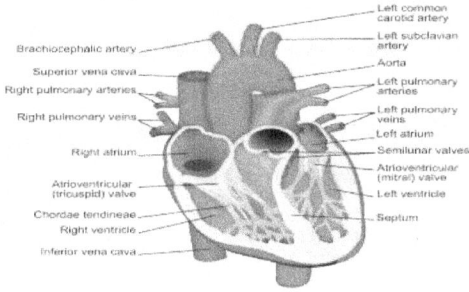
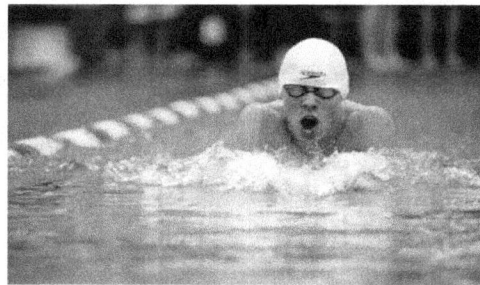

Fun Activities in Supreme Aquatic Exercise Programs.

Side-of-Pool Activities

A variety of activities can be done while holding onto the side of the pool with one or both hands. These activities range from simply moving your legs to the side, front, or back to practicing a variety of kicks that ultimately can be used while swimming. ROM movements in the pool are a good way to warm up before undertaking the more vigorous activities of walking or jogging across the pool.

Walking and Jogging Across the Pool

If you have low functional capacity, you can begin an aquatic program by simply walking across the shallow end of the pool. The water resists the movement while supporting your body weight, reducing the downward load on your ankles, knees, and hips. Your arms can be involved by simulating a swimming motion, which increases the ROM of your arms and shoulder girdle.

The speed and form of the walk can change as you become accustomed to the activity. You can take long strides with your head just above the water or you can sidestep across the pool.

Last, you can jog across the pool with the water at chest height.

Remember to check whether your THR has been achieved.

Using Flotation Devices

If you have limited skill, you can use flotation devices (e.g., a life jacket or kickboard). The extra resistance of the jacket compensates for the extra buoyancy it provides. Remember to check periodically determine whether your THR has been reached.

Lap Swimming

You must be (or should be) skilled to substitute swimming for running or cycling.

An unskilled swimmer operates at a very high energy cost, even when moving slowly, and may become too fatigued to last the whole workout.

But being unskilled at swimming doesn't mean that it should be eliminated as an option in personal fitness programs. You can easily learn to swim over a few weeks, while gradually adjusting to the exercise. After learning to swim, you can use swimming as your primary activity, even if using elementary strokes.

Lap swimming should be approached the same way as lap running: warming up with stretching activities, starting slowly, taking frequent breaks to check the pulse rate, and gradually increasing the distance.

Remember, the caloric cost of swimming compared with the cost of running the same distance is about 4:1…….. If jogging 1 mi (1.6 km) is a reasonable goal in a physical activity program, then swimming 400 m (0.25 mi) is equivalent in terms of energy expenditure.

The stages in the swimming program are not discrete steps that must be followed in a particular order. Two stages can be combined or games can be introduced to make the walk-and-jog and width swims more enjoyable. The ultimate goal is to gradually increase the intensity and duration of the aquatic activities.

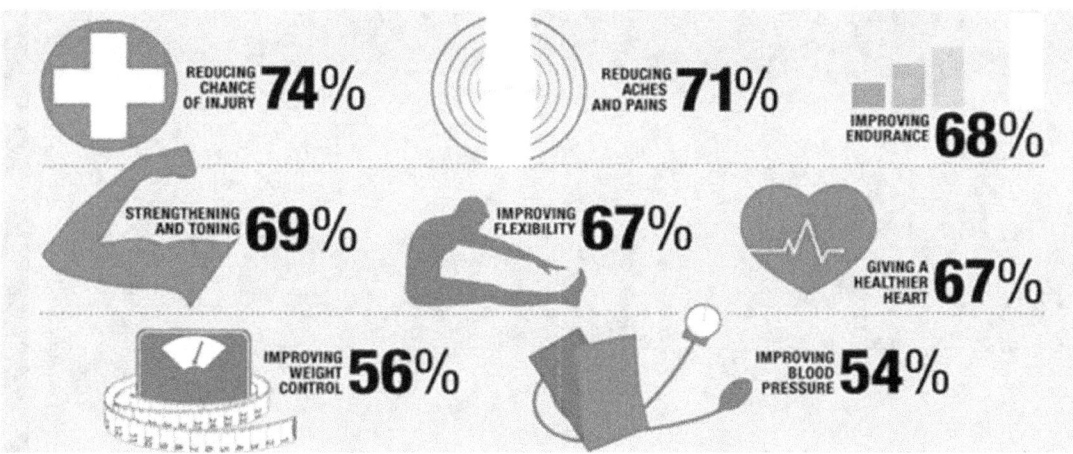

Swimming Program Rules & Stages

1. Start at a level that is comfortable for you.

2. Don't progress to the next stage if you are not comfortable with the current one.

3. Monitor and record your HR.

***All stages assume that a warm-up has preceded the activity and that a cool-down follows.*

* *Stage 1* In chest-deep water, walk across the width of the pool four times and see if you are close to THR. Gradually lengthen the walk until you can do two 10 min walks at THR.

* *Stage 2* In chest-deep water, walk across and jog back. Repeat twice and see if you are close to THR. Gradually lengthen the jogging until you can complete four 5 min jogs at THR.

* *Stage 3* In chest-deep water, walk across and swim back (any stroke). Use a kickboard or flotation device if needed. Repeat this cycle twice and see if you are at THR. Keep up this pattern for 20 to 30 min of activity.

* *Stage 4* In chest-deep water, jog across and swim back (any stroke); repeat and check THR. Gradually shorten the jog and lengthen the swim until four widths can be completed within the THR zone. Accomplish 30 to 40 min of activity per session.

* *Stage 5* Increase the duration of continuous swimming until you can accomplish 30 to 40 min without a rest.

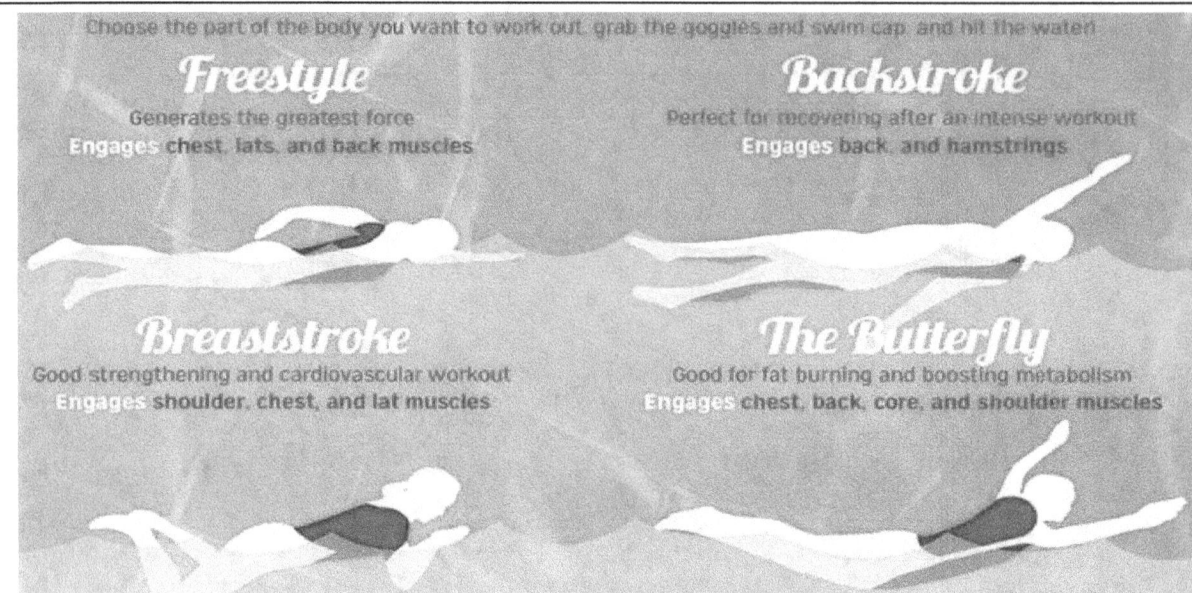

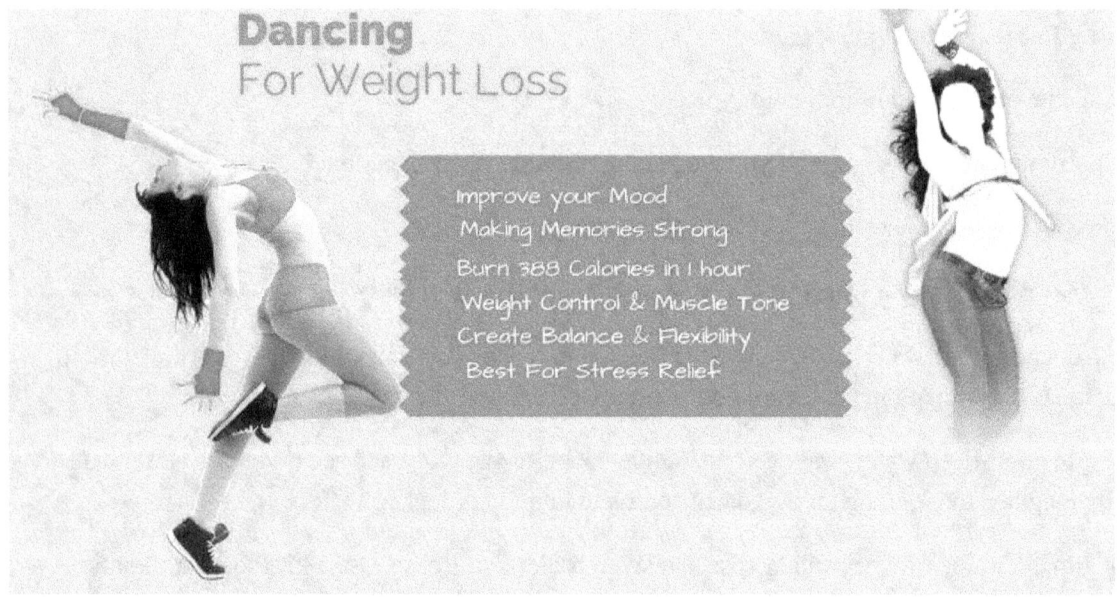

Dance Your Way Into Healing, Health and Abundant Life!

Don't be sad if you can't burn the dance floor with your dancing. But a dancing session of at least a half an hour on a daily basis can help you create the environment for your healing, while improving your health and helping to Build and increase your Energy and Power.

Dancing is considered to be the **best cardio for weight loss**.

Health benefits of dancing:

Dancing can be a way to stay fit for people of all ages, shapes and sizes. It has a wide range of physical and mental benefits including:

- improved condition of your heart and lungs
- increased muscular strength, endurance and motor fitness
- increased aerobic fitness
- improved muscle tone and strength
- weight management
- stronger bones and reduced risk of osteoporosis
- better coordination, agility and flexibility
- improved balance and spatial awareness
- increased physical confidence
- improved mental functioning
- improved general and psychological wellbeing
- greater self-confidence and self-esteem
- better social skills.

Getting started with dancing

You can dance in a group, with a partner, or on your own. There are lots of different places where you can enjoy dancing, for example, at dance schools, social venues, community halls and in your own home.

Dancing can be a great recreational and sporting choice, because anyone of any age can take part. It doesn't matter whether it is cold or raining, as dancing is usually done indoors.

The gear you need for dancing will depend on the style of dancing you choose. For example, tap dancing will involve buying tap shoes, whereas ballet will need ballet slippers and ballet clothing. To get started, simply choose a style you enjoy, or would like to try, look in the *Yellow Pages* or online for dance schools in your local area and join a class.

Move Something!

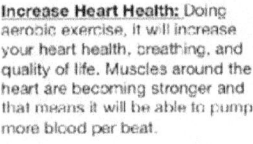

Increase Heart Health: Doing aerobic exercise, it will increase your heart health, breathing, and quality of life. Muscles around the heart are becoming stronger and that means it will be able to pump more blood per beat.

Improves Self Esteem: In a dance class, you will meet new people. You will gain confidence in yourself. You will also improve your self esteem, build new social skills, and will be able to communicate well in a group. Just from exercising will make you a happier person.

Improves Memory: By memorizing dances and aerobic respiration, it can reverse the loss of memory in the hippocampus, which is part of the brain that holds memory.

Improves Mental Health and Stress: When you are dancing, the stress levels are reduced when a chemical is released and burned off by the nervous system. This helps you appreciate strength, and Flexibilty.

Improves Flexibility: By stretching before dancing, it can reduce the risk of injuries. Flexibility releases tension and pressure on joints. It also improves posture.

Improves Immune System: When you are dancing and exercising regularly, your immune system gives you a boost in production to fight off bacteria, and also temporarily increases the number of white blood cells to fight off infections.

Keep Your Bone Mass: By staying active, the bones and bone tissue will stay healthy. Dancing will keep you constantly moving so your bones can stay strong.

Increases Stamina: By dancing, you can increase your stamina from all the movements. Increasing your stamina will let you work out longer, and it will make you stronger in the long run.

Helps Prevent Diabetes: Just by dancing and exercising, you can reduce your risk of getting diabetes. It helps control your cholesterol, blood pressure, and regulates insulin production.

Helps Your Balance: Dance requires a lot of fast movement and good posture. By this, your body will learn how to stabilize and gain control of your body.

Types of dance

There are many styles of dance to choose from, each with its own attractions. Popular styles of dancing include:

- **Ballet** – mostly performed to classical music, this dance style focuses on strength, technique and flexibility.

- **Ballroom dancing** – this involves a number of partner-dancing styles such as the waltz, swing, foxtrot, rumba and tango.

- **Belly dancing** – originating in the Middle East, this dance style is a fun way to exercise.

- **Hip-hop** – performed mostly to hip-hop music, this urban dance style can involve breaking, popping, locking and freestyling.

- **Jazz** – a high-energy dance style involving kicks, leaps and turns to the beat of the music.

- **Salsa** – involving a mixture of Caribbean, Latin American and African influences, salsa is usually a partner dance and emphasizes rhythms and sensuality.

- **Square-dancing** – a type of folk dancing where four couples dance in a square pattern, moving around each other and changing partners.

- **Tap dancing** – focuses on timing and beats. The name originates from the tapping sounds made when the small metal plates on the dancer's shoes touch the ground

General tips for dancing

If you are thinking of taking up dancing, suggestions include:

- See your doctor for a check-up if you have a medical condition, are overweight, are over 40 years of age or are unfit.
- Wear layers of clothing that you can take off as your body warms up.
- Do warm-up stretches or activities before you begin a dance session.
- Drink plenty of water before, during and after dancing.
- Make sure you rest between dance sessions.
- Don't push yourself too far or too fast, especially if you are a beginner.
- Wear professionally fitted shoes appropriate to your style of dance.
- Sit and watch new dance moves first. Learning new moves increases your risk of injury, especially if you are already tired.
- Move as fluidly and gracefully as you can.
- Cool down after a dance session, including stretching.
- HAVE FUN!!!!!

With Dancing, you can Move YourSelf and have FUN!

Exercise should be Fun ... You are getting yourself Healthier .... You are creating the environment for your Healing ... and you are setting the stage for the Successful Enjoyment of your Abundant Life!

All you have to do is

Move SomeThing!

What are You Moving?

YourSelf!

Where are You going?

Your abundant Life!

Climbing Stair
For Weight loss

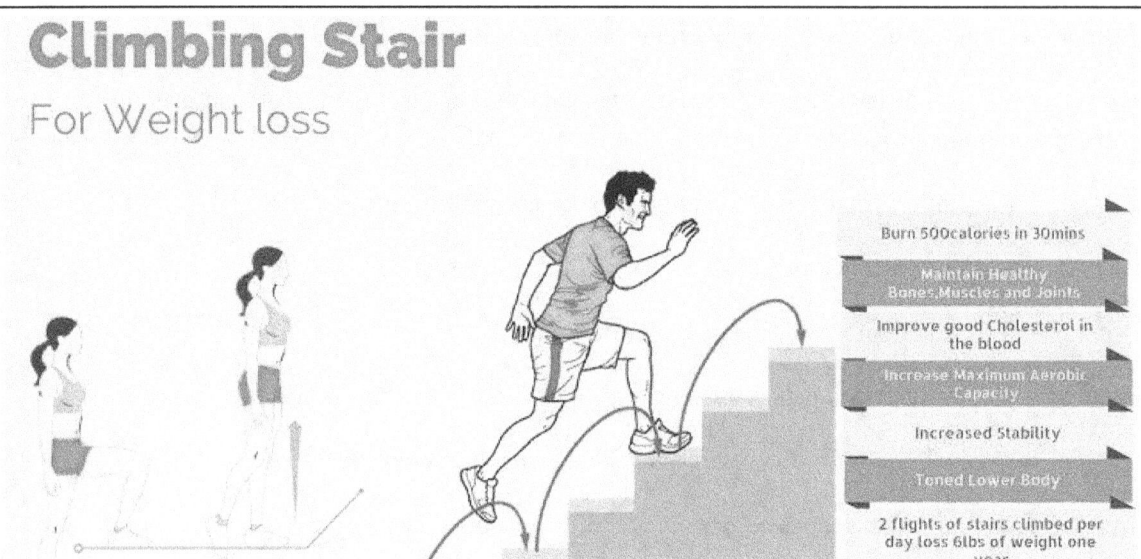

Supreme Stair Climbing - Climb Your Way into Healing & Abundant Your Life!

You must be a lucky chap if your office or home is located on the third or fourth floor of the building.

How? Climbing stairs on a regular basis are itself a great cardiovascular workout which helps you maintain a safe distance from the fatal obesity even if you enjoy the pizza party once in a month.

You can burn more than 500 calories per day once you reach the level of the 60-minute session of climbing stairs.

It's hard but you can achieve the same level with sheer dedication and determination.

Is Climbing stairs a good exercise?

Yes… it is a great exercise!

In addition, stair climbing also raises your heart rate immediately thus maximizing your cardio benefits.

It also increases your core muscle strength: Climbing stairs is a great way to amp your core muscle strength. — glutes, hamstrings, quadriceps, abs and calves to exercise and thus tones your body better.

Benefits of climbing stairs:

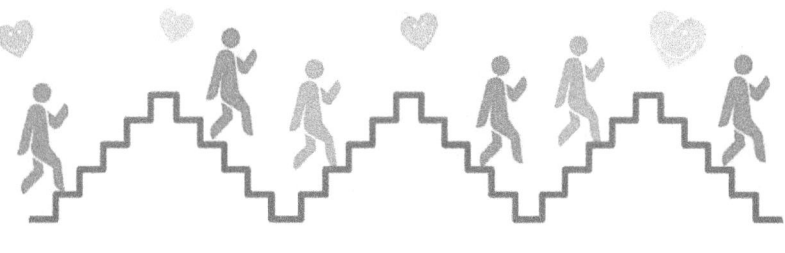

- Excellent to eliminate cellulite burning fat cells and also to reduce bad cholesterol.

- Climbing stairs burned on average 500 calories in one hour.

Stair climbing **exercises our bones and muscles**, improving strength, bone density and muscle tone.

Men who climb an average of eight or more flights of stairs a day have a 33% lower mortality rate than men who were sedentary.

Taking the stairs causes our bodies to release endorphins, these so-called feel good hormones in turn **improve our mental wellbeing.**

- It helps to increase the proportion of muscle mass to total body weight.

- It is a very effective aerobic activity to work the leg muscles, to burn fat in the lower part of our body and to expend energy.

- This exercise will help you to burn the macronutrients of the foods.

- Burns more calories per minute than jogging.

- Reduces cardio risk by more than 30%

- Helps control weight and builds muscle tone.

- Saves up to 15 mins a day and cuts carbon.

- Easy to build into your life and make it habit.

How many calories do you burn walking upstairs for 10 minutes?

Effects. A person weighing 160 lbs. will burn 102 calories walking up and down stairs for 10 minutes. By running, the calories burned will increase to 191.

For a person who weighs 200 lbs., walking up and down stairs burns 127 calories in 10 minutes, while running the stairs burns 239 calories.

Climbing stairs is an aerobic exercise that also strengthens the muscles of your lower body. ... You will burn more calories climbing stairs than you will walking because it is a more vigorous aerobic activity.

How many stairs do I need to climb to lose weight?

Add time and try climbing stairs for **60 minutes**, **four days** a week.

Each 60-minute session could burn roughly 532 calories per session, which will equate to about 2,218 calories burned in a week's time. With that pace, you'd be able to burn about one pound in a week and a half.

Is it better to walk or climb stairs?

Both are good for you but because **stair climbing** requires you to pull your weight against gravity, its health benefits accrue much more rapidly. Even when **climbing stairs** at a normal pace, you will burn two to three times more energy **than walking** on the flat at a brisk pace.

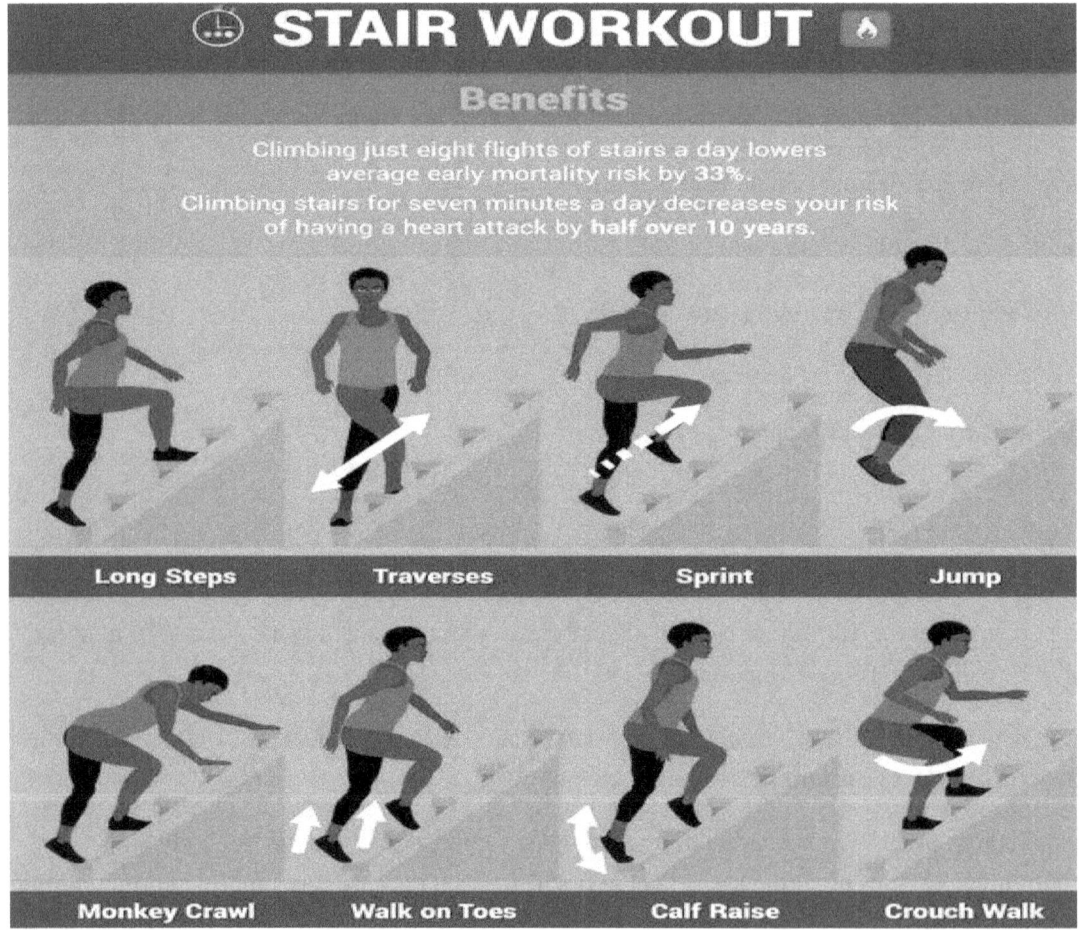

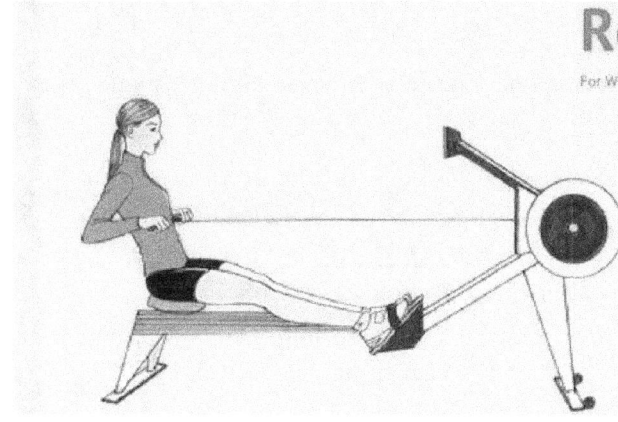

Supreme Rowing - Fall in Love & Row YourSelf into Abundant Life!

The science of rowing machines says- more time you spend on the machine, more fat you lose.

But you will have to be a miser in the calorie intake to experience the weight loss through rowing; else your sweat will go in the vain.

Eating high fiber food with no intake of saturated fat is the secret to losing weight along with the cardiovascular programs like rowing.

Rowing with the correct technique is safe and puts very less strain on your body.

A Rowing Machine Provides a Full-Body Workout

One of the rowing machine's excellent qualities is it's fantastic at working out your whole body

This is a Good Thing and a Better Thing ….. for Building and Maintaining your Supreme Health and Wellness.

Your upper and lower body are required to complete a full rowing stroke. This is a **Good Thing** because you'll be getting a solid workout that's guaranteed to get you sweating.

It's a **Better Thing** because unlike an elliptical, you can't cheat! Meaning, on an elliptical you can let go of the handles to give your arms a rest but still "keep going".

On a rowing machine, you must use your entire body to complete a full stroke every time!

A rowing machine is one of the few machines on the market that truly works out your entire body.

Your Muscles Worked on Rowing Machine

The images below highlight the phases of a rowing motion and oury muscles engaged during a single rowing stroke:

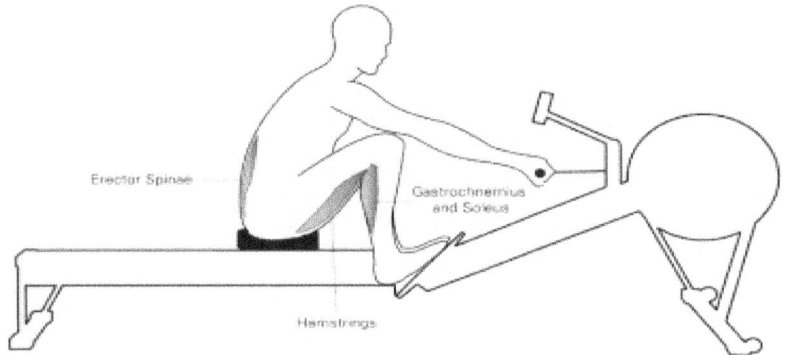

The "Catch"- Your Muscles worked: Erector Spinae, Gastrochnemius and Soleus, and Hamstrings.

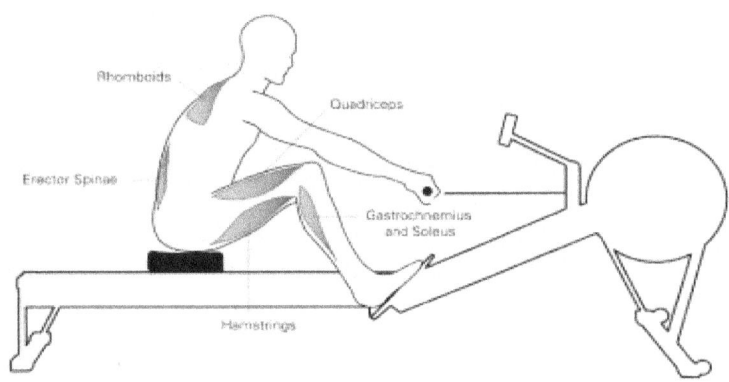

Start of The "Drive"- Your Muscles worked: Erector Spinae, Rhomboids, Quadriceps, Gastrochnemius and Soleus, and Hamstrings.

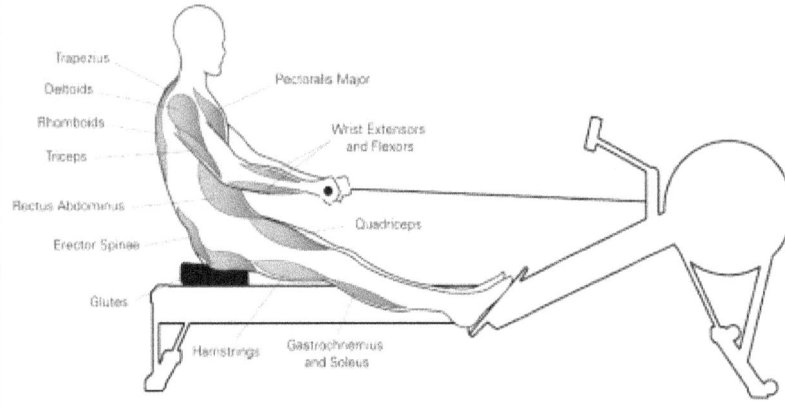

The "Drive"- Your Muscles worked: Erector Spinae, Rectus Abdominus, Triceps, Rhomboids, Deltoids, Trapezius, Pectoralis Major, Wrist Extensors and Flexors, Quadriceps, Glutes, Hamstrings, and Gastrochnemius and Soleus.

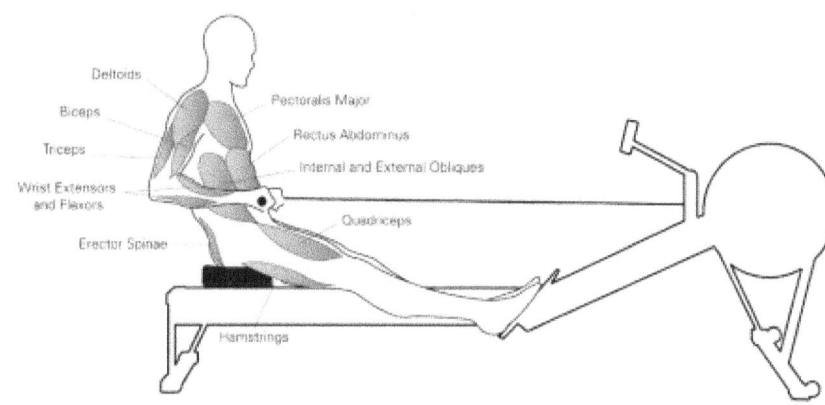

The "Finish" Your Muscles worked: Erector Spinae, Wrist Extensors and Flexors, Triceps, Biceps, Deltoids, Pectoralis Major, Rectus Abdominus, Internal and External Obliques, Quadriceps, and Hamstrings.

Because the Rowing machine exercise is a total body activity, it Builds your Whole Body and prepares your Whole Body to Successful Move You into your Abundant Life!

A Rowing Machine Provides Your Ultimate Cardiovascular Exercise

In a nutshell, cardiovascular or aerobic exercise is an activity that raises your heart rate and keeps it at that elevated heart rate for a period of time.

According to Dictionary.com, aerobic exercises are "any of various sustained exercises, such as jogging, rowing, swimming, or cycling, that stimulate and strengthen the heart and lungs, thereby improving the body's utilization of oxygen."

Anyone who uses a rowing machine knows that they stimulate and strengthen the heart and lungs!

Whether it's when you push off with your legs or use your upper-body to pull the handle to your midsection, a rower requires use of all muscle groups. Your entire body is working which will easily get your heart rate up and keep it there.

This makes rowing extremely efficient at burning calories and shedding fat, since your whole body has to work – **the entire time!**

Rowing Is Low Impact and Non-Weight Bearing

Another less known claim to fame for a rower is it's low-impact and non-weight bearing because rowing is performed while sitting down.

Rowing is ideal for everyone, but this makes a rowing machine even more beneficial. Especially for people with weak joints and people rehabilitating after surgery.

High-impact activities such as playing sports that involve a great deal of running and jumping put a lot of stress on your joints and is weight bearing since you have to support the weight of your body.

These activities are terrible for people with bad knees and ankles.

Even if you currently don't have any bad joints, you might eventually. Especially if you always participate in high-impact activities. So, mix your workout up with a low-impact / high results exercise like rowing!

The rowing machine, also known as rower and ergometers, is a new-found trend in the fitness world. And it has rocked the fitness world with its calorie-incinerating benefits. The science supports that using a rowing machine burns approximately **10-15% more** calories than either running or cycling!

Benefits Of Using A Rowing Machine:

Here are the reasons why you should hop on a rowing machine and ditch that treadmill.

1. Rowing is an effective aerobic exercise with excellent cardiovascular benefits that help to keep your heart and lungs healthy.

2. You get a total body workout with the rowing machine. Rowing works on all the major muscle groups. It is one of those few exercises, which work on both the upper and lower body.

3. Only a few exercises burn calories the way rowing machine does. Rowing machine is effective for weight loss as the exercise provides both strength training and cardio workout. Rowing creates the condition where you can burn fat and builds muscles simultaneously!

4. It is great for endurance conditioning, training and improvement.

5. Vigorous rowing engages all the major muscles in your body and tones and strengthens them.

6. It provides you the ability to create and expand a broader range of motion.

7. Rowing machine provides greater resistance than cycling. The continuous pull and push motion of rowing provides resistance in two opposite directions – building total body strength.

8. It is low impact in nature and can be used by people with joint problems. It is also suitable for elderly people.

9. Rowing helps in improving the flexibility of your body as well as your stamina.

10. It has lower risk of injury.

11. Rowing machine is a good option for cross-training.

12. Rowing machine is convenient and efficient. It burns more calories in less time.

Move Something!

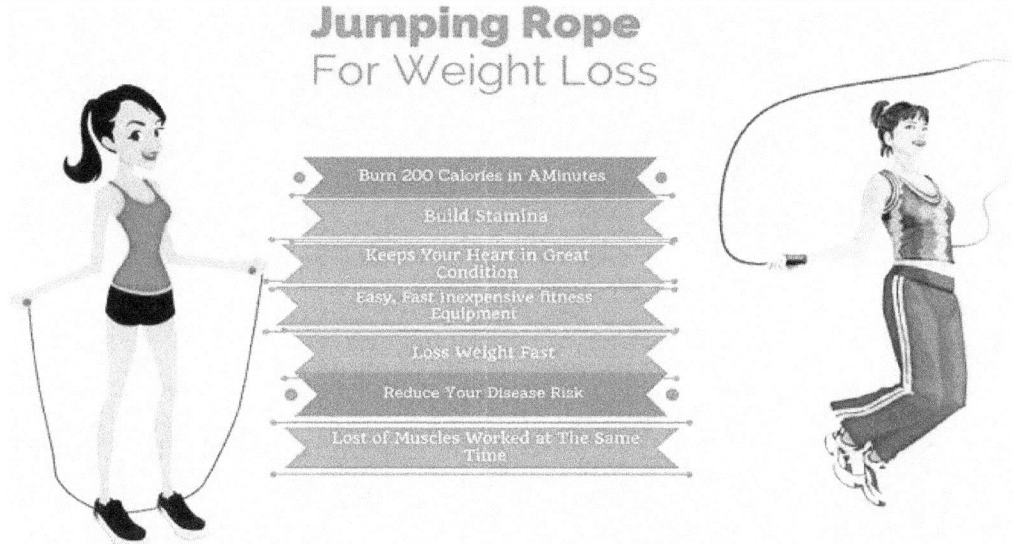

Supreme Rope Jumping – Jump over Disease and Pre-Mature Death!

You can burn 600-960 calories per hour with a jumping rope even at a moderate rate. Doesn't such an effective calorie burning rate make it a great cardio for fat loss?

The jump rope workout divided into the 6 sets of 10-minute not only burns the calories but gives the mammoth power and stamina to your whole body.

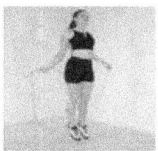
Basic Bounce

You won't believe that each 10-minute session of skipping rope is equal to the running of approximately 8 miles.

Expert says that jumping rope is better for your heart, muscles, and joints because that is good calorie burner in short period and more efficient than running.

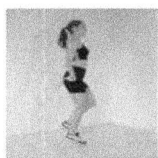 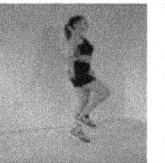 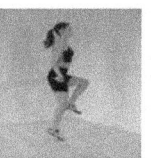
Alternate Foot Step   High Knees

The major benefits of jumping rope are:

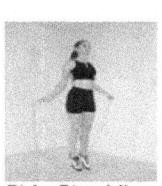 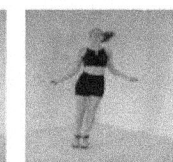 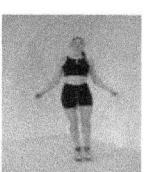
Side Straddle   Skier's Jump

- Stronger Heart. Jumping up and down increases your blood flow. ...
- Lower Blood Pressure. Jumping rope helps control high blood pressure, also known as hypertension. ...

Supreme Health & Fitness!   Health & Wellness Series ... Vol 3!

benefits of jumping rope!

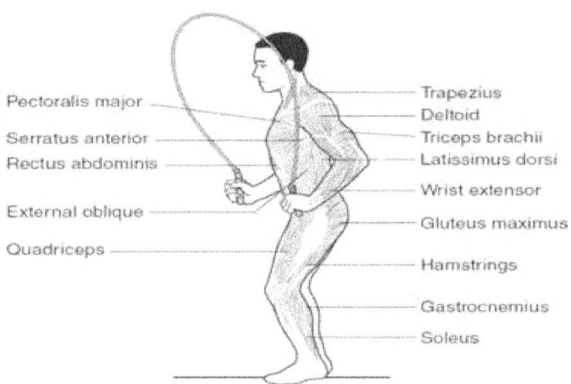

Figure 3.1 Muscles used during the load phase.

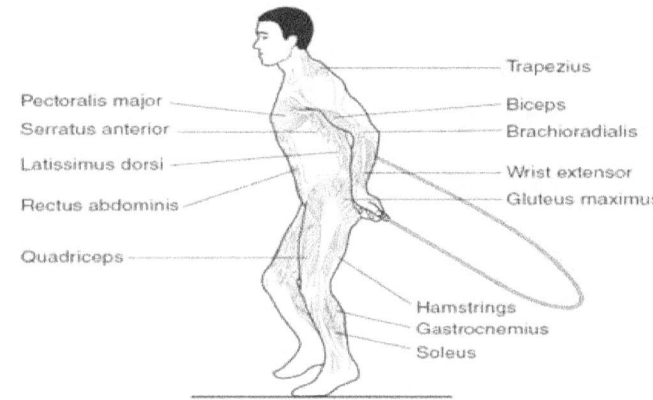

Figure 3.3 Muscles used during the landing phase.

- Lower Cholesterol. ...
- Weight Control. ...
- Stronger Arms. ...
- Healthier Bones. ... Improves bone density
- Stress Relief.
- Effectual calorie burner
- Remarkable boost in agility and swiftness
- Enhances memory power and brain functioning

Exercise & Fitness Games for Health, Wellness & Recapturing Your Youth!

Alternative Physical Activity

- Recreational Sports: Noodle Hockey, Paddle, Jumping Ropes,
- Bodymind Activities: Pilates, Yoga, Taichi, BodyFlow, Relaxation
- Weight lifting, Bodypump.
- Fitness Walking, Jogging, Hiking
- Traditional Games
- Alternative Games and Sports: Floor Ball, Indiaca, Frisbee, KingBall, Ultimate, Flag Football…
- Music Activities: Aerobic, Dance
- Cycling, Swimming, Skating, Sailing, kayaking
- Wii Sports
- School, Gym, Outdoor, Clubs …

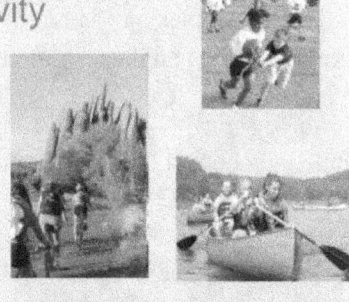
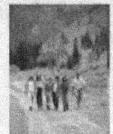
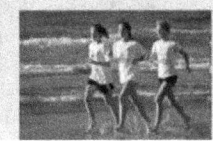

One of the wonderful characteristics of children that is often lost in adulthood is playfulness. A child does not feel the need to justify spending time playing a game just for fun.

One of the attributes that seems to be present in coronary-prone behavior is the inability to appreciate play for its own sake.

A good fitness program can provide you with activities that increase both fitness and playfulness.

Games can involve diverse muscle groups and use your body weight as resistance.

Simultaneously, games develop greater balance and coordination, which are not necessarily outcomes of walking, jogging, or exercising with fixed equipment.

For games to be an effective part of a fitness program, certain elements must be present:

- *Competition*. Competition is not to be avoided, but little to no emphasis should be put on winning. The game should be all about Building Health and Wellness!

- *Cooperation*. Having small groups solve problems together to accomplish fitness tasks can be enjoyable and healthy.

- *Enjoyment*. Enjoyment requires a balance of cooperation and competition, continued participation by everyone, as well as the chance for everyone to be a winner = Healthier and Fit!

- *Inclusion*. A key ingredient for a fitness game is including everyone. This may mean modifying the rules so that everyone can participate and build and improve their Health and Wellness!

- *Skill*. Some fitness games require minimum levels of certain skills that can be taught as part of the fitness program.

- *Vigor*. The main workout should include games in which all participants are continuously active in their specific THR range.

Fitness Games and Activities

- **Skills and games with balls of various sizes**. The size and type of ball can lead to innovative use—for instance, a cage ball can substitute for a basketball. Examples of other balls include tennis balls, volleyballs, playground balls, basketballs, medicine balls, handballs, softballs, mush balls, and foam balls.

- **Activities with apparatuses**. Examples include hula hoops, Frisbees, paddle rackets, skip ropes, skittles, quoits, surgical tubing, culverts, and play buoys.

- **Chasing games**. Examples include tag, chain tag, fox and geese, and dodgeball.

- **Relays with and without apparatuses**. Examples include running, hopping, rolling, crawling, and dribbling with hands and feet.

- **Stunts and contests**. Examples are dual activities such as balancing stunts, forward rolls, backward rolls, strength moves, push-ups, sit-ups, and limited combat games such as rooster fights and partner sparring.

- **Lead-up games for major sport games**. Examples are soccer, tennis, basketball, volleyball, handball, and football, often with rules adjusted to fit the abilities of the participants.

- **Children's games**. Activities include kick ball, foursquare, dodge ball and bounce ball.

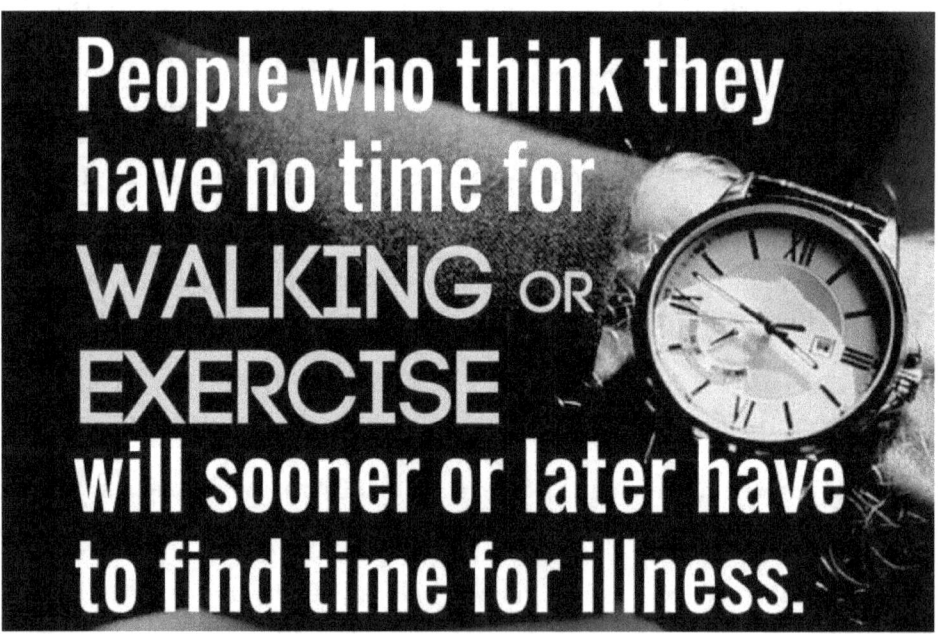

5 Primary Benefits of Aerobic Exercise

The benefits of aerobic exercise come from positive changes in your heart, blood vessels, muscle cells, lungs and nervous system. Cardio training causes your body as a whole to operate more efficiently, so that you can exercise or work at a higher intensity with less effort.

Though the current trend toward high intensity interval training has caused traditional steady state cardio to fall out of fashion, the benefits of aerobic exercise remain scientifically proven and significant, as you will see below.

#1 Enhance your cardiovascular capacity.

Aerobic exercise causes your breathing muscles to strengthen, which improves your ventilation. Capillaries multiply in your lungs, making it easier to pass oxygen into your bloodstream. Your heart becomes stronger so that it can deliver more blood per heart beat to your working muscles. As a result of these changes, you will improve your VO2 Max, which is the ability of your body to absorb and consume oxygen to fuel physical activity.

#2 Reduce your cardiovascular & general health risks.

If you average 30 minutes of moderate intensity exercise (or physical activity) per day, rather than remaining sedentary, you will reduce your risk of premature death, heart disease and stroke by 20-30%. Exercise reduces risk of 3 major forms of cancer by 25-35% and diabetes risk reduction is estimated at 80%. Aerobic exercise even reduces depression, anxiety and dementia risk by 20-35%.

#3 Improve cellular energy and your muscular endurance.

Cardio exercise stimulates muscle cells to produce more receptors for insulin. This makes it easier for cells to pick up glucose for energy from your blood stream. Cells are also triggered to build more internal energy centers (mitochondria). The enhanced energy production from the mitochondria strengthens muscle cells, allowing them to recover from stress and remove waste products more efficiently. Cardio exercise also trains your muscles to be more relaxed at rest. All of these changes at the cellular level result in improved muscular endurance.

#4 Improve your stress tolerance and immunity.

Cardio exercise raises your stress threshold, so that it takes a higher level of perceived stress to cause a physical reaction, such as increased heart rate or rapid breathing. If you are under stress, cardio exercise will reduce the feelings of stress so that the damaging effects of stress on your body will be limited. Because of the improved response to stress in your body, the benefits of aerobic exercise include lowering your risk of developing stress and immune related disorders, such as chronic fatigue, fibromyalgia, and arthritis.

#5 *Improve the functioning of your brain.*

Aerobic exercise increases production of brain-derived neurotrophic factor (BDNF), which is a hormone that stimulates growth of new nerve cells throughout the brain. Your brain will grow in response to exercise just as muscles will grow. Studies have shown a 20% greater rate of learning immediately following aerobic exercise.

Cardio exercise as a safe starting point for beginners

In addition to the above benefits of cardio exercise, steady aerobic training is easier to manage for anyone who is out of shape or new to exercise. Moderate effort walking, biking, hiking, stair climbing and similar activities are a great place to start when you are acclimating to exercise training. Aerobic exercise will help you get used to physically exerting yourself and it will help you get familiar with your physical ability level and your limitations.

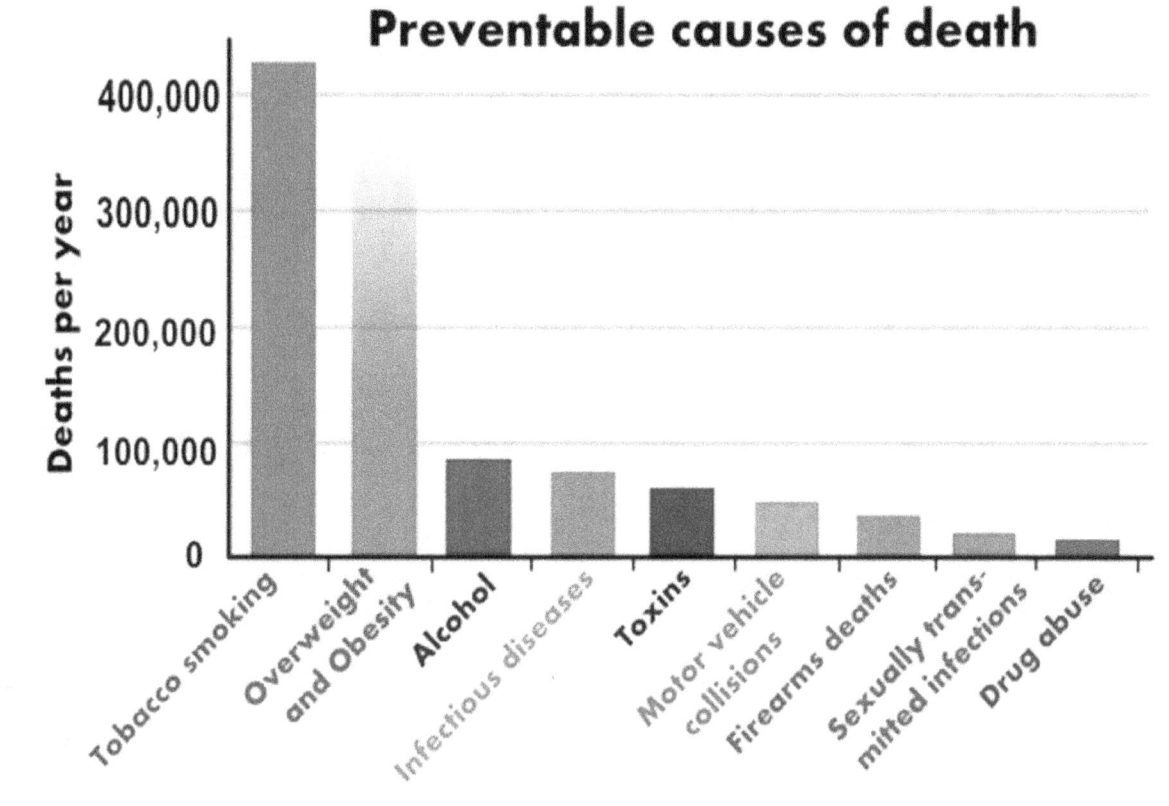

Move Something!

Chapter Fifteen

5 Leading Causes of Death

******

Each year, nearly 900,000 Americans die prematurely from the five leading causes of death – yet 20 percent to 40 percent of the deaths from each cause could be prevented, according to a study from the Centers for Disease Control and Prevention.

The five leading causes of death in the United States are heart disease, cancer, chronic lower respiratory diseases, stroke, and unintentional injuries. Together they accounted for 63 percent of all U.S. deaths in 2010, with rates for each cause varying greatly from state to state. The report, in this week's issue of CDC's weekly journal, Morbidity and Mortality Weekly Report, analyzed premature deaths (before age 80) from each cause for each state from 2008 to 2010. The authors then calculated the number of deaths from each cause that would have been prevented if all states had same death rate as the states with the lowest rates.

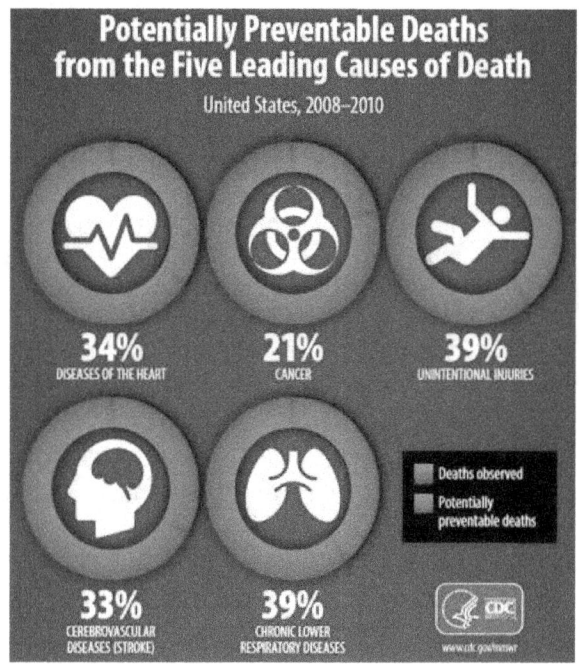

The study suggests that, if all states had the lowest death rate observed for each cause, it would be possible to prevent:

- 34 percent of premature deaths from heart diseases, prolonging about 92,000 lives

- 21 percent of premature cancer deaths, prolonging about 84,500 lives

- 39 percent of premature deaths from chronic lower respiratory diseases, prolonging about 29,000 lives

- 33 percent of premature stroke deaths, prolonging about 17,000 lives

- 39 percent of premature deaths from unintentional injuries, prolonging about 37,000 lives

The numbers of preventable deaths from each cause cannot be added together to get an overall total, the authors note. That's because prevention of some premature deaths may push people to different causes of death. For example, a person who avoids early death from heart disease still may die prematurely from another preventable cause, such as an unintentional injury.

Modifiable risk factors are largely responsible for each of the leading causes of death:

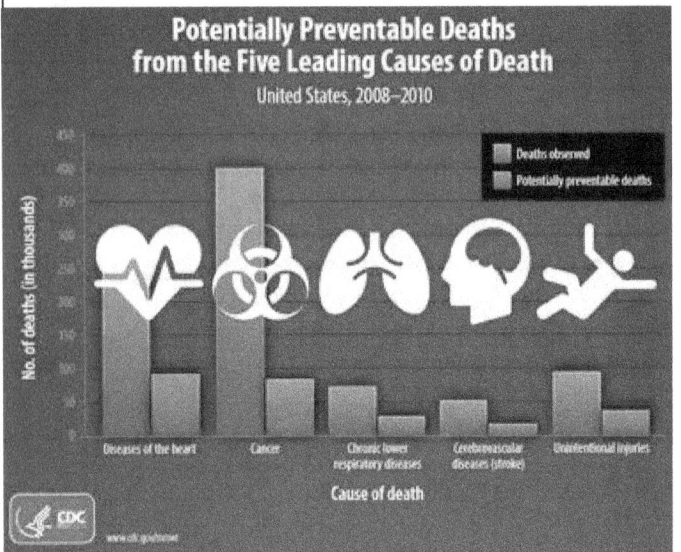

Potentially Preventable Deaths from the Five Leading Causes of Death

- Heart disease risks include tobacco use, high blood pressure, high cholesterol, type 2 diabetes, poor diet, overweight, and lack of physical activity.

- Cancer risks include tobacco use, poor diet, lack of physical activity, overweight, sun exposure, certain hormones, alcohol, some viruses and bacteria, ionizing radiation, and certain chemicals and other substances.

- Chronic respiratory disease risks include tobacco smoke, second-hand smoke exposure, other indoor air pollutants, outdoor air pollutants, allergens, and exposure to occupational agents.

- Stroke risks include high blood pressure, high cholesterol, heart disease, diabetes, overweight, previous stroke, tobacco use, alcohol use, and lack of physical activity.

- Unintentional injury risks include lack of seatbelt use, lack of motorcycle helmet use, unsafe consumer products, drug and alcohol use (including prescription drug misuse), exposure to occupational hazards, and unsafe home and community environments.

Many of these risks are avoidable by making changes in personal behaviors. Others are due to disparities due to the social, demographic, environmental, economic, and geographic attributes of the neighborhoods in which people live and work. The study authors note that if health disparities were eliminated, as called for in Healthy People 2020, all states would be closer to achieving the lowest possible death rates for the leading causes of death.

Southeastern states had the highest number of preventable deaths for each of the five causes. The study authors suggest that states with higher rates can look to states with similar populations, but better outcomes, to see what they are doing differently to address leading causes of death.

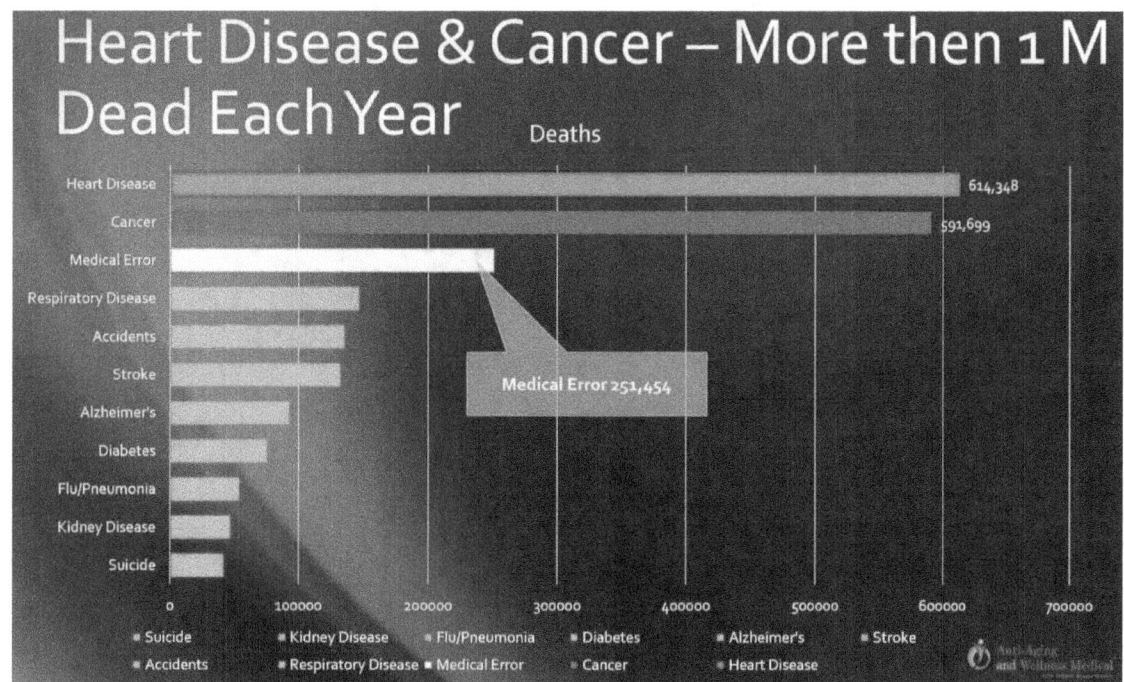

Medical Errors are now the 3rd Cause of Death …. Surpassing Respiratory diseases.

This means that it is imperative for you to take control of your Health and Wellness by applying the Sciences of Eating To Live and Moving YourSelf!

The list of incurable diseases are growing. Obesity is an epidemic. Hypertension is the Silent Killer – meaning you could die from it at any time.

Add Medical Errors to these and you should clearly see the writing on the wall …… That You Must Take Control Of Your Health!

Move Something!

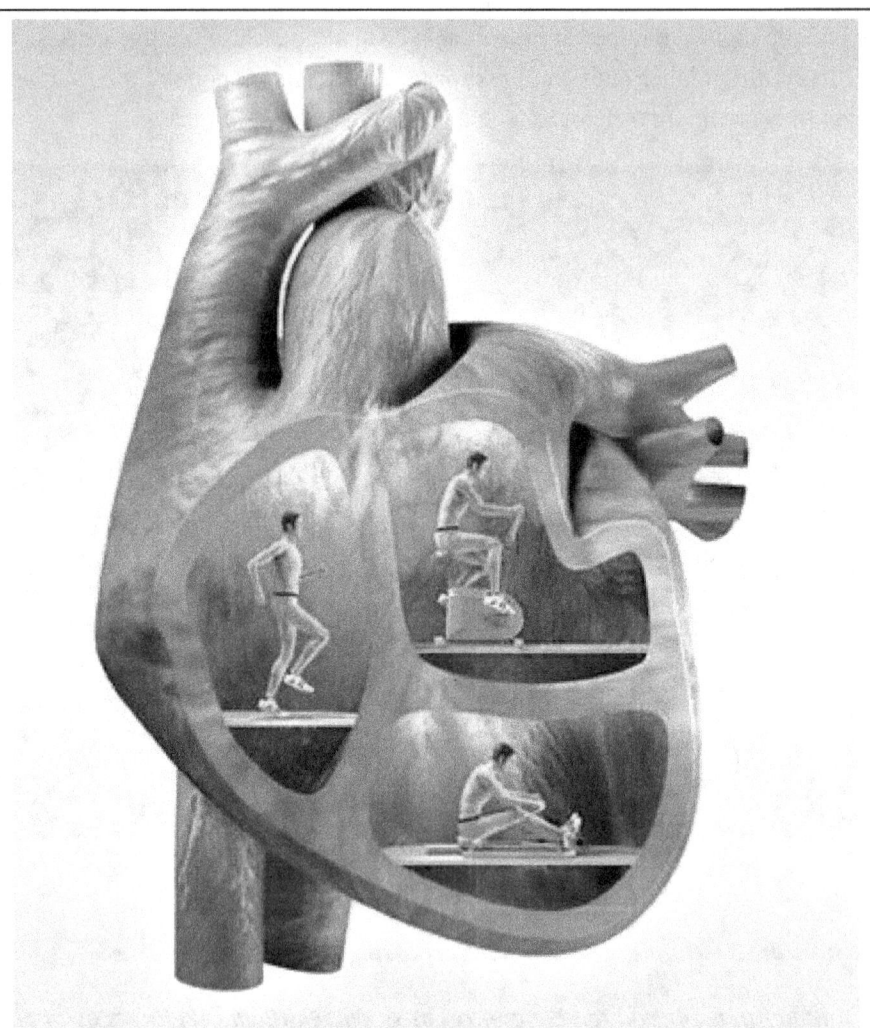

Exercise and Heart Disease

Moderate to intense physical activity for 30-45 minutes on most days of the week is recommended

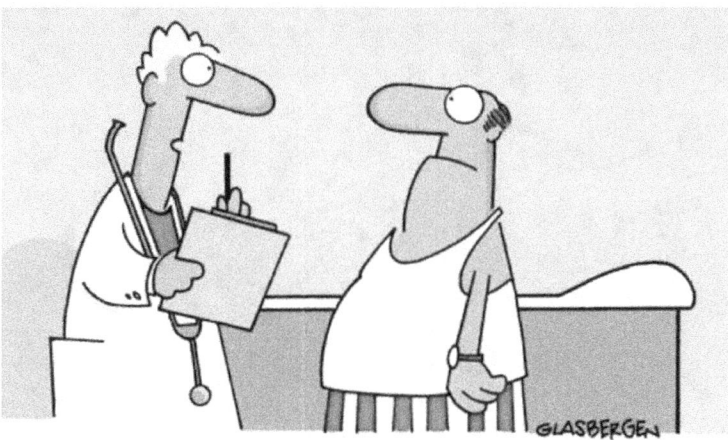

"What fits your busy schedule better, exercising one hour a day or being dead 24 hours a day?"

Exercise

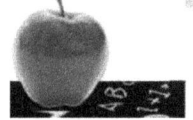

Blood vessels supplying active skeletal muscle fibers

℞
1. Whole body exercise
2. Combined aerobic and resistance exercise
3. Modulate exercise mode and intensity to ↑ skeletal muscle fiber recruitment

Chronic adaptations

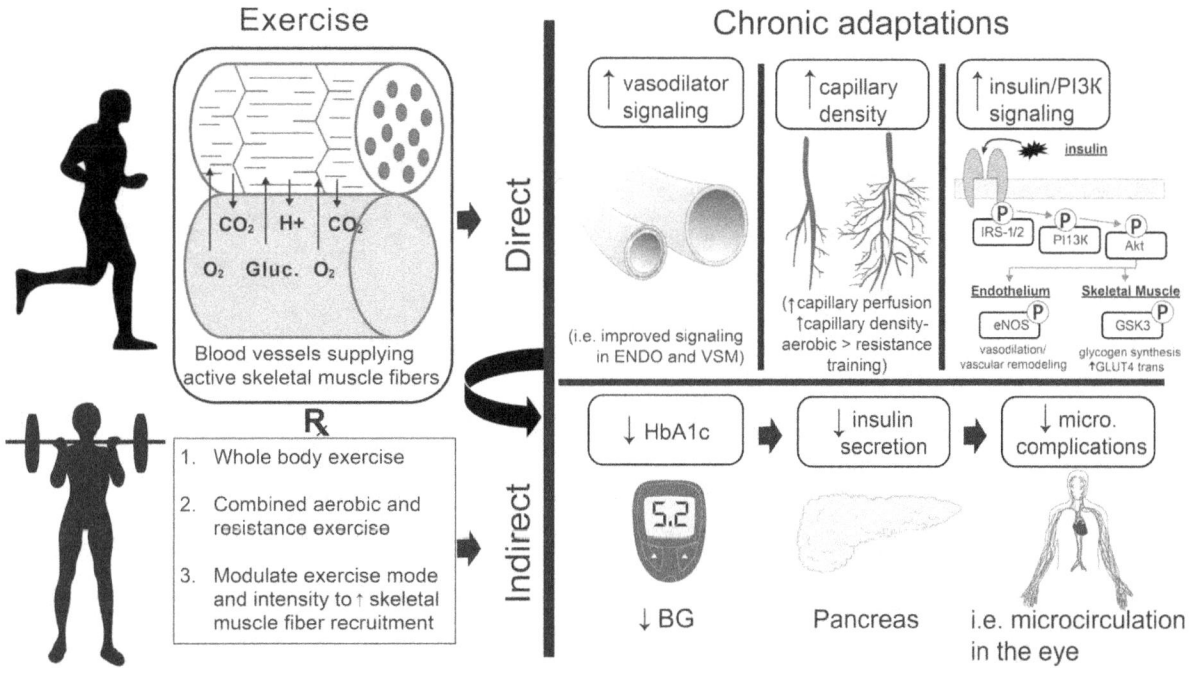

Chapter Sixteen

Exercise & Heart Disease

*****

Unless you are born with a condition - Almost every heart disease is preventable and/or controllable!

Coronary heart disease (CHD) is a major problem in the United States and other industrialized nations. This chapter provides you with a basic understanding of the development of CHD, the benefits of exercise for a cardiac population, and the special considerations for exercise prescription for those in this group.

Atherosclerosis

Atherosclerosis is defined as an accumulation of lipid deposits in the large and medium-sized arteries, a process that provokes fibrosis and calcification.

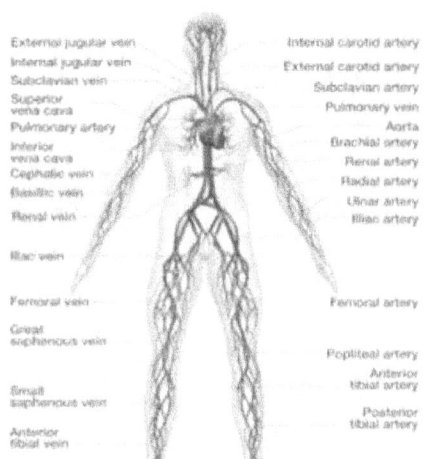

Cardio-Vascular Disease

- Cardiovascular diseases (CVDs) are a group of disorders of the heart and blood vessels.

➢ Coronary heart disease/ Coronary artery disease
➢ Cerebrovascular disease
➢ Peripheral arterial disease
➢ Rheumatic heart disease
➢ Congenital heart disease
➢ Deep vein thrombosis and pulmonary embolism.

Atherosclerosis starts to develop early in life … but isn't noticed until a level of accumulation had developed – but by this tie it is almost too late.

Early development of atherosclerosis means that poor dietary choices are being taught and developed in us from childhood.

It is believed that the atherosclerotic process begins when the **endothelial cells** lining the artery become damaged because of smoking, toxic agents, or high BP. When lipoproteins are deposited at the damaged site, plaque formation (or atherosclerosis) occurs. Eventually, these deposits impede blood flow in the affected arteries, sometimes to the point of complete occlusion.

Consequences of Atherosclerosis

Atherosclerosis can occur in various arteries throughout your body and have various results. Blockages in your coronary arteries lead to **myocardial ischemia** (reduced blood flow to the heart) and in severe cases to **myocardial infarction (MI).** If the blood vessels in your brain become occluded, a **stroke** will result.

Blockages in your peripheral leg vessels can result in **claudication,** or intermittent muscle pain that occurs with exertion.

Cardiovascular Disease

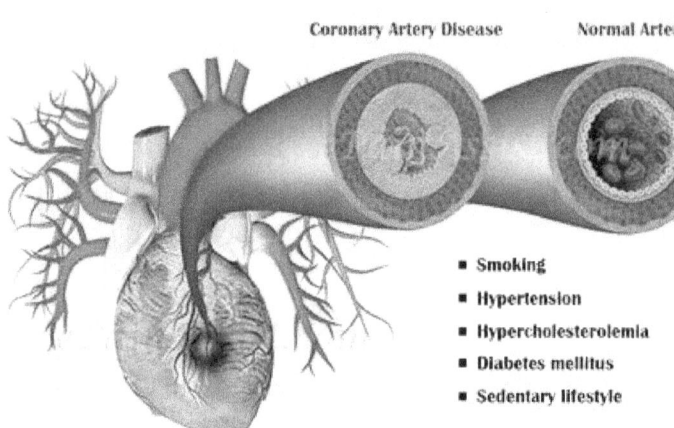

In the United States, CVD is the **leading cause of death**, with 831,272 people dying from CVD (including congenital cardiovascular defects) in 2006. CHD accounts for 51% of these deaths, with stroke (17%), hypertensive disease (7%), and CHF (7%) making up most of the other leading causes. (CVD refers to any disease of the heart and the blood vessels or circulation, while CHD is a more specific condition resulting from reduced blood flow in the coronary arteries.)

The death rate attributable to coronary artery disease (CAD) has declined in recent decades, but it remains a problem of huge proportions, **ESPECIALLY IN THE BLACK COMMUNITY**.

According to the AHA, approximately 1,255,000 Americans will have a coronary attack this year. About 785,000 of these will be first heart attacks, and the rest will be recurrent attacks. Of those experiencing a heart attack, 80% will survive, and some of the survivors will be referred to cardiac rehabilitation programs.

Although CVD is often thought of as a man's disease, it is the leading cause of death in women as well as men.

These numbers of death were/are completely PREVENTABLE!

You have to create the condition that causes your heart to become dis-eased!

Your hearts main function is to disperse the Breath of Life throughout your body.

Cholesterol

Cholesterol is an oil-based substance and does not mix with the blood, which is water-based. It is carried around the body by lipoproteins.

There are 2 types of lipoproteins that carry the parcels of **cholesterol**: Low-density lipoprotein (LDL) - **cholesterol** carried by this type is known as "bad" **cholesterol**.

High-Density Lipoprotein is known as "good" cholesterol.

Total Cholesterol Level	Category
Less than 200mg/dL	Desirable
200-239 mg/dL	Borderline high
240mg/dL and above	High

LDL (Bad) Cholesterol Level	LDL Cholesterol Category
Less than 100mg/dL	Optimal
100-129mg/dL	Near optimal/above optimal
130-159 mg/dL	Borderline high
160-189 mg/dL	High
190 mg/dL and above	Very High

HDL (Good) Cholesterol Level	HDL Cholesterol Category
Less than 40 mg/dL	A major risk factor for heart disease
40—59 mg/dL	The higher, the better
60 mg/dL and higher	Considered protective against heart disease

Weight loss and exercise are shown to decrease total cholesterol while increasing levels of HDL, the good cholesterol. Smoking cessation decreases LDL levels plus smoking is a primary risk factor for heart disease and stroke. One drink of alcohol a day may help increase HDL levels, but too much alcohol can damage the liver and increase the risk of elevated LDL.

Cholesterol in cell membranes

Cholesterol is a type of lipid with the molecular formula $C_{27}H_{46}O$.

Cholesterol is very important in controlling membrane fluidity. It binds to hydrophobic tails of the phospholipids, packing them more closely together. The more cholesterol, the less fluid (more stable) – and the less permeable – the membrane.

Cholesterol is also important in keeping membranes stable at normal body temperature – without it, cells would burst open.

What is cholesterol?

Cholesterol is a chemical compound that your body requires as a building block for cell membranes and for hormones like estrogen and testosterone.

Your liver also produces about 80% of your body's cholesterol and the rest comes from dietary sources like meat, poultry, eggs, fish, and dairy products.

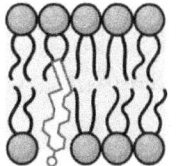

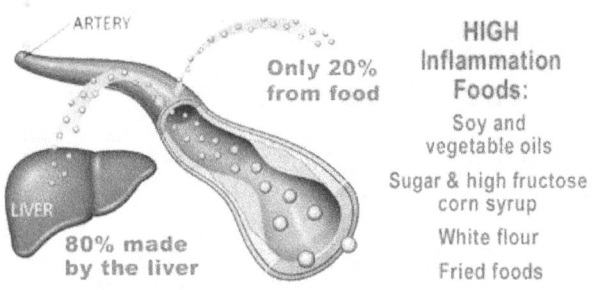

CHOLESTEROL SOURCES REALITY CHECK
- Only 20% from food
- 80% made by the liver

HIGH Inflammation Foods:
- Soy and vegetable oils
- Sugar & high fructose corn syrup
- White flour
- Fried foods

LESSON: Avoid foods causing an inflammtion response in the liver!

Foods derived from plants contain no cholesterol.

The Cholesterol content in your bloodstream is regulated by your liver. After a meal, cholesterol in the diet is absorbed from your small intestine and metabolized and stored in your liver. As your body requires cholesterol, it may be secreted by your liver.

When too much cholesterol is present in your body, it can start to build up in deposits that are called plaque along the inside walls of arteries, which ultimately causes them to narrow.

What are the different types of cholesterol?

Cholesterol does not travel freely through your bloodstream. Instead, it is attached or carried by lipoproteins (lipo = fat) in your blood. Let's look at the 2 types lipoproteins that are categorized based upon how much protein there is in relation to the amount of cholesterol.

Low-density lipoproteins (LDL) contain a higher ratio of cholesterol to protein and are thought of as the "bad" cholesterol. Having Elevated levels of LDL lipoprotein increase your risk of heart disease, stroke, and peripheral artery disease, by helping form cholesterol plaque along the inside of your artery walls.

Over time, as this plaque build-up (plaque deposits) increases, your artery begins to narrow (atherosclerosis) and this action causes your blood flow to decrease. If this plaque ruptures, it can cause a blood clot to form that prevents any blood flow. If the clot occurs in one of your coronary arteries in your heart then this clot is the cause of a heart attack or myocardial infarction.

HDL Raise	HDL Lower	LDL Raise	LDL Lower
Alcohol			
Niacin		Niacin	
Fibrates		Fibrates	
Statins	Certain Drugs	Statins	
		Dietary Fats	Fat Reduction
Smoking Cessation	Smoking		
Estrogen	Progesterone		Estrogen
	Diabetes	Diabetes	
Weight loss	Obesity	Obesity	Weight Loss
	Metabolic Syndrome	Thyroid Disease	
		Renal Disease	
		Liver Disease	
Exercise	No Exercise	Genetics	Resins
	High Triglycerides		Bile Acid Sequestrants

High-density lipoproteins (HDL) are made up of a higher level of protein and a lower level of cholesterol. These tend to be thought of as "good" cholesterol.

The higher the HDL to LDL ratio, the better it is for the individual because such ratios can potentially be protective against heart disease, stroke, and peripheral artery disease.

Why is high cholesterol dangerous?

Elevated cholesterol levels are one of the risk factors for heart disease, stroke, and peripheral artery disease. The mechanism involving cholesterol in all three diseases is the same; plaque buildup within arteries decreases blood flow affecting the function of your cells and organs that these blood vessels supply.

- Atherosclerotic heart disease or narrowed coronary arteries in the heart can cause the symptoms of angina, when your heart muscle is not provided with enough oxygen to function.

- Decreased blood supply to your brain may be due to narrowed small arteries in your brain or because the larger carotid arteries in your neck may become blocked. This can result in a transient ischemic attack (TIA) or stroke.

- Peripheral artery disease describes gradual narrowing of the arteries that supply your legs. During exercise, if the legs do not get enough blood supply, they can develop pain, called claudication.

Where does cholesterol come from?

Your liver is responsible for managing the levels of LDL in your body. It manufactures and secretes LDL into your bloodstream and there are receptors on your liver cells that can "monitor" and attempt to adjust your LDL levels as needed. Unfortunately, if there are fewer of your liver cells available or if they do not function effectively, your LDL level may rise.

Both your Diet and Genetics play a factor in a your cholesterol levels. There may be a genetic predisposition for familial hypercholesterolemia (hyper = more = cholesterol + emia = blood) where the number of liver receptor cells is low and your LDL levels rise causing the potential for atherosclerotic heart disease at a younger age.

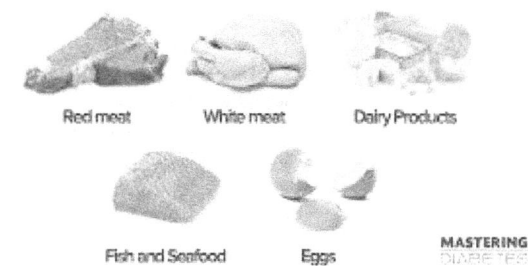

In your diet, cholesterol comes from saturated fats that are found in meats, eggs as well as dairy products. Excess intake can cause the LDL levels in your blood to rise.

Some vegetable oils made from coconut, palm, and cocoa are also high in saturated fats.

Which foods can help lower cholesterol?

The American Heart Association has developed diet guidelines to help lower cholesterol levels. The 1st step is to STOP eating manufactured and processed foods which often contain preservatives, high sodium or sugar contents, among other dangerous ingredients that are harmful to your health.

It may be a challenge to read the nutritional contents on food packaging and on restaurant menus or to do the math, but IF you are going to consume such food-like items, then the benefit will decrease the risk of heart attack and stroke = *Saving Your Own Life!*

- Limit total fat intake to less than 25% to 35% of your total calories each day.

- Limit saturated fat intake to less than 7% of total daily calories.

- Limit trans-fat intake to less than 1% of total daily calories.

- The remaining fat should come from sources of monounsaturated and polyunsaturated fats that are found in unsalted nuts and seeds and vegetable oils.

- Limit cholesterol intake to less than 300 mg per day, for most people. If you have coronary heart disease or your LDL cholesterol level is 100 mg/dL or greater, limit your cholesterol intake to less than 200 milligrams a day.

Some food groups may be beneficial in directly lowering cholesterol levels and include foods with plant sterol additives, high fiber foods like bran, oatmeal, and fruits like apples and pears and olive oil.

Some of these foods like nuts and fruits are also high in calories, so moderation is always advisable.

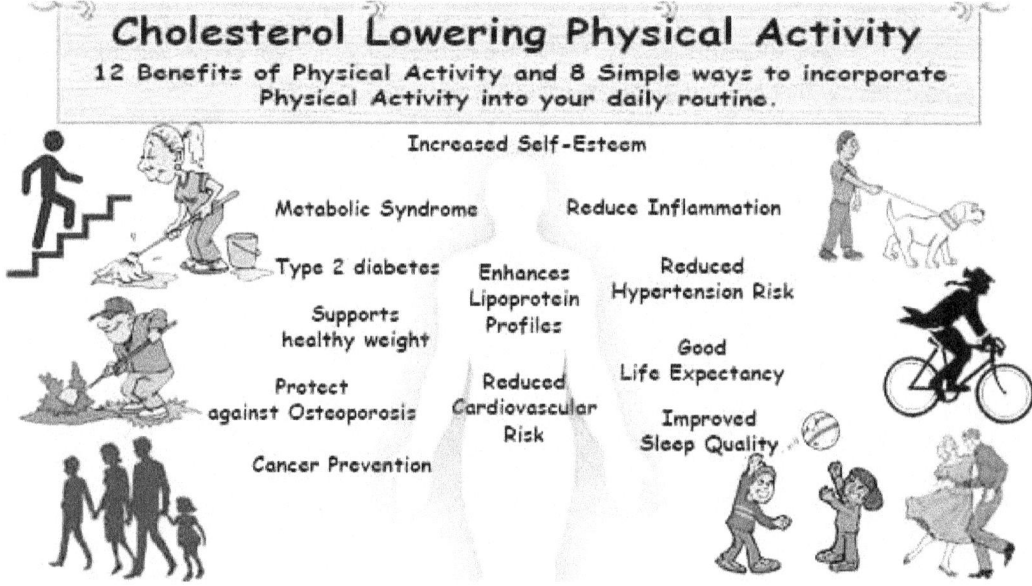

How does exercise lower lipid profile?

Exercise makes your heart beat faster and breathes harder, thus burns more calories. Lungs expand more and energize the whole body.

The mechanisms of lipid lowering effect of exercise and its suggested pathways:

1. During exercise, your skeletal muscles start utilizing lipids instead of glycogen that decreases plasma lipid levels.

2. Exercise stimulates the production and actions of certain enzymes that help move cholesterol from your blood to your liver (reverse cholesterol transport). Then cholesterol is converted into bile for fat digestion or excreted out.

3. Exercise will lower the levels of an enzyme (cholesteryl ester transfer protein) that decrease HDL level in your plasma. That is why exercise proportionally increases HDL cholesterol level.

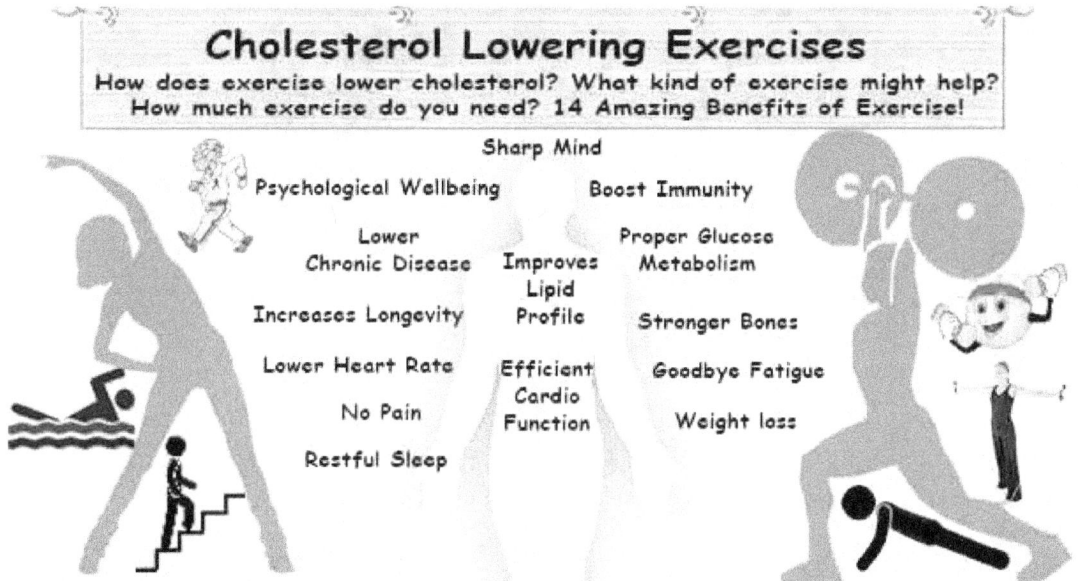

What kind of exercise might help lower cholesterol?

Exercise has positive impacts on the pathogenesis, symptomatology and physical fitness of individuals with dyslipidemia, and to reduce cholesterol levels.

Numerous studies prove the effectiveness of both aerobic exercise and resistance training in controlling/improving cholesterol levels and your cardiovascular health.

Aerobic and resistance training combination might produce even better improvement in cholesterol levels.

How much exercise do you need to lower cholesterol level?

Start exercising in intervals of 10 to 15 minutes and increase slowly to 60 minutes over time.

Your Exercise intensity should be low or moderate level as your endurance increases.

You want to strive to perform and complete at least 60 minutes of moderate intensity exercise 7 days a week to improve cholesterol levels, lower blood pressure and reduce your heart attack or stroke risk.

A minimum of at least **250 minutes of moderate intensity** exercise or **90 minutes of vigorous intensity** exercise per week is recommendable for overall cardiovascular health.

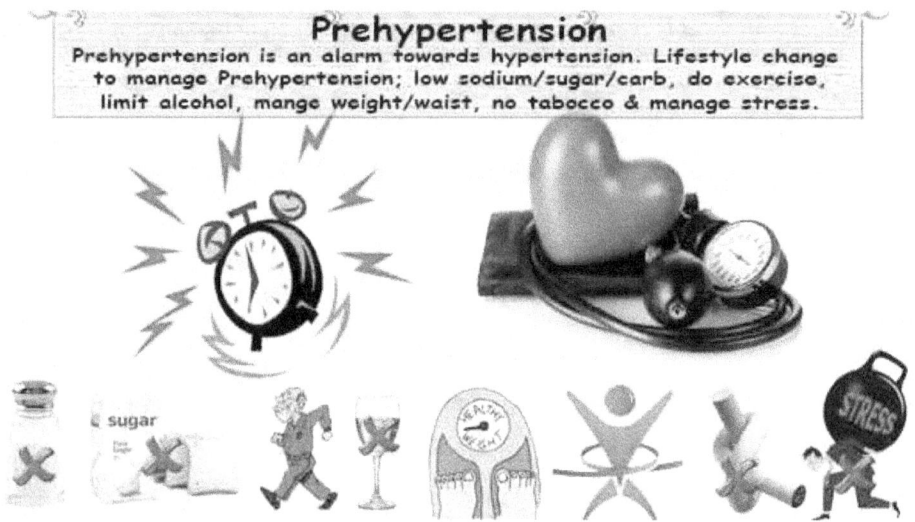

Hypertension

Hypertension, or high Blood Pressure (BP), greatly increases the risk of developing CVD.

Hypertension is also known as the Silent Killer because you normally do not know that you suffer from it until it manifests and then it is usually too late.

Hypertension is especially prevalent among Black and poor minorities with approximately 42% of Black Men and 47% of Black Women being diagnosed as suffering from hypertension.

It is estimated that 75 million people in the United States have hypertension, which is defined as having a BP of **140/90 or higher**.

High Blood Pressure

The greatest risk factor for heart disease.

Uncontrolled, can injure or kill you.

The "Silent Killer" because it often has no symptoms.

1:3 Adults has HBP **AND** 21% don't know they have it.

Of those with HBP, 69% are receiving treatment,
--and only 45% have blood pressure under control.

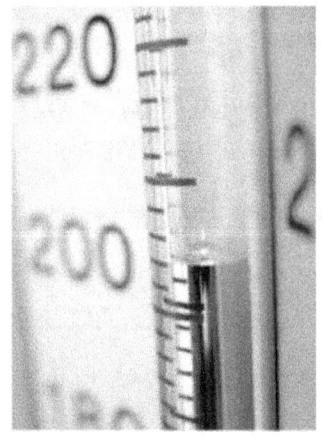

Stage 1 hypertension is defined as having a **SBP** of **140 to 159 mmHg** or **a DBP** of **90 to 99 mmHg**. For those who have this type of hypertension, a variety of nonpharmacological approaches to reducing BP are often recommended at first; however, if their BP is not normalized with lifestyle changes, medications may be prescribed.

Dietary change includes reducing sodium intake, which has been shown to independently lower SBP and DBP by 5 and 3 mmHg, respectively (13,15). Obesity is linked to hypertension, and research shows that a loss of 1 kg of body weight decreases SBP and DBP by 1.6 and 1.3 mmHg, respectively.

Also, Moving YourSelf and participating in endurance activities have been shown to decrease the SBP and DBP by **7 and 6 mmHg**, respectively, in those dealing with hypertension.

Stage 2 hypertension (SBP of 160-179 mmHg or DBP of 100-109 mmHg) is more serious, and it is typically controlled through medication.

Stage 3 hypertension refers to a persistent elevation in BP (SBP >180 mmHg or DBP >110 mmHg) with target-organ damage. This may include damage to the heart (such as enlargement of the left ventricle), damage to the kidneys leading to renal insufficiency, and damage to the eyes caused by small hemorrhages in the blood vessels.

All stages of hypertension are preventable and/or controllable!

Performing endurance exercise at moderate intensities (40%-60% VO2 Max) has been shown to reduce BP.

Moderate-intensity exercise should be done frequently and for durations long enough to expend a large number of calories.

Applying the science of Eating To Live, changing or stopping detrimental activities like smoking, and Moving YourSelf to control your body weight contribute to the successful control and maintenance an appropriate BP once it has been normalized.

- **Blood Pressure**
Pressure under which the blood travels as it is ejected from the left ventricle
Blood vessel constriction increases BP; dilation reduces BP

1. **DIASTOLE:**
Heart is relaxed, BP is reduced
2. **SYSTOLE:**
Heart contracts, BP is increased

BP during aerobic exercise;
- Systolic BP increases in direct proportion to increased exercise intensity
- Diastolic BP changes little if any during endurance exercise, regardless of intensity

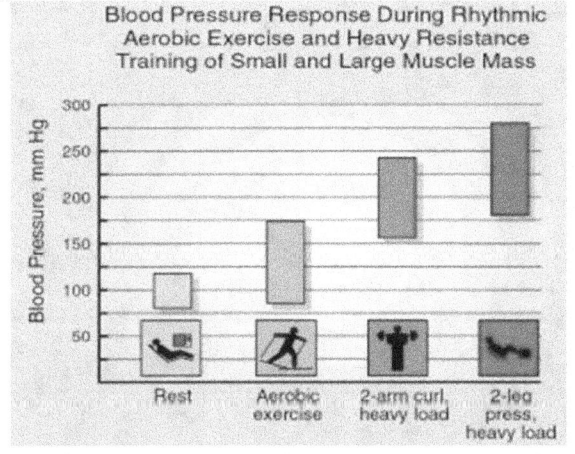

Blood Pressure Response During Rhythmic Aerobic Exercise and Heavy Resistance Training of Small and Large Muscle Mass

Evidence for Exercise Training

Fifty years ago, the most common advice given to patients who had experienced an MI was to take several weeks of complete bed rest. Today, however, exercise training is an ordinary part of treatment for people with CHD. …..

That's right – Move SomeThing ….. Move YourSelf into Heart Health and Wellness!

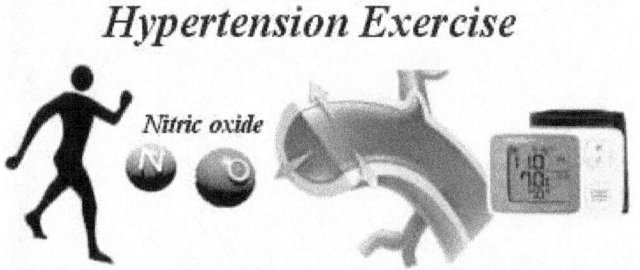

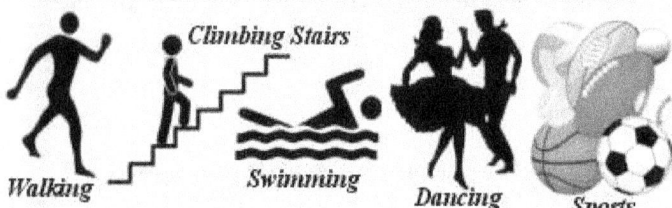

a good Cardiac rehabilitation program is designed with the use a multidisciplinary approach of education and exercise to help clients with heart disease return to normal function within the limits of their disease.

There is no question that patients with CHD have improved cardiovascular function as a result of exercising.

Moderate reductions in body fat, BP, total cholesterol, serum triglycerides, and LDL-C have been shown to occur with regular exercise, along with increases in HDL-C.

A major focus of cardiac rehabilitation programs is to reduce the occurrence of subsequent MIs. This is referred to as **secondary prevention** of CHD. The Framingham Heart Study has shown that people who have experienced one heart attack are at increased risk of a second heart attack.

Also, the likelihood of recurrence clearly is associated with many of the same risk factors that caused atherosclerosis in the first place.

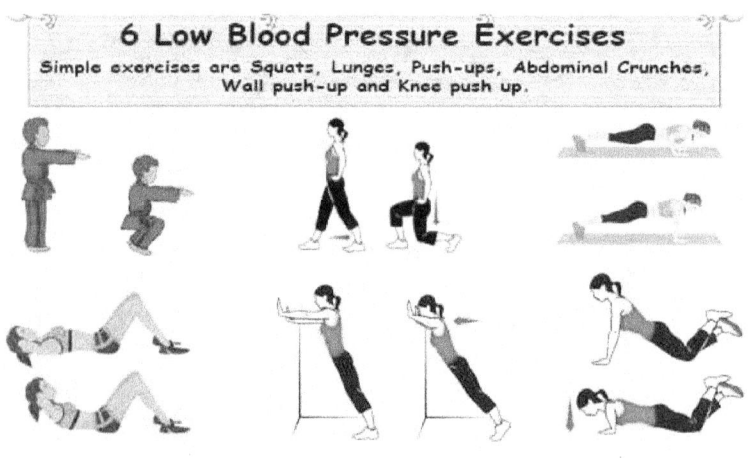

In general, the research has shown that a cardiac rehabilitation program involving exercise results in a 20% to 25% reduction in all-cause and cardiovascular mortality after an MI. This is good news, because it indicates that such patients derive a substantial benefit from participating in cardiac rehabilitation. In addition, patients gain an improved sense of well-being.

Several of the patients in the Farmington study showed actual **reversal** of blockages in their coronary arteries, which reinforced the knowledge that this condition can, in some cases, be treated with nonsurgical interventions.

Cardiac rehabilitation programs help people with heart disease regain their fitness and return to normal, everyday activities. The benefits of such programs include increased work capacity and reduced cardiovascular risk factors. ***Cardiac rehabilitation programs also generally lower the risk of a second heart attack.***

One of the most exciting developments in cardiac rehabilitation in recent years is the demonstration that lifestyle modification CAN reverse CAD.

Science and research studies show that a program consisting of Eating To Live, Moving YourSelf, meditation, smoking cessation, and Breathing properly all contributed to the successful control and/or prevention of the atherosclerosis.

All you have to do is …….

Move SomeThing!

What are you Moving?

YourSelf!

Where are you going?

Abundant Life!

Exercise!

Among Americans age 20 and older, 145 million are overweight or obese (BMI of 25.0 kg/m2 and higher).

76.9 million men and 68.1 million women.

Increased body fat — especially if a lot of it is at your waist — increases risk of health problems including high blood pressure, high blood cholesterol and diabetes.

Those overweight/obese can significantly reduce risk for heart disease by weight loss.

When coming up with a fitness and nutrition plan to lose weight, one must understand calorie intake and amount of energy calories you're burning off with different levels of physical activity.

It's a matter of balancing healthy eating (caloric energy) with the (molecular) energy that leaves your body through a healthy level of exercise.

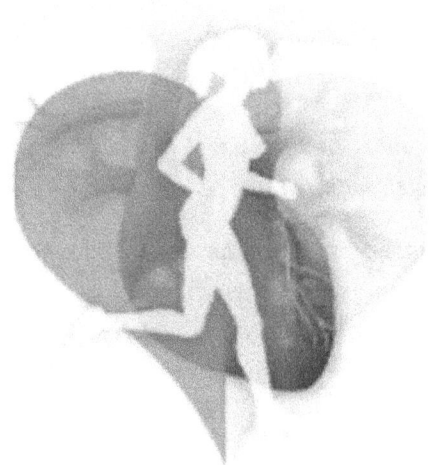

CENTRAL ILLUSTRATION: Metabolically Healthy Obese and Incident Cardiovascular Disease

Normal Weight Metabolically Healthy
- BMI 18.50-24.99 kg/m^2
- No Dyslipidemia
- No Hypertension
- No Type 2 Diabetes

Obese Metabolically Healthy
- BMI ≥30.00 kg/m^2
- No Dyslipidemia
- No Hypertension
- No Type 2 Diabetes

↓

Cardiovascular Disease

- 49% Increased Risk of Coronary Heart Disease
- 7% Increased Risk of Cerebrovascular Disease
- 96% Increased Risk of Heart Failure

THE 10 MOST OBESE COUNTRIES ON EARTH
According To The World Health Organization | % Obesity rate

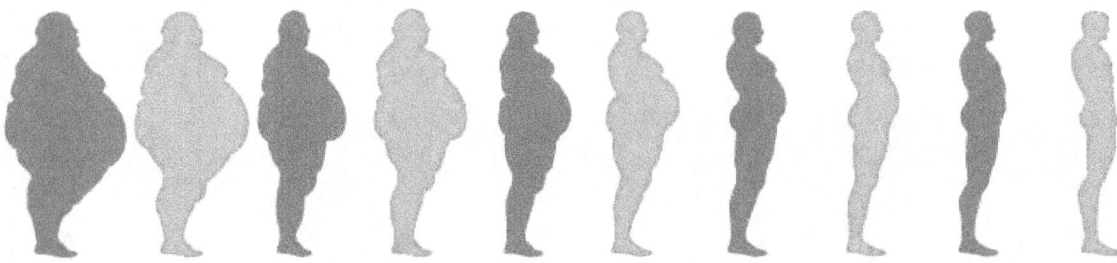

United States of America	New Zealand	Australia	Czech Republic	United Arab Emirates	Slovakia	Norway	Canada	Germany	Hungary
33.8%	26.5%	24.6%	24.2%	23%	23%	22.4%	22%	20.2%	18.8%

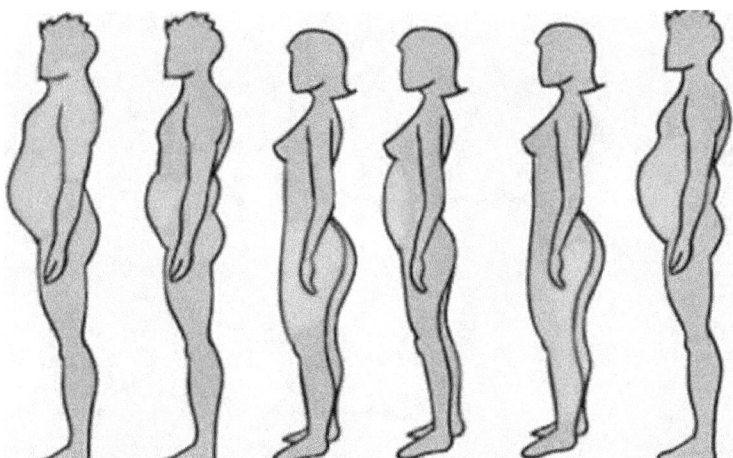

Estimated (Age-Adjusted) Percentage of US Adults with Obesity by Race/Ethnicity, 2013–2014 NHANES Data

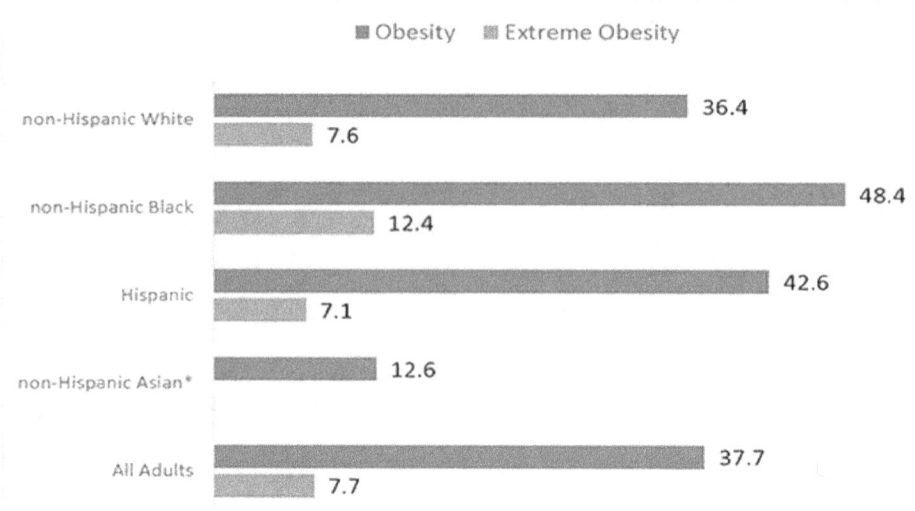

*data for extreme obesity in Asians were not reported since the numbers are close to zero.

America Is Fatter Than Ever
Obesity prevalence among adults and youths in the U.S.'

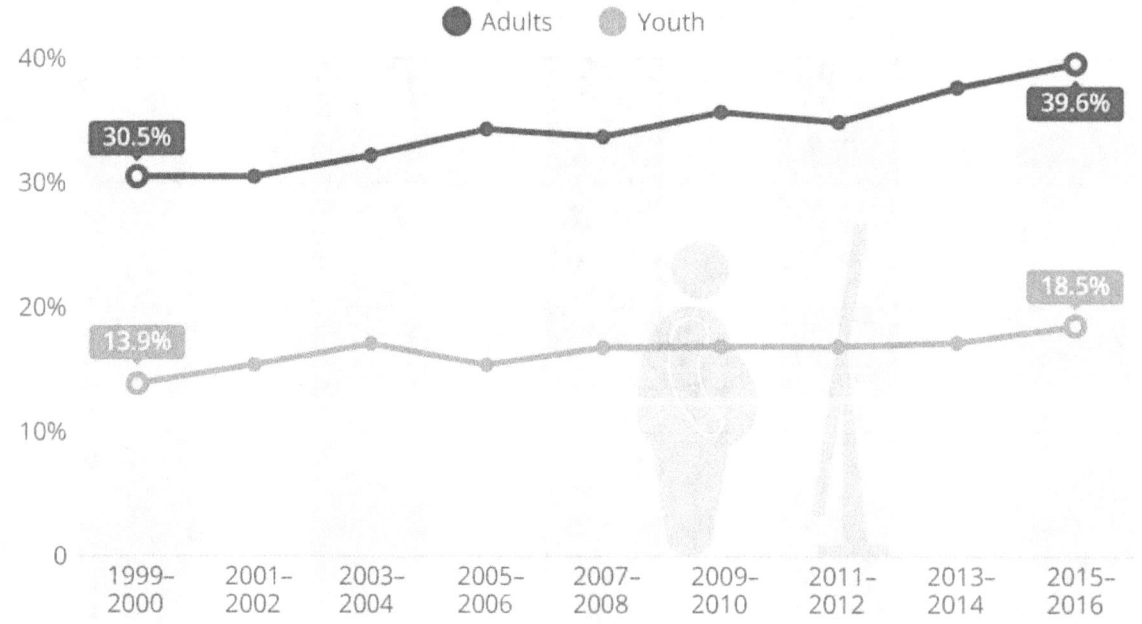

OBESITY AT A GLANCE

Adult obesity rate

32% nationwide **24%** Minnesota

19 states have a lower rate than Minnesota

Obese or overweight children

Rate in children ages 10-17

#1 Mississippi **44%**

#50 Minnesota **23%**

IN THE UNITED STATES

Obesity rate by race

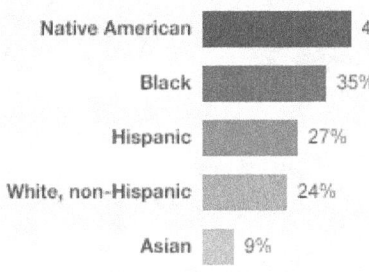

- Native American — 42%
- Black — 35%
- Hispanic — 27%
- White, non-Hispanic — 24%
- Asian — 9%

IN MINNESOTA

Growing concerns about children

14% of children in the state's Women, Infants and Children (WIC) program are overweight.

35% of Minnesota students receive school lunch at for free or at a reduced cost.

28% the increase in the number of students receiving free and reduced lunch since the 2002-03 school year.

OBESITY COSTS

In 2000, **$117 billion** was spent on obesity and associated health care costs. Based on national estimates, Minnesota's financial burden for obesity in 2004 was **$1.3 billion.**

Causes of Obesity

There's usually not just one cause of obesity. Multiple factors may interact and contribute to the condition.

- **Eating** more calories than the body requires
- **Pregnancy** difficulty losing weight after childbirth
- **Environment** demanding work schedule, easy access to inexpensive high-caloric processed food, high cost of gym membership
- **Emotional or psychological factors** such as stress, depression or low self-esteem
- **Certain medical conditions** such as polycystic ovary syndrome, a hormonal disorder
- **Lack of sleep** imbalance of hormones that control appetite
- **Genes and family history** families share diet and lifestyle habits
- **Medications** such as some antidepressants
- **Lack of exercise**

Chapter Nineteen

Exercise and Obesity

*****

Obesity characterized by excessive adiposity. It can be documented by examining the relationship between height and weight (e.g., BMI) or by evaluating percent body fat (%BF). Because BMI requires simple measurements and, for the majority of adults, closely relates to body fatness, it has become the clinically preferred method of assessing obesity. Generally accepted guidelines classify a BMI of 30 kg · m^{-2} or higher as obese.

The following are the current subclasses of obesity:

- **Class I obesity**—30.0 to 34.9 kg · m^{-2}

- **Class II obesity**—35.0 to 39.9 kg · m^{-2}

- **Class III (extreme) obesity**—40 kg · m^{-2} or higher

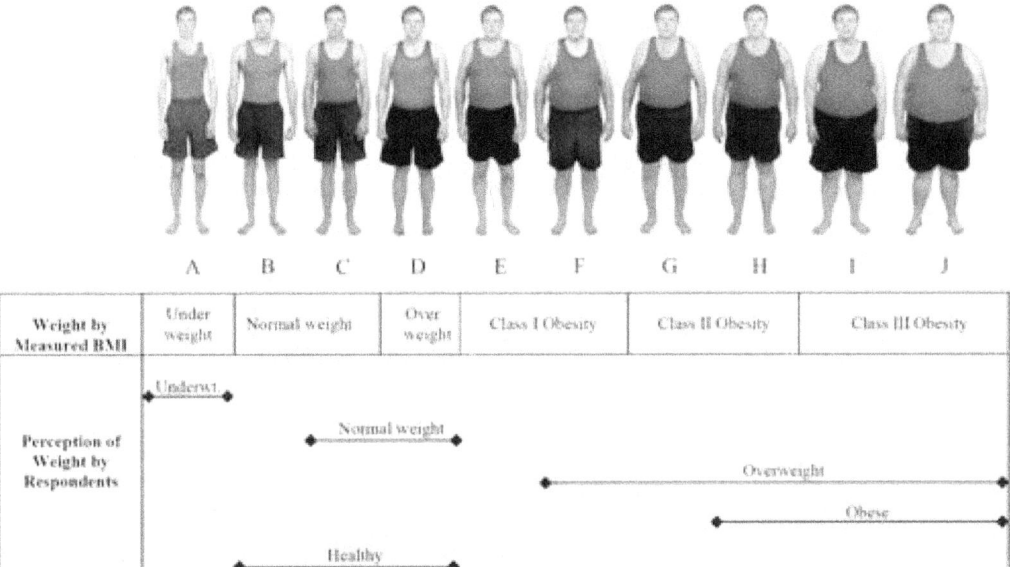

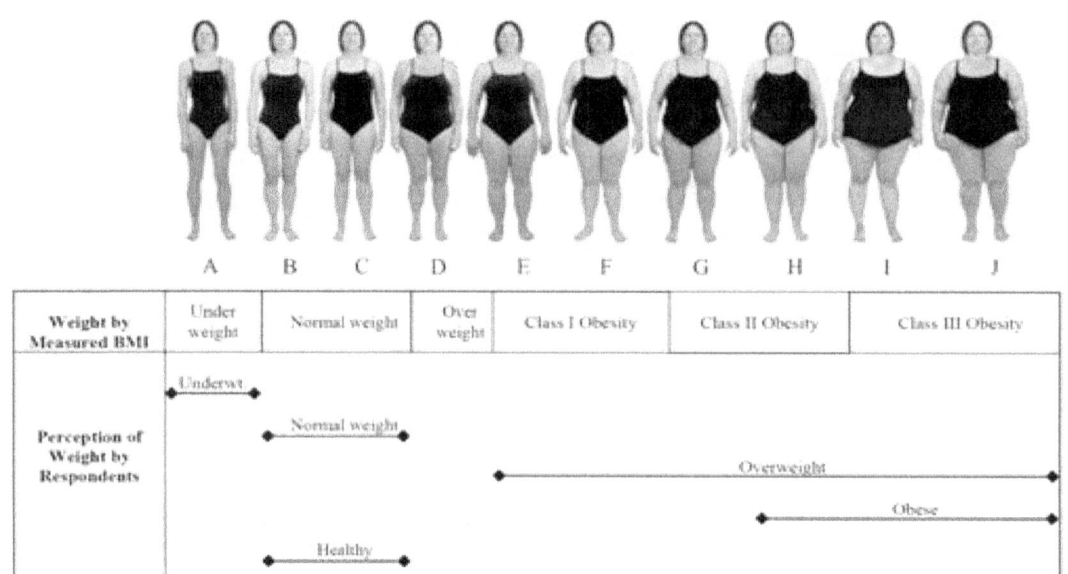

Although there are no universally agreed-upon standards for classifying obesity from %BF, a %BF of >38% for females and >25% for males generally is considered to be obese.

Another tool used to screen for obesity is Waist Circumference (WC).

Adiposity located in the abdominal region is strongly linked with chronic disease risk; therefore, a WC of ≥102 cm (40 in.) in men or ≥88 cm (35 in.) in women is used to classify individuals with abdominal obesity.

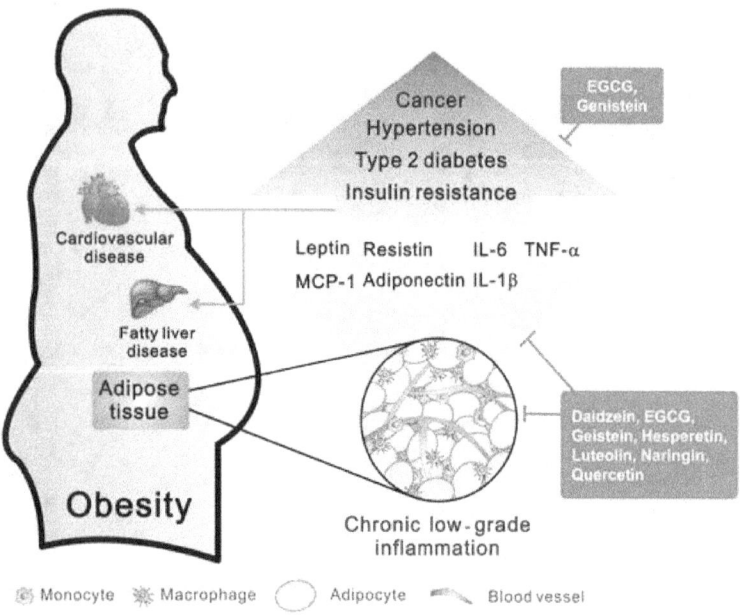

Causes of Obesity

Although consuming calories in excess of daily caloric need is an easily identified culprit in the etiology of obesity, this condition is much more complex than suggested by that simple explanation. Both biological (e.g., genetic predisposition attributable to lower-than-normal metabolic rate) and psychological (e.g., poor body image) factors can and do also contribute to obesity and they also pose significant obstacles when a person attempts to lose weight.

Some studies show that genetics contribute around 25% to 40% of the variation in body composition. There are many biological factors have been identified as possible mechanisms that predispose a person to obesity. These factors include production of leptin (a protein), activity of your sympathetic nervous system, in addition to several neuropeptides as well as the production and function of some of your hormones.

Why is obesity an issue?

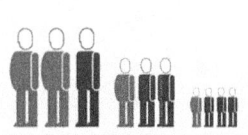

It's widespread

Two thirds of adults, **a quarter** of 2–10 year olds and **one third** of 11–15 year olds are overweight or obese

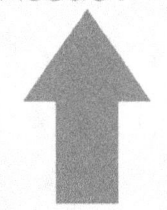

Prevalence remains high

Overweight and obesity in adults is predicted to reach **70% by 2034**

More adults and children are now severely obese

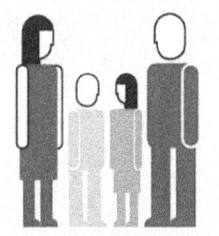

Consequences are costly

A high BMI...
- is costly to health and social care
- has wider economic and societal impacts

Suggested pathways through which these factors work include lowering your resting metabolic rate, influencing your eating behaviors, and slowing the rate of your fat oxidation.

Although some biological factors clearly contribute to the condition of obesity, the imbalance between **energy intake** and **expenditure** ultimately leads to fat accumulation.

Education on the role of applying the Sciences of Eating To Live and Moving YourSelf to maintain a healthy weight is an important aspect of building your Supreme Health and Fitness!

The unfortunate prevalence of obesity here in the United States and in many countries around the world has increased dramatically during the last part of the 20th century. Here in the U.S., the prevalence of obesity rose from 13.4% in the early 1960s to 33.8% in 2007. Recent national surveys reveal that 68% of American adults now have a BMI of 25 kg $\cdot$ m^{-2} or higher and therefore are classified as **overweight** or **obese**.

Unfortunately, Black people and Mexican Americans are groups who lead in and that are particularly at risk for overweight and obesity, with having prevalence rates of **73.8%** and 78.8%, respectively, for BMI $\geq$25 kg $\cdot$ m^{-2}.

According to the criteria for waist circumference, there are approximately **38.3%** of men and **59.9%** of women in these population groups that have abdominal obesity.

Another disturbing trend is the increasing rate of obesity among children, also known as childhood obesity. Recent national surveys reveal that over 40% of American children are overweight (at or above the 85th percentile for BMI), over 30% are obese (at or above the 95th percentile for BMI), and over 20% are extremely obese (at or above the 97th percentile for BMI).

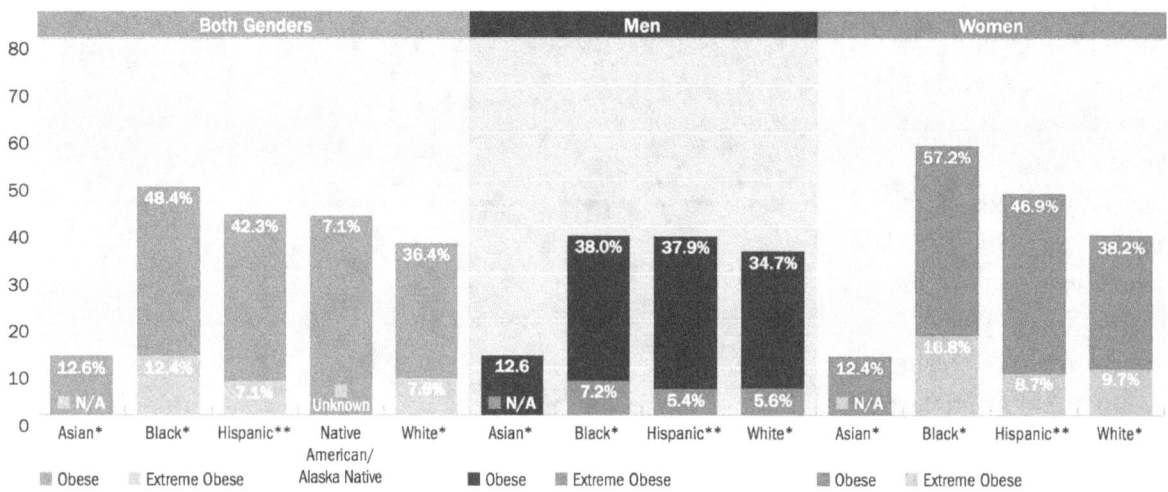

The rapid increase in obesity in the United States over the last four decades supports the contention that lifestyle choices (i.e., diet and physical activity), not genetics, are primarily responsible for the increasing prevalence of obesity.

Obesity is linked with increased mortality and morbidity rates. The diseases and conditions associated with obesity include CHD, CHF, stroke, type 2 diabetes, hypertension, dyslipidemia, gallbladder disease, osteoarthritis, some cancers (e.g., breast, colon), sleep apnea, and respiratory problems.

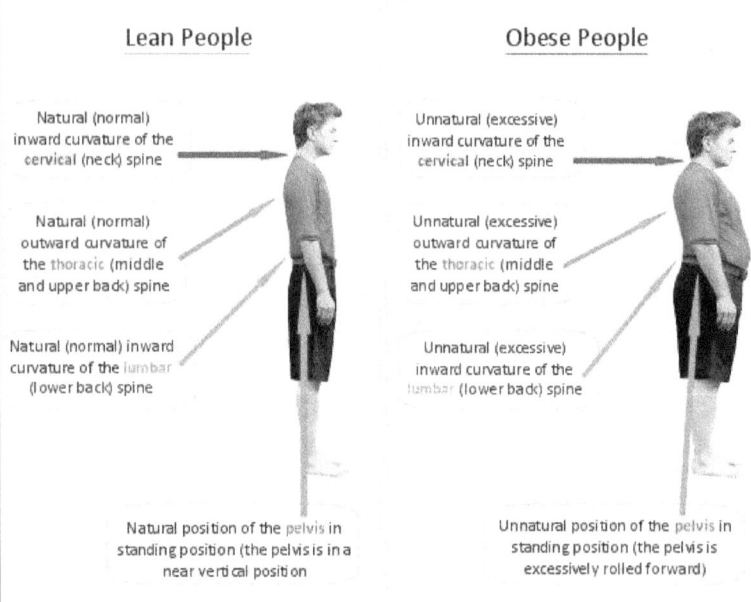

Women who are obese are more likely to experience menstrual irregularities and complications with pregnancy. Estimates of annual U.S. deaths attributable to obesity range from 112,000 to 300,000. Deaths due to CVD, diabetes, and kidney disease are particularly related to obesity. Recent reviews of the costs related to obesity reveal the toll this condition places on the economy.

It is estimated that the medical costs of an obese person are 30% higher than those of a person of normal weight.

Here in the United States, it is estimated that the cost of treating those with the conditions of overweight and obesity is approximately $114 billion and accounts for over 10% of health care spending.

Physical Activity in Prevention and Treatment of Obesity

The rapid increase in obesity prevalence appears linked to both low physical activity and excessive energy intake. This suggests that increasing physical activity and reducing caloric intake will lower rates of obesity. Prospective studies suggest that active people are less likely to be obese, and those who maintain an active lifestyle are least likely to become obese over time.

The data from the National Weight Control Registry (NWCR) suggest that regular aerobic exercise is common among those who successfully maintain significant weight loss.

REASONS TO MAINTAIN A HEALTHY WEIGHT AND KEEP ACTIVE

The adenocarcinoma subtype of esophageal cancer, colorectal, endometrial, gallbladder, kidney, pancreatic, and postmenopausal breast cancers have been causally linked to being overweight or obese.

7 TYPES OF CANCER

Sedentary behavior may increase the risk for developing colorectal, endometrial, ovarian, and prostate cancers.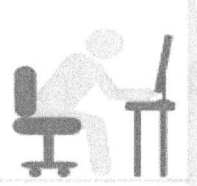

About one in every three new cases of cancer diagnosed in the United States is related to being overweight or obese, being inactive, and/or eating poorly. **33% CANCER CASES**

Regular physical activity can decrease an individual's risk of developing colon, endometrial, and postmenopausal breast cancers.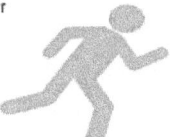

Obesity, lack of regular physical activity, and sedentary behavior are linked to worse outcomes, including increased risk for death, for patients with a number of types of cancer. 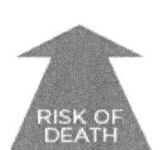 **RISK OF DEATH**

Also, in a recent international consensus meeting concluded that 45 to 60 min of daily moderate activity is needed to prevent obesity.

A number of studies have used exercise as a means for treating obesity, with research showing that greater weight loss and management is accomplished when a person applies Eating To Live in conjunction with Moving SomeThing.

There is also evidence that a combination of dietary restriction and exercise is better at helping maintain weight loss than is either method alone. This is understandable because both POOR dietary habits and LACK of movement are BOTH the #2 Actual Cause of Death.

Active people are less likely to be overweight or obese. Exercise can be an important part of a weight-loss program and is a key to maintaining weight loss.

6 Major Types of Obesity & EASY Solutions!

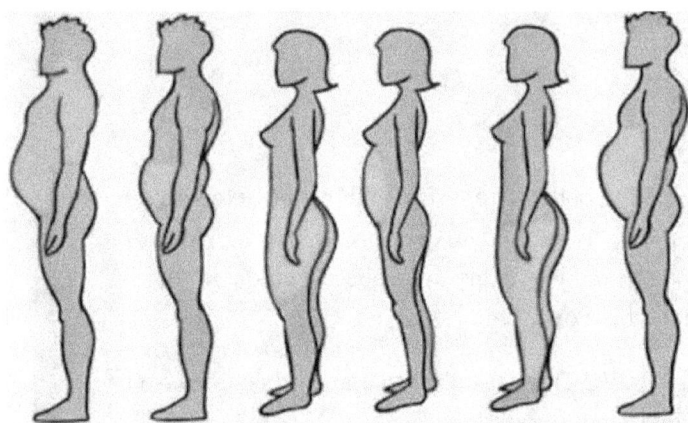

- **Obesity from food** – this is the most common type of obesity in the world and is the manifestation of excessive intake of processed and manufactured food-like items and sugars.

To solve this, You simply have to apply the Science of Eating To Live!

You will have to make some changes in your diet - discarding the 'FAKE' sugars and food-like items and Moving YourSelf at least 60 minutes daily. Over-eating creates an Energy Imbalance of Too Much Energy IN vs Too Little Energy Expended.

By Moving for at least 60 minutes a day, you create the Energy/Nutrition deficit so when you eat, you don't consume MORE Calories than you expended.

- **Obesity caused by venous circulation** – this is genetically inherited obesity and occurs during pregnancy and in people who suffer from swollen legs. Your genetics are influenced by your dietary choices as well as your level of activity. Both of these are classified as Epigenetics- the Outside influence of your Gene Expression.

To solve this, You must apply the science of Eating To Live and Moving YourSelf for at least 60 0minutes a day. Eating To Live can set the environment for your body to heal or correct a Gene imbalance.

Moving YourSelf increases your circulation which improves the health of your arteries and veins, as well as increasing the amount of Oxygen and Nutrition to your Cells that need repair. You must Move YourSelf at least 60 minutes a day and incorporate activities Exercises like climbing stairs and running are the best MoveMents for this issue.

- **Obesity caused by "nervous stomach"** – this is caused by stress, anxiety and depression which causes these people to intake an excessive amount of sweets a lot.

To solve this, You must understand that your Emotions are energy frequencies and the best way to control these frequencies is by Moving YourSelf to USE the energy of stress, anxiety and depression and converting it into Endorphins.

The endorphins is your Positive Energy that will allow you to Rise above negative/low emotional frequencies and increase your ability to THINK.

You must apply the science of Eating To Live and control it your mental state through implementing physical activities – Moving YourSelf! The foods you eat provide energy and there are certain emotional frequencies associate with foods. Eating To Live helps you to control your external influences from food.

- **Metabolic obesity** – these people have stomach bloated like a balloon and have accumulated fat in that part. This condition appears in people who consume alcohol, have psychological issues as well as problems with breathing.

  To solve this, you must STOP the consumption of alcohol, as well as the consumption of manufactured/processed sugars. Your metabolism is based-on, balanced and maintained by Moving YourSelf for at least 60 minutes a day!

- **Gluten obesity** – this is common in women who are going through menopause and those with impaired imbalance.

  To solve this, You must understand that it is very significant to avoid prolonged sitting, smoking and alcohol, and practice exercises with weights instead.

- **Obesity from inactivity/sedentary** – it affects the parts of your body which used to be active in the past. Being sedentary creates a USE or LOSE effect your body – from your cells, tissues, muscles and organs. You are created from Motion ….. Life Is The Science of Motion.

  To solve this, You must simply begin to…..

Move SomeThing!

What are You Moving?

YourSelf!

Where Are You Going?

Abundant Life!

Exercise Testing

Typically, your initial intensity as well as your incremental increases should reflect your current fitness and activity level.

This is particularly important because of the severe deconditioning that often exists with obesity. With severe obesity or when ambulation is problematic, it may be preferable to use cycle or arm ergometry for performing activities.

The physiological response to exercise is found to be typically similar in people who are obese and people who are normal weight, except that excessive weight often reduces cardio-respiratory function.

However, comorbidities, especially hypertension and type 2 diabetes, can also significantly alter their exercise or post-exercise response.

Exercise Prescription

Weight loss, greater fitness and improved chronic disease risk factors are the primary focus of exercise programs for those who are suffer from the condition of obesity. These 3 categories are the main factors for creating or losing your ability to Heal and Healthy.

If you are obese, you should strive to begin to exercise on most, if not all, days of the week for a minimum of 250 min · wk^{-1} in order create the environment in self that helps to protect against chronic disease.

Now remember, this is just the beginning. When first beginning an exercise program, participants may be unable to exercise this long, so an initial focus of Moving YourSelf is to build enough endurance to sustain aerobic activity to reach your duration goals.

Accumulating activity in shorter bouts throughout the day is also an option.

Evidence indicates that an even greater caloric expenditure (i.e., 300-420 min · wk^{-1}) may be most beneficial for long-term weight control.

To gain maximum benefits, if you are obese, then you should strive to increase your activity to at least **45 to 60 minutes** of daily moderate activity to prevent weight **gain** and **60 to 90 minutes** for those who in order to prevent weight **regain**.

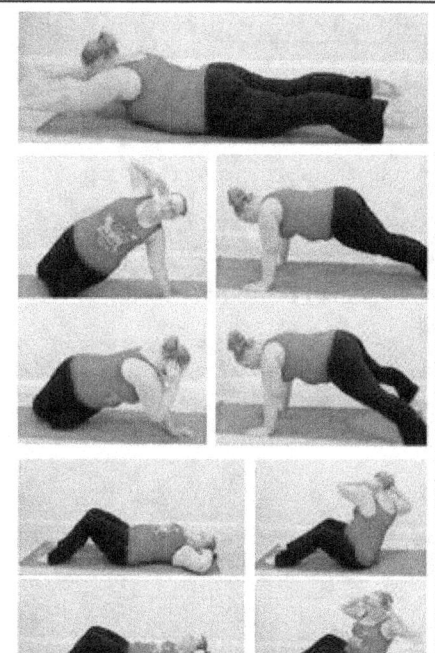

Here at Supreme Health and Fitness, I encourage people who are using exercise for weight loss or weight control to accumulate **420 min · wk^{-1}** of moderate-intensity exercise, or **250 min · wk^{-1}** of vigorous-intensity activity.

Recommendations for approaching exercise for weight loss:

- **Frequency**: 5 to 7 days · wk^{-1}.

- **Intensity**: initially moderate (40%-60% HRR), with progression to higher intensity (50%-75% HRR).

- **Duration**: progress from short, easily tolerated bouts to 45 to 60 min · day^{-1}. Multiple daily bouts can be used with bout duration of 10 min or longer.

- **Type**: aerobic exercise targeting your large muscle groups. Resistance exercise is recommended as a supplement to aerobic activity.

Special considerations:

Designing exercise programs for individuals who are obese does require some special considerations. One of the primary aims of any exercise program should be your safety. For those who are obese, avoiding orthopedic injuries is a particular concern because of the additional loading to joints. Therefore, performing low-impact activities (water exercise, cycling, and walking) are preferable when individuals who are obese begin to exercise regularly. After some weight loss and conditioning occur, they may then begin performing and participating in higher impact sports and activities.

Modification of Exercise

Several exercises may need to be modified in order to work around the excess weight and any other physical or medical limitations. Here are just a few ideas of how to modify an exercise:

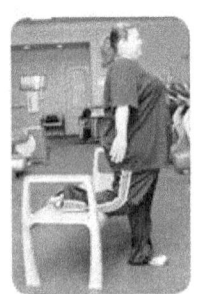
Modified Quadriceps Stretch

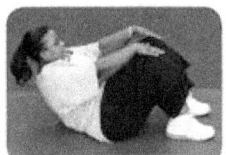
Seated Leg Lift

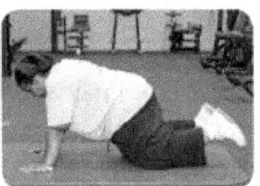
Modified Push-up

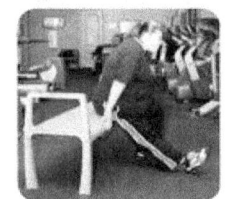
Knee Taps

Seated Hamstrings Stretch

Photos provided by the author

Another safety concern is your thermoregulation (discussed in Chapter 14 – Regulating Your Body Temperature). Because of excessive body fatness taken in conjunction with the increased energy demands of activity, keeping your body cool during exercise can be problematic if you have a lot of body fat.

Anyone with excess body fat should be encouraged to exercise at cool times of the day or in temperature-controlled environments. You should also maintain your hydration by drinking adequate amounts of water.

Resistance training should also be included and be an important component of your overall exercise program. Although resistance training typically does not burn off a large number of calories, it can serve important functions in weight loss.

During the process of weight loss, both your lean and fat tissues typically diminish. However, your lean tissue can be maintained, or at least your muscle loss can be minimized, by using resistance training during your caloric restriction.

Maintaining muscle mass benefits both your functional capacity and metabolic rate. Compared with fat, muscle is a metabolically active tissue, so maintaining lean mass helps minimize potential decreases in your metabolic rate.

A well-planned, low-fat diet with a caloric deficit of 500 to 1,000 kcal · day^{-1} gradually reduces your weight without sacrificing your nutritional needs. An appropriate distribution of macronutrients along with the necessary amounts of vitamins and minerals should be included in the dietary planning.

Diets that are low in fat, particularly saturated fat, not only are effective for weight loss but also are associated with your long-term weight maintenance.

If you are suffering from being overweight or obese, you strive to should reduce your body weight by at least 5% to gain health benefits such as lower BP and a more favorable blood lipid profile. For some individuals, an even greater reduction in body weight may optimize their health improvement.

Long-term adherence to exercise is problematic for people who have been sedentary and are obese. The most commonly reported barriers are feeling too fat to exercise, believing that their health is too poor for exercise, and believing that an injury or disability precludes participation in exercise.

Look for opportunities to increase energy expenditure through structured exercise (e.g., taking brisk 30 min walks) and lifestyle activity (e.g., substituting active for sedentary leisure pursuits).

The ability for you to manage your weight, get in-shape and significantly improve your health is Fun, Easy and simply starts with you Moving SomeThing!

You can Move YourSelf into the Successful Enjoyment of Your Abundant Life!

Modern Western Living

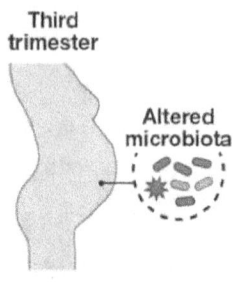
Third trimester
Altered microbiota

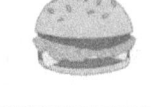
Diet

Increased Obesity Risk
Low/Neutral Risk

Epigenetics

Exercise
Low inflammation,
Normoglycemia,
Normal GWG

GUT Microbiota

Normal B/F ratio?
Low LPS,
Butyrate-SCFA,
Microbial diversity, richness

Metabolome

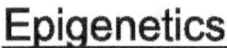 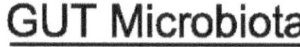

NEONATE in Utero

Smoking, Excessive
GWG, Inflammation,
High-fat diet, Fasting
glucose, HOMA-IR

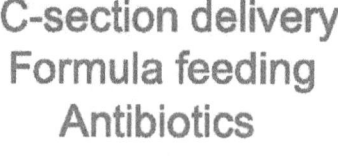
C-section delivery
Formula feeding
Antibiotics

Altered B/F ratio,
Low butyrate, SCFA,
Low microbial diversity,
High n-6:n-3 ratio,
High leptin?

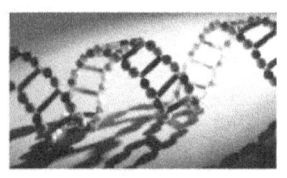 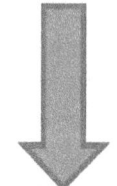 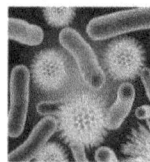

High Lactobacillaceae
Low Staphylococcus aureus
Other species?

Genetically Susceptible Host
- Methylation
- Acetylation
- miRNA
- ncRNA

Rapid weight gain
First 1,000 days of Life

Infant Gut Metagenome
- Lipid Metabolism
- Amino Acid Synthesis
- Inflammation
- Appetite Regulation

Move Something!

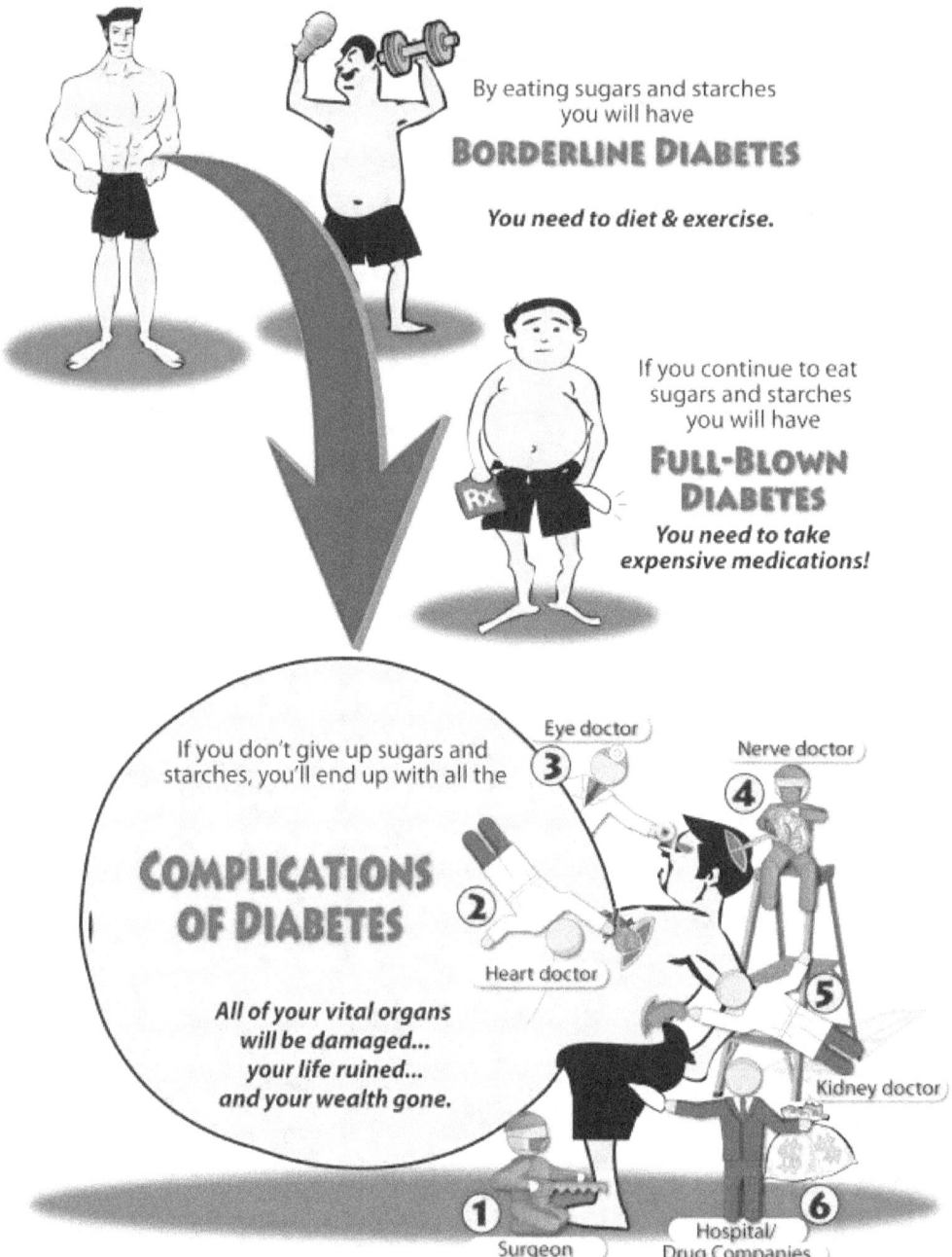

DIABETES INFOGRAPHICS #3

DIABETES
RISK FACTORS

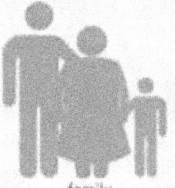
family history

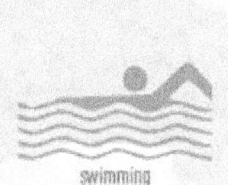
lack of exercise

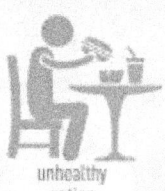
unhealthy eating

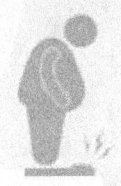
overweight

10 million people are diagnosed with type 2 diabetes each year. If you think you are at risk GET TESTED.

DIABETES INFOGRAPHIC #4

DIABETES
REDUCE YOUR RISKS

swimming

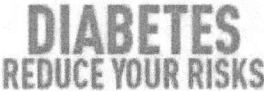
cycling

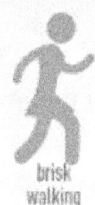
brisk walking

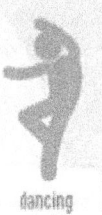
dancing

30 minutes of exercice a day can reduce your risk of developing type 2 diabetes by 40%

Move Something!

Chapter Eighteen

Exercise and Diabetes

*****

We must first understand that diabetes is a food-related condition …. You can be born with a gene abnormality …. BUT YOU CANNOT BE BORN WITH DIABETES!

Diabetes is an Imbalance that can be Solved and BALANCE Restored!

If you have created this condition or imbalance …. IT IS UP TO YOU TO CHANGE OR RE-CREATE A NEW CONDITION AND REGAIN YOUR BALANCE!

Diabetes mellitus refers to metabolic diseases that are characterized by **hyperglycemia** (i.e., elevated plasma glucose). The criteria used to diagnose diabetes are developed from your fasting blood glucose levels, your blood glucose response to ingesting carbohydrate, and/or your hemoglobin A1c (i.e., glycosylated hemoglobin) level. Hemoglobin A1c is a form of hemoglobin that is typically found in low concentrations but exists in higher concentrations when blood glucose is constantly higher than normal. Therefore, hemoglobin A1c reflects the overall blood glucose control during the past 2 to 3 months.

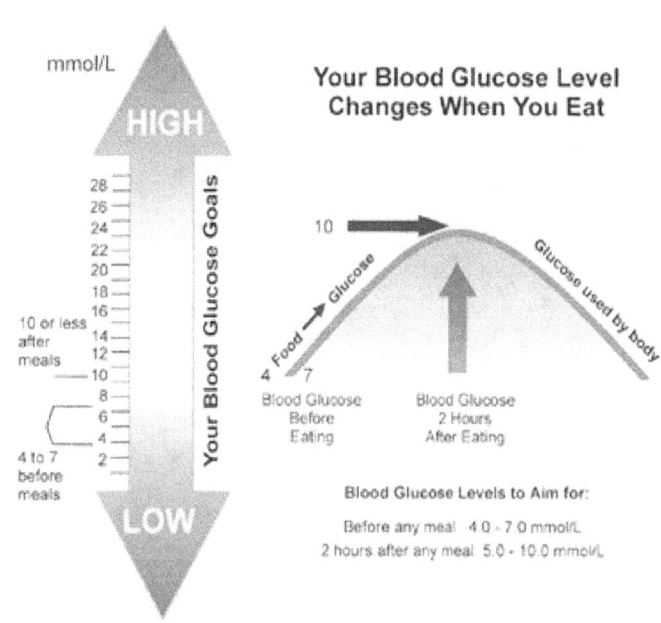

The cause of hyperglycemia has been shown to vary and depends on the form of diabetes present, with the most common forms being type 1 and type 2 diabetes.

Type 1 diabetes accounts for approximately 5% to 10% of cases of diabetes and is characterized by a deficiency of insulin often attributable to an autoimmune destruction of the insulin-producing beta cells of the pancreas.

Type 1 diabetes results from a lack of insulin. The most common cause is autoimmune destruction of the insulin-producing beta cells of the pancreas, leading to lack of insulin.

Without insulin, your cells are unable to take in glucose. Unlike type 2 diabetes, type 1 diabetes often appears early in life and is more closely linked to genetic than lifestyle factors. People with type 1 diabetes require insulin injections.

There are many types of insulin, and they vary by how rapidly they begin working, their peak time of action, and how long they continue to work

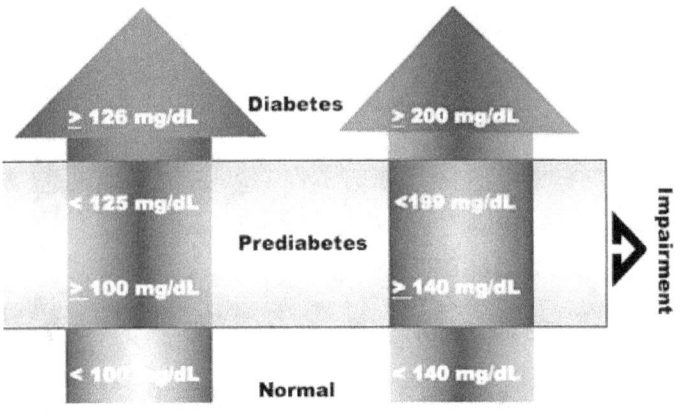

In **Type 2 diabetes,** the insulin receptors become insensitive or resistant to insulin and, because glucose cannot move readily into the cells, hyperglycemia results. This form of diabetes has both lifestyle and genetic roots. Many of those that are diagnosed with type 2 diabetes are mostly inactive and overweight or obese, with particular excessive abdominal fat.

Type 2 diabetes frequently coexists with other conditions such as hypertension and dyslipidemia. Although type 2 diabetes can appear at any age, the highest rates are seen among people aged 60 years and older. However, there is an increasing prevalence of type 2 diabetes among children, and this trend seems to be linked to increasing obesity rates. Other risk factors include a family history of type 2 diabetes (which is related to the lifestyle and diet of the family), older age and belonging to an ethnic minority – with an abnormally higher prevalence among, Black people, Hispanics and Native Americans when compared with/to Caucasians.

Although there are other forms of diabetes mellitus (e.g., gestational diabetes), type 1 and type 2 account for the vast majority of cases.

Regardless of the type, a number of complications may result from diabetes. These complications typically affect the blood vessels and nerves and include vision impairment, kidney disease, peripheral vascular disease, atherosclerosis, and hypertension.

Which underlines WHY obesity is at the root of almost every Cause of Death.

Approximately 30 million Americans have diabetes, and unfortunately, approximately 6 million of them are people who are unaware that they are diabetic. Between 90% and 95% of the cases are type 2 diabetes.

Symptoms of type 1 and type 2 diabetes may include:

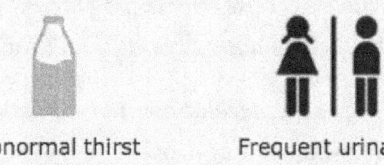

Abnormal thirst | Frequent urination | Extreme tiredness

Type 2 diabetes usually develops over time, first appearing as

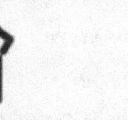

Sudden weight loss | Constant hunger | Blurred vision

impaired fasting glucose (100-125 mg · dl^{-1}) or **impaired glucose tolerance (IGT)**. Impaired glucose tolerance is a condition in which the increase in blood glucose after ingestion of carbohydrate is higher than normal and remains elevated longer than normal.

A glucose level of 140 to 199 mg · dl^{-1} 2 hr after an oral glucose tolerance test indicates impaired glucose tolerance.

A person with either impaired fasting glucose or impaired glucose tolerance is classified as having **prediabetes**.

Without intervention, prediabetes generally evolves into type 2 diabetes. It is estimated that at least 57 million Americans have prediabetes.

KEY Knowledge

Diabetes mellitus is characterized by hyperglycemia. Approximately 24 million Americans have diabetes mellitus, and the economic cost is approximately $174 billion each year.

Type 1 diabetes results from a lack of insulin production.

Type 2 diabetes, the most common form of diabetes, is characterized by the cells becoming insensitive to insulin. Risk factors for type 2 diabetes include older age, a family history of type 2 diabetes, excess weight, and inactivity.

Exercise Precautions and Safety

Medical clearance should be required if you have been diagnosed with diabetes mellitus to ensure that they can safely perform exercise.

You should discuss with their physicians how to modify their insulin dosage and/or other diabetes medications with exercise. Because exercise increases glucose uptake from peripheral tissues regardless of insulin levels, hypoglycemia may result if insulin intake is not adjusted.

Diabetes is a primary risk factor for the development of CVD, so anyone with diabetes should be screened carefully for signs and symptoms of disease.

If the exercise prescription you perform is to be more vigorous than brisk walking, it is recommended that you, particularly if you were formerly sedentary and older people, undergo a GXT with ECG monitoring and a full medical screening with particular attention to diabetes-related complications (e.g., CAD, retinopathy, nephropathy) before beginning an exercise program.

People with type 2 diabetes frequently are overweight and hypertensive and have a poor blood lipid profile; therefore, they may be taking a number of medications that can influence their exercise response.

For people who have had diabetes for a number of years, peripheral neuropathy may be a problem. Damage to the sensory nerves in the feet can lead to ulcerations, and if there is damage to blood vessels, healing can be slow. Because of these and other issues, conducting a thorough medical history is particularly important with those seeking exercise remedies.

Guidelines for Higher-Risk Clients With Diabetes

Diabetic individuals who meet one of the following criteria should undergo diagnostic exercise tests (e.g., ECG stress testing) before beginning any exercise programming:

- Older than 40 yr

- Older than 30 yr with diabetes more than 10 yr

- Older than 30 yr and hypertensive

- Older than 30 yr and a smoker

- Older than 30 yr and dyslipidemic

- Older than 30 yr with retinopathy

- Older than 30 yr with nephropathy, including microalbuminuria

- Anyone with known or suspected CAD, cerebrovascular disease, peripheral artery disease, autonomic neuropathy, or advanced nephropathy with renal failure

Because of the increased risks for exercise-related complications associated with diabetes mellitus, physician clearance should be obtained before exercise testing.

The type of tests will depend on the person's health needs and type of exercises.

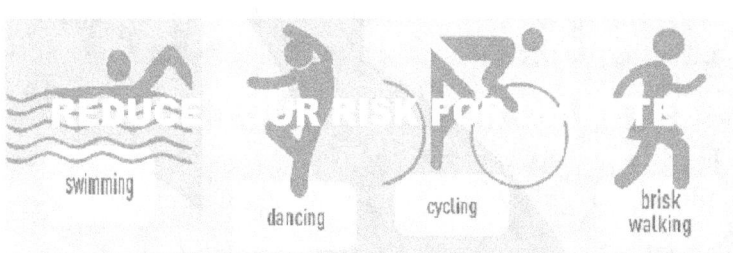

Understanding Exercise Programs for Those With Diabetes

Exercise can provide many benefits to individuals with type 1 or type 2 diabetes. This is particularly true because of the strong link between diabetes and CVD and the role that exercise plays in reducing CVD risk. Remember, CVD is the #1 Leading Cause of Death.

Unfortunately, research and studies show that people with diabetes are much less likely to exercise than their nondiabetic peers.

Type 1 Diabetes:

Although research is still being conducted on the prevention and cure of Type 1 diabetes, exercise is being proven to be a major component in the methods of prevention and/or cure of Type 1 diabetes and presents several other health benefits that underscore WHY exercise should be encouraged in this particular population.

Exercise improves insulin sensitivity and reduces disease risk for people with diabetes, much like in the population without diabetes. Because of the high rate of CVD among people with diabetes, exercise can promote overall well-being. Exercise protects against CAD, dyslipidemia, hypertension, and obesity.

Increased physical activity and improved physical fitness also promote psychological health and quality of life.

A person with type 1 diabetes must carefully consider modifying insulin dosage and carbohydrate ingestion before beginning an exercise program.

Increasing the intake of carbohydrate or reducing insulin dosage is often necessary to maintain glucose control and to avoid hypoglycemia that can result from exercise. The adjustment in carbohydrate intake and insulin dosage depends on the intensity and duration of activity.

Your Glucose should be measured before initiating an exercise session. If your glucose is <100 mg · dl^{-1}, then you should ingest carbohydrates (20-30 g) before beginning exercise.

If your glucose is >300 mg · dl^{-1} but without ketosis, then it is conventionally safe and can undertake moderate-intensity exercise only if you are feeling well and are well hydrated; otherwise exercise should be delayed.

If you have type 1 diabetes and was previously inactive, your progression should be slow, with careful monitoring of your blood glucose and symptoms of cardiovascular and metabolic distress.

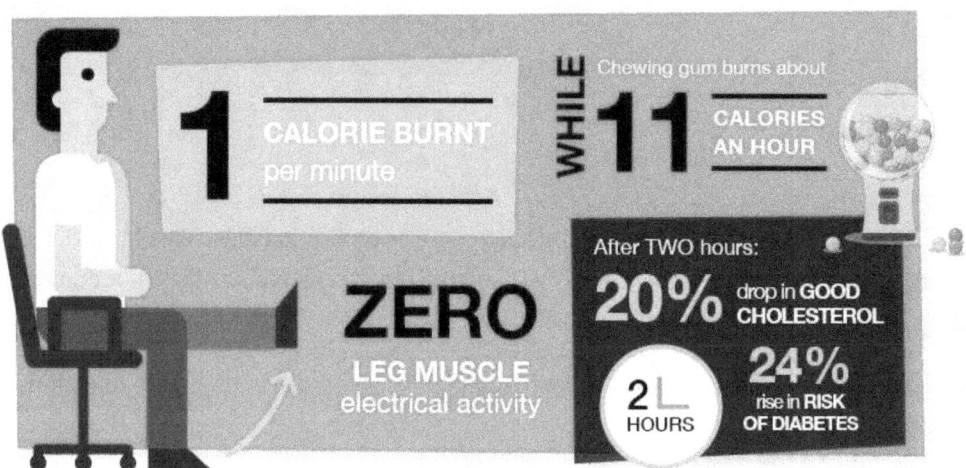

Type 2 Diabetes:

Exercise helps prevent and treat Type 2 diabetes. Inactivity and obesity are common characteristics shared by people with type 2 diabetes. Research has shown that individuals who are regularly active are 30% to 50% less likely to develop type 2 diabetes compared with their inactive counterparts.

Additionally, people who have impaired glucose tolerance are significantly less likely to develop type 2 diabetes if they begin to exercise regularly.

Exercise is highly recommended—for most people with type 2 diabetes, including those with complications.

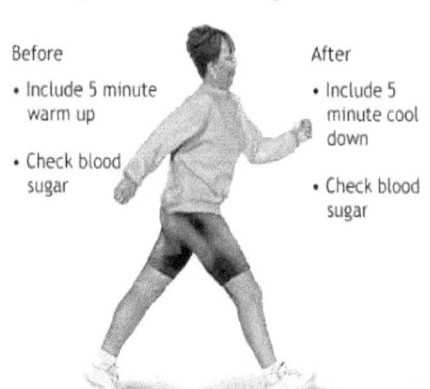

A person with type 2 diabetes can use exercise to help control their blood sugar levels and provide energy their muscles need to function throughout the day.

Evidence is mounting that people with type 2 diabetes experience better glucose tolerance and improved insulin sensitivity through regular exercise.

This means that you significantly control yourself by constantly and consistently Moving YourSelf!

You can literally Move YourSelf into Healing, Health and your Abundant Life!

There are a number of reasons why exercise can benefit the treatment of type 2 diabetes, including the following:

- *Lower fasting blood glucose concentrations*
- *Better glucose tolerance (less of a spike in glucose after eating)*
- *Improved insulin sensitivity (more glucose uptake with a given amount of insulin)*
- *Weight control (increased lean mass and reduced fat mass)*
- *Improved lipid profiles*
- *Reduction in BP for those with hypertension*
- *Lower risk of CVD*
- *Stress management (stress can affect glucose control via increased levels of catecholamines)*

As I previously stated, exercise has been shown to be effective in preventing and treating type 2 diabetes.

I want you to Understand that regardless of the type of diabetes, exercise benefits people with diabetes in several other ways.

Diabetes is an Energy Imbalance ….. And your body is created to BALANCE itself and achieve Homeostasis. Diabetes is a Self-Imposed IMBALANCE ….. The Solution is to restoring BALANCE is Self-Imposed!

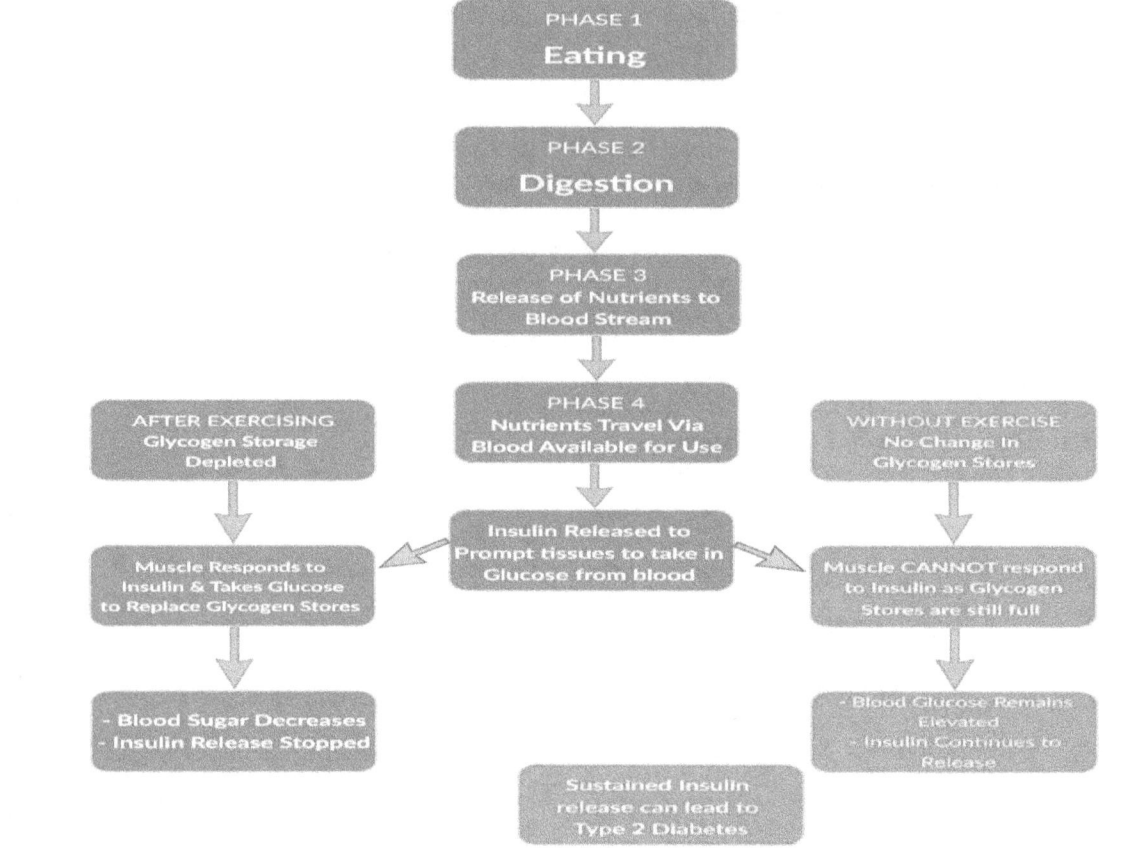

EATING …. Following the ingestion of food, your body begins to works hard to break down (digest) the food to the core nutrients that can be used to keep your body healthy. After the food is digested, the nutrients are released into your blood to be transported around your body.

GLUCOSE (SUGAR) …. One of the most prominent nutrients that is released following digestion of carbohydrates is glucose (also known as sugar). Glucose is your #1 fuel source and helps provide energy to your muscles, organs and especially your brain. Once in your blood, glucose travels around and can be accepted into your cells for use.

INSULIN …. Once your body receives a fresh supply of glucose, your pancreas releases insulin which helps inform your body's cells that there is plenty of glucose that is available for use. The release of insulin is vital to keep your body's vital cells working by ensuring they have glucose available for energy.

GLYCOGEN …. Glycogen is the storage form of glucose. When there is extra glucose, glycogen is formed and the glucose is preserved for later use. The liver and muscles are the main locations where glycogen can be stored.

Move Something!

MUSCLES .... Muscles are one of the biggest users of glucose. They need it so often that they have plenty of storage space for extra glucose (glycogen) that can be saved for when the muscle needs to work.

AFTER EXERCISE ..... As your Move YourSelf and exercise or engage in any physical activity, your muscles use glucose as energy to keep your muscle working = You Moving. Once the glucose runs out, your muscle takes the glycogen out of storage and uses that for energy. The muscle is then able to take more glucose from your blood (if it's available) and replenish the storage - ready for your next movement.

WITHOUT EXERCISE ..... The health epidemic issue that has arisen in our society revolves around SEDENTARY. This means that your aren't Moving enough and your muscles are not being used for large portions of the day. When your muscle isn't used, the glycogen stores in them remain full. If you continue to eat & digest and have excess glucose you create the environment of there being nowhere left to store it. With nowhere to go, the glucose remains IN your blood and continues to circulate waiting to be taken by your cells. With the copious amounts of blood glucose, your pancreas continues to release insulin to keep your cells aware that there is plenty of glucose that can be used.

EFFECT ON TYPE 2 DIABETES ..... Without regular exercise, blood glucose levels remain consistently elevated. Your pancreas continues to produce and release insulin in an attempt to reduce your blood sugar and promote glucose to be taken from your blood by your muscles & organs. This may contribute to Type 2 Diabetes by straining your pancreas' ability to produce insulin. Performing regular exercise also improves the efficiency of your muscles in accepting glucose from your blood, which creates double benefits of managing and preventing Type 2 Diabetes.

Regular exercise and physical activity are vital in regulating your blood glucose levels whether you have the imbalance of diabetes or not. Through participation in regular exercise, your muscle glycogen is depleted enabling your muscle to take in glucose lowering your blood glucose levels.

Pair your regular exercise with appropriate diet & nutrition and you create the condition for maximal benefits.

A Lowered blood glucose level take pressure off your pancreas' production of insulin, which also helps you to prevent or manage type 2 diabetes.

Exercise Precautions, Safety & Prescriptions for Those with Diabetes:

The goals of exercise programming for those with diabetes include: increasing aerobic power, reducing disease risk, increasing flexibility, increasing muscular strength and endurance and they are similar to those who do not have diabetes, with the exception of increased attention to improving glucose control.

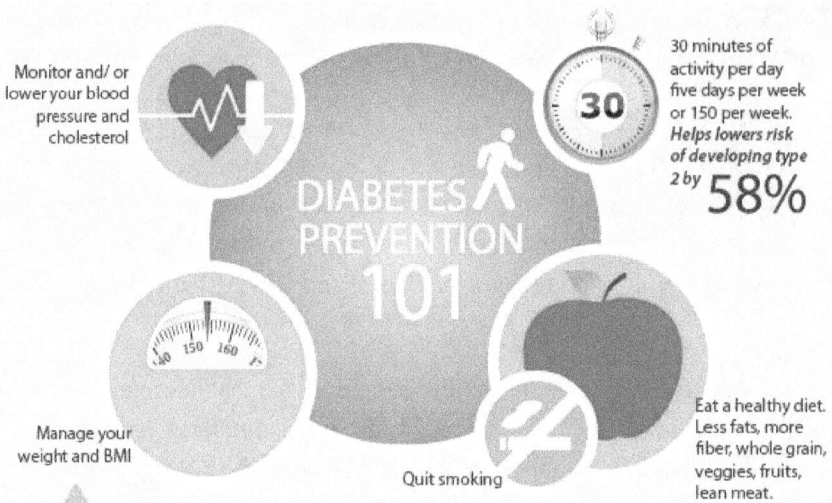

Initially, supervised exercise is recommended.

Once you have become able to maintain your glucose control with exercise, then you performing unsupervised exercise is acceptable.

Please note that it is always preferable that anyone with diabetes DO NOT exercise alone because of the need to have someone nearby in case of a hypoglycemic event. Symptoms of hypoglycemia include dizziness, nausea, headache, confusion, and irritability.

The following precautions should be observed for avoiding exercise-induced hypoglycemia:

- Measure blood glucose immediately before and 15 min after exercise (also during exercise if the exercise lasts longer than 30 min).

- Consume carbohydrate if glucose is <100 mg $\cdot$ dl^{-1}.

- Avoid exercising during times of peak insulin action.

- Reduce insulin dose (and inject into inactive areas) on days of planned exercise.

- Consume carbohydrate (5-30 g) after exercise, particularly after high-intensity, glycogen-depleting exercise. Hypoglycemia can appear several hours after exercise, so monitoring after exercise is crucial.

- Avoid exercise late at night, because hypoglycemia could occur while sleeping.

- Extend the warm-up and cool-down if needed.

Moving YoursSelf in a regular (4 or more times a week) aerobic exercise is recommended to maximize your blood glucose control. The intensity of the exercise should match your characteristics.

Although moderate-intensity resistance exercise is safe for most people with diabetes, those with advanced complications (e.g., kidney disease, vision impairment) should avoid heavy lifting, where extreme BP elevation is possible.

Dehydration due to polyuria can be problematic for diabetic clients. Dehydration can lead to a number of complications, including poor thermoregulatory control. Diabetic persons should be encouraged to maintain adequate hydration and watch for signs of heat or cold illness.

Because peripheral neuropathy can lead to ulcerations of your feet, good foot care is essential. Properly fitting and supportive shoes are particularly important for those with diabetes who are engaging in weight-bearing exercise. For those with advanced peripheral neuropathy, performing low-impact and potentially non-weight-bearing exercises are more appropriate.

Diabetes: Risk Factors and Prevention

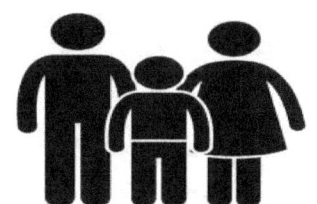
Family History

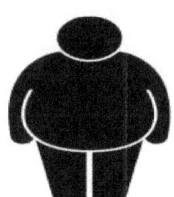
Obesity

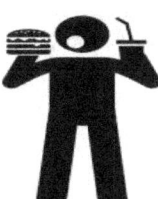
Poor Diet

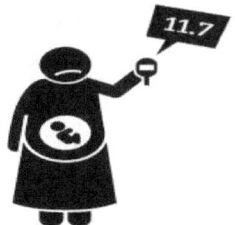
Gestational Diabetes

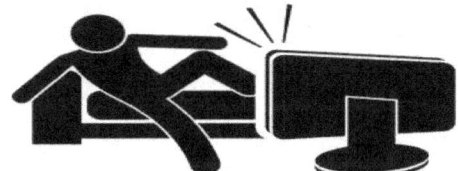
Physical Inactivity

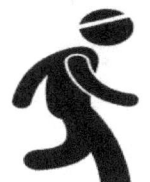
Regular Exercise

Eating Healthy

General recommendations for aerobic exercise with diabetic patients are as follows:

- **Type**: Rhythmic, large-muscle-group activities dependent on personal preferences and needs
- **Intensity**: 50% to 80% VO2 Max or HRR; RPE 12 to 16
- **Frequency**: 3 to 7 days · wk^{-1}
- **Time**: 20-60 min in bouts of at least 10 min

In the absence of retinopathy, recent laser treatments, or other contraindications, then the performing of resistance exercise is also recommended for diabetic patients.

General guidelines are as follows:

- **Type**: Based on individual needs, with particular emphasis on avoiding major increases in blood pressure (avoid static contractions and sustained gripping; avoid Valsalva maneuver)

- **Intensity**: 2 to 3 sets of 8 to 12 repetitions (60%-80% of 1RM)

- **Frequency**: 2 to 3 days $\cdot$ wk^{-1}

- **Time**: 8-10 complex (multi-joint) exercises with major muscle groups (upper and lower body) stressed

Type 2 Diabetes

In both the ADA and ACSM, they recommend that individuals with type 2 diabetes engage in both endurance and resistance training, unless they have significant complications or limitations exist to prevent Motion.

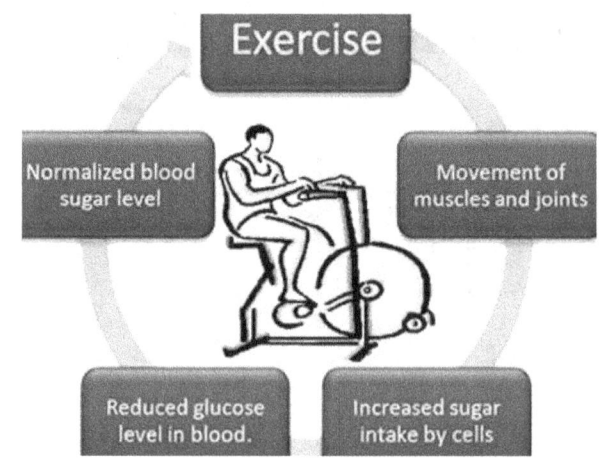

You should strive to accumulate at least **300 min $\cdot$ wk^{-1}** in **moderate-intensity** exercise. When possible, additional minutes (e.g., 300 - 420 min $\cdot$ wk^{-1}) should be encouraged in order to achieve additional benefits.

If you are overweight or obese, then your aerobic activity should focus on caloric expenditure and weight control. Although at least 3 nonconsecutive days of exercise per week are recommended for those with Type 2 who are just beginning, you may choose to engage in daily physical activity to maximize your glucose control and caloric expenditure.

Moderate-intensity exercise is generally recommended, although your characteristics should ultimately be considered when determining your level of intensity. Activity at higher intensities are acceptable for those who are conditioned and choose more vigorous exercise.

Because of the possibility of autonomic neuropathy, using your HR to monitor your exercise intensity may be problematic. Therefore, using your RPE may be a better choice for self-monitoring your exercise intensity.

Your exercise **intensity** and **duration** should be balanced to achieve your goals for caloric expenditure as well as cardiovascular conditioning and health.

Typically, exercise sessions lasting at least 10 min are suggested, with physical activity accumulating to 30 to 60 min each day.

The mode of aerobic exercise should fit your **needs** and **abilities** and should never exceed what you are capable of doing – mentally or physically.

Walking is the mode of choice for many, but for those with peripheral nerve damage, other modes (e.g., swimming, nonimpact exercise equipment) may be preferable.

General recommendations for aerobic exercise with type 2 diabetic patients are as follows:

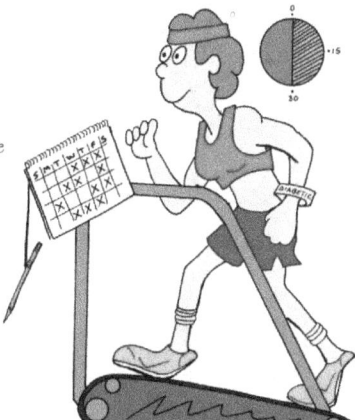

EXERCISE GUIDE FOR DIABETIC FITNESS

F Frequency
Regular (3x to 4x Per Week)

I Intensity
60-80% Of Maximal Heart Rate

T Time
Aerobic Activity
20-30 Min.
With 5-10 Min.
Warm Up

- **Type**: Rhythmic, large-muscle-group activities dependent on personal preferences and needs

- **Intensity**: 60% to 80% VO2 max or HRR; RPE 12 to 16

- **Frequency**: 3 to 7 days $\cdot$ wk^{-1}

- **Time**: 20 to 60 min in bouts of at least 10 min

Resistance training also is suggested and is very effective for many people with type 2 diabetes.

Resistance training maintains or even increases muscle mass and assists with glucose tolerance and insulin sensitivity.

The program should focus on your major muscle groups – with 8-10 exercises and consist of 2 to 3 sets of 8 to 12 repetitions. This routine should be performed at least 2 days $\cdot$ wk^{-1}.

If you are without advanced complications, then you can follow more aggressive programs. However, for those with eye or kidney damage resulting from diabetes, particular caution should be taken to avoid extreme BP elevations.

In the absence of retinopathy, recent laser treatments, or other contraindications, then resistance exercise is recommended for diabetic patients.

General guidelines are as follows:

- **Type**: Based on individual needs, with particular emphasis on avoiding major increases in blood pressure (avoid static contractions and sustained gripping; avoid Valsalva maneuver)

- **Intensity**: 2 to 3 sets of 8 to 12 repetitions (60%-80% of 1RM)

- **Frequency**: 2 to 3 days $\cdot$ wk^{-1}

- **Time**: 8 to 10 complex (multi-joint) exercises with major muscle groups (upper and lower body) stressed

Benefits Of Moderate Exercise And Diabetes

Benefits Of Exercise

1) Weight Loss
2) Lower Blood Pressure
3) Reduce Risk for Heart Disease
4) Improve Cholesterol Ratios
5) Control Blood Sugar
6) Reduce Back and Joint Pain
7) Improve Balance
8) Reduce Medications
9) Increase Self Confidence
10) Reduce Risk For Fall

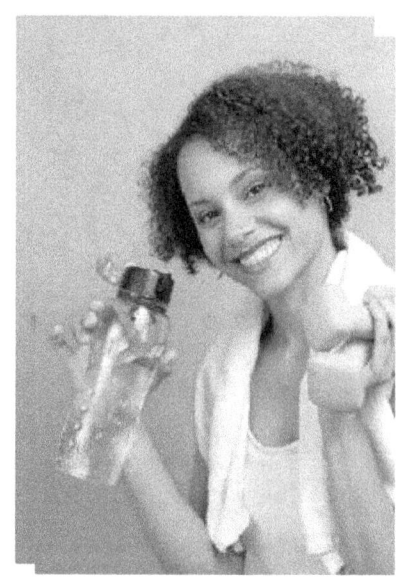

Because many clients with type 2 diabetes have a history of being relatively inactive and are often overweight, beginning and then maintaining an active lifestyle presents particular challenges. Creating a supportive environment is critical to your Success.

Early in the exercise program, it is particularly important for you to understand the information on the benefits of a lifetime commitment to exercise.

Careful monitoring of blood glucose levels is needed to help avoid any potential hypoglycemic events. For individuals with type 2 diabetes, a minimum goal for aerobic activity should be **300 min $\cdot$ wk^{-1}** of **moderate-intensity** exercise.

Resistance training can be used with clients who have diabetes as long as the client avoids damage to already weakened blood vessels.

The main thing is to create Motion …. Life is based on Motion and the ability to maintain and sustain your Motion!

Once you begin the process of starting your exercise routine, then you begin the process of creating the environment in you to facilitate your Healing and that will improve the condition and quality of your Health and Life!

It's as EASY and FUN as …….

Moving SomeThing!

What are You Moving?

YourSelf!

Where are You Going?

Abundant Life!

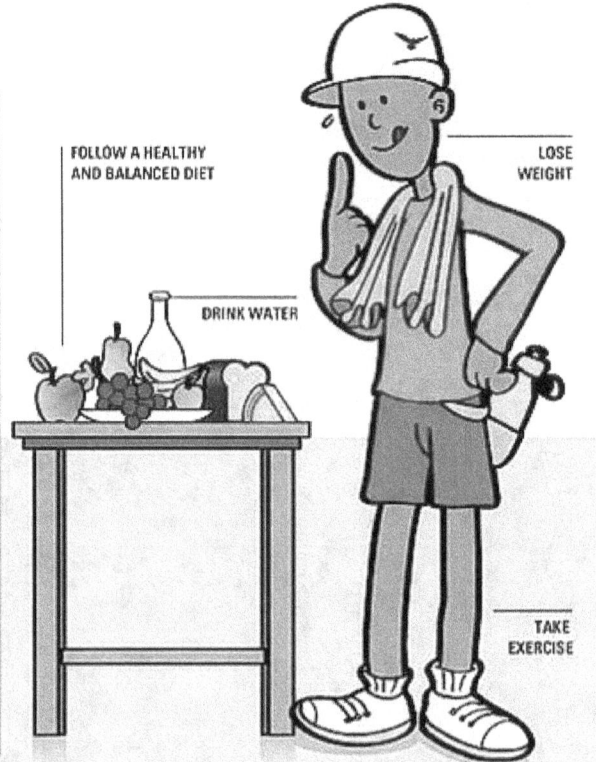

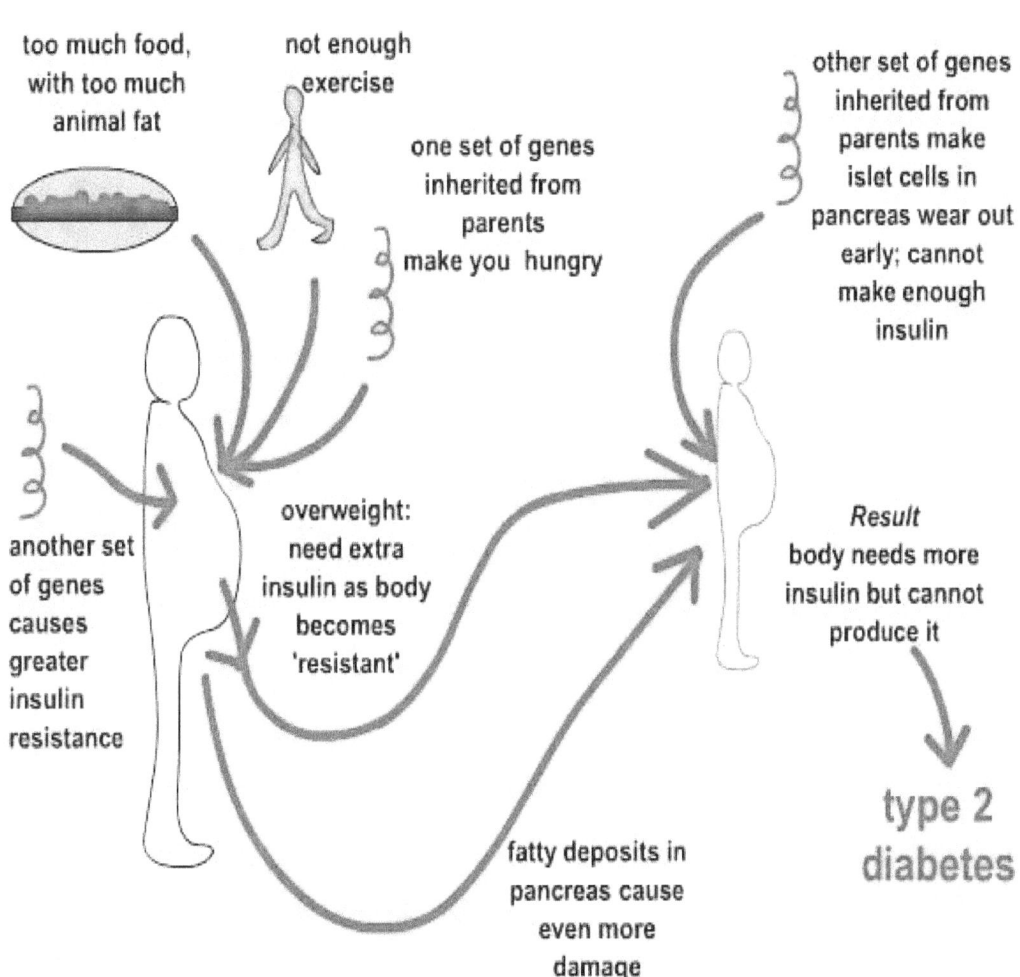

Chapter Nineteen

Exercise and Pulmonary Disease

*****

Pulmonary diseases are usually subdivided into two major categories. Chronic Obstructive Pulmonary Diseases and Restrictive Lung Diseases.

In **chronic obstructive pulmonary diseases (COPDs),** the airflow into and out of your lungs is impeded.

In **restrictive lung diseases,** the expansion of your lungs is reduced because of conditions involving your chest cavity or parenchyma (lung tissue).

There are some pulmonary diseases that are genetically inherited (e.g., cystic fibrosis), but in most cases there is involvement of external factors that include: cigarette smoking, environmental pollutants and occupational exposure to silica, coal dust, or asbestos, which are the major primary contributing factors.

All pulmonary diseases show a disruption in the exchange of gases between the ambient air and the pulmonary capillary blood. As a result, your VO2max becomes reduced, which makes the work of breathing become increased and your ability to Move YourSelf is limited.

OBSTRUCTIVE VS. RESTRICTIVE

Obstructive disorders	Restrictive disorders
• **Characterized by:** reduction in airflow. • So, shortness of breath → in exhaling air. (the air will remain inside the lung after full expiration) 1. COPD 2. Asthma 3. Bronchiectasis	• **Characterized by** a reduction in lung volume. • So, Difficulty in taking air inside the lung. (DUE TO stiffness inside the lung tissue or chest wall cavity) 1. Interstitial lung disease. 2. Scoliosis 3. Neuromuscular cause 4. Marked obesity

Chronic Obstructive Pulmonary Diseases

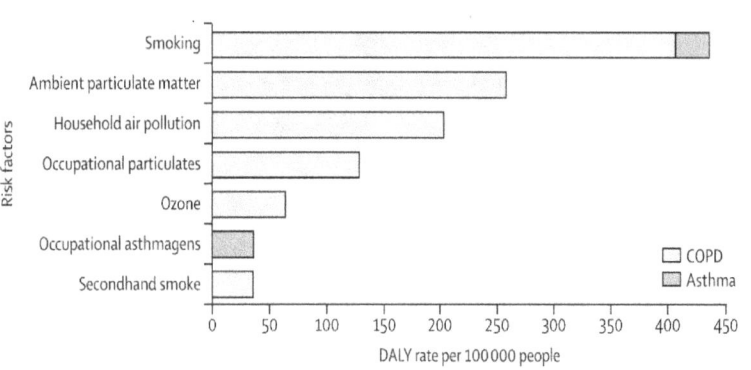

COPDs cause a reduction in airflow that can dramatically affect your ability to perform your basic and daily activities.

Characteristics of COPDs include expiratory flow obstruction and shortness of breath on exertion. These diseases include chronic bronchitis, emphysema, and bronchial asthma. All of these diseases obstruct airflow, but the underlying reason for obstruction differs for each:

- **Bronchial asthma** is caused by bronchial smooth muscle contraction and increased airway reactivity.

- **Chronic bronchitis** results from persistent production of sputum which is attributable to a thickened bronchial wall with excess secretions.

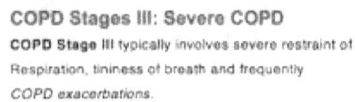
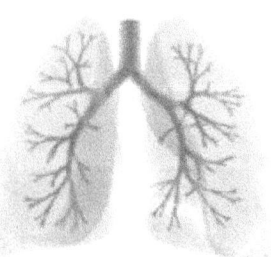
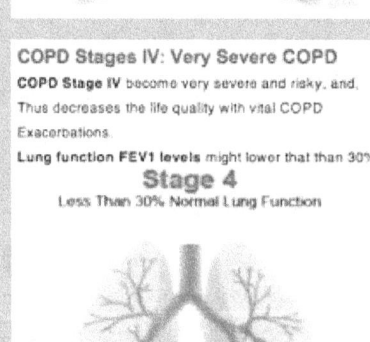

- **Emphysema** is caused by loss of elastic recoil of alveoli and bronchioles and enlargement of those pulmonary structures.

- **Cystic fibrosis** is a genetic disorder that results in excessive mucous production in your airways, which hinders ventilation of the lungs.

In 2016, approximately 18.1 million Americans reported that they were diagnosed to have COPD. Unfortunately, the mortality rates associated with COPDs have increased over the past two decades.

Unfortunately, Chronic bronchitis and emphysema are currently considered by allopathic or western medicine as being not reversible.

In 2015, COPD was the 3rd Leading Cause of Death accounting for over 130,000 deaths in 2016.

Types of exercise in COPD

Endurance Training
(Walking, Cycling, Stair climbing)

Interval Training
(Cycling)

Water-based Training
(Swimming, Aquasize)

Nordic Walking Training
(Walking with diagonal locomotion)

Conventional Exercise Types

Alternative Exercise Types

Resistance Training
(Weight lifting of light loads)

Ground Walking Training
(Walking)

T'ai Chi Training
(Circular movements, Balance, Light weights)

Nonlinear Periodized Training
(Mix of Aerobic, Anaerobic & Resistance exercise)

Asthma

There are an estimated 20.5 million people in the US that have been diagnosed with asthma; and of this number, approximately 30% are children under the age of 18.

Fortunately, Asthma is a condition that can reverse itself, and it varies from wheezing and slight breathlessness to severe attacks that may result in suffocation.

The causes of asthma include allergic reactions to antigens such as dust, pollen, smoke and air pollution.

Why asthma makes it hard to breathe

Air enters the respiratory system from the nose and mouth and travels through the bronchial tubes.

In an asthmatic person, the muscles of the bronchial tubes tighten and thicken, and the air passages become inflamed and mucus-filled, making it difficult for air to move.

In a non-asthmatic person, the muscles around the bronchial tubes are relaxed and the tissue thin, allowing for easy airflow.

Inflamed bronchial tube of an asthmatic

Normal bronchial tube

There are also Nonspecific factors such as emotional stress and exercise as well as viral infections of the bronchi, sinuses, or tonsils that can also result in asthma.

People with exercise-induced asthma may have normal resting pulmonary function but experience bronchospasms during exercise. In some cases, there are no specific cause of the asthma that can be identified.

Modern medicine treatments involve bronchodilators (often administered by inhalers) and other drugs that thin the mucous secretions and help eject them (expectorants).

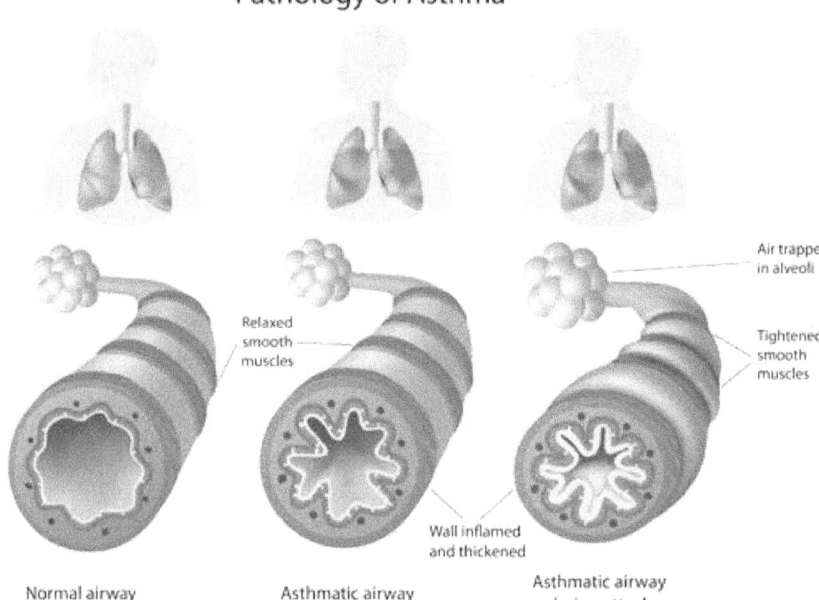

Exercise-induced asthma is a reactive airway disease affecting between 4% and 20% of the U.S. population. With this condition, exercise tends to cause your bronchioles to constrict.

Fortunately, those diagnosed with exercise-induced asthma can usually engage in exercise training. In fact, notable Olympian Jackie Joyner-Kersee (gold medalist in heptathlon, 1988 and 1992) has this condition.

Natural strategies to improve exercise tolerance include exercising in warm, moist environments rather than in cold, dry ones. Many people with asthma tolerate swimming better than running. In addition, a long warm-up can lessen the airway constriction that is more likely to occur with sudden, strenuous exercise.

Chronic Bronchitis

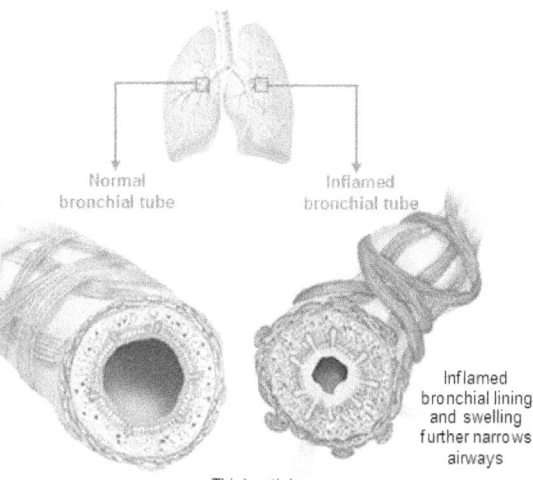

According to data from the U.S. National Center for Health Statistics, there are approximately 11.5 million Americans who are diagnosed with chronic bronchitis in 2016.

Bronchitis is characterized by the inflammation of your bronchi which are your anatomical structures that carry air from your trachea to your lungs.

Symptoms of chronic bronchitis include a cough, often with the production of sputum (i.e., mucous that is coughed up from your respiratory tract).

Airflow into your lungs is restricted due to inflammation of your airways and excess mucous production and build-up. Upon exertion, a person with chronic bronchitis may experience wheezing and dyspnea or shortness of breath.

The most common risk factor for chronic bronchitis is cigarette smoking. Chronic bronchitis can also be caused by air pollution, secondhand smoke, occupational exposure to airborne irritants, and in some cases genetic factors.

Chronic bronchitis is much more serious than acute bronchitis. About 90% of the time, acute bronchitis results from an acute virus such as the common cold or flu. Over time, acute bronchitis goes away and it normally does not pose a problem for long-term health.

The most important treatment for bronchitis is to stop smoking, if the patient is a smoker. This helps relieve symptoms and halt the progression of the disease.

Breathing as created is the #1 remedy for Asthma. By inhaling through your mouth is how you get all the external triggers INSIDE of your respiratory system.

By inhaling properly, you successfully are able to prevent an asthma attack and you create the environment in yourself that allows your body to Heal or correct the deficiency in your Respiratory system that is known as Asthma.

OBSTRUCTIVE CHRONIC BRONCHITIS AND/OR EMPHYSEMA

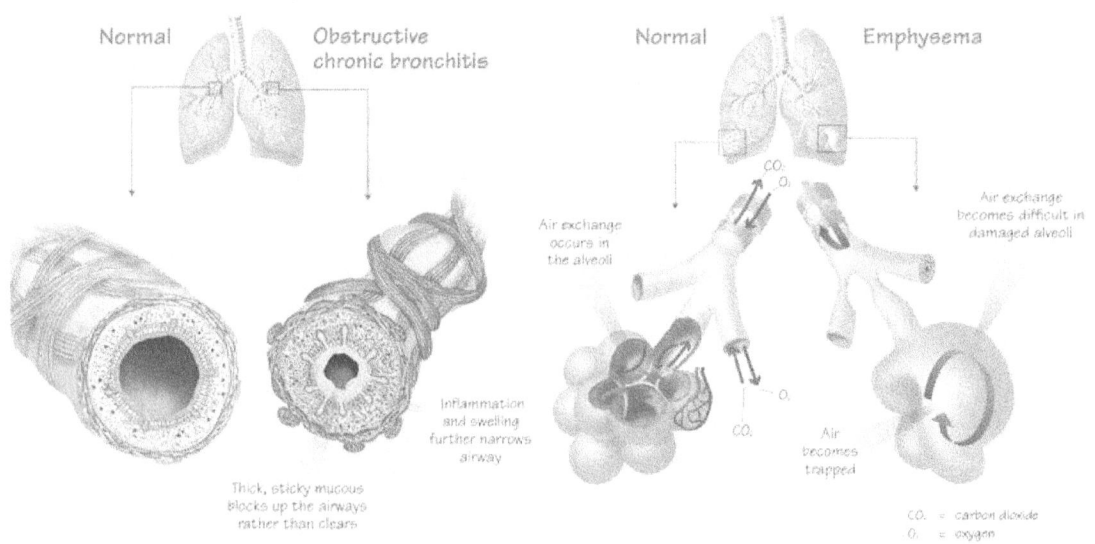

Emphysema

There are an estimated 4.1 million Americans that have reported being diagnosed with emphysema. Emphysema is characterized by destruction of your alveolar walls and enlargement of air spaces distal to your terminal bronchioles. As a result, your lung loses their elasticity and your airways tend to collapse on exhalation.

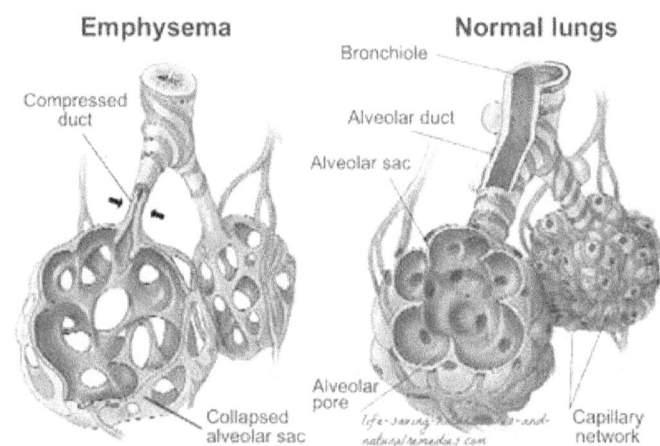

Symptoms include coughing and severe shortness of breath upon exertion.

The inability of your lungs to saturate your arterial blood with oxygen leads to hypoxemia.

Cigarette smoking is the most common cause of emphysema, just as with chronic bronchitis.

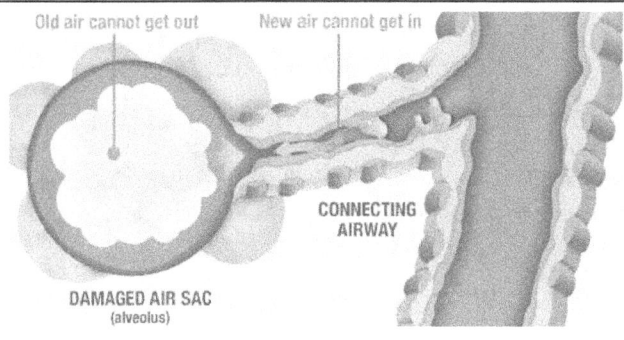

Other causes of emphysema include environmental air pollutants and, in rare cases, a hereditary deficiency of alpha-1 antitrypsin - a compound that breaks down the fibroelastic network of the lungs.

Someone with emphysema can usually be recognized because they may have a barrel-shaped chest due to hyperinflation of the lungs. Their breathing rate is also often rapid and their tidal volume is found to be smaller than normal.

Unfortunately, the current treatment for emphysema offered by western medicine cannot cure or reverse the existing lung damage. In western philosophy, smoking cessation and prevention of respiratory infections with antibiotics are important in allopathic medical management of emphysema. Supplemental oxygen is also often needed administered for approximately 18 to 24 hr · day^{-1}.

Bronchodilators are sometimes given to relax and open the airways, and corticosteroids are used to reduce inflammation of the respiratory tract. Expectorants can help loosen the mucous secretions, enabling the patient to cough them up.

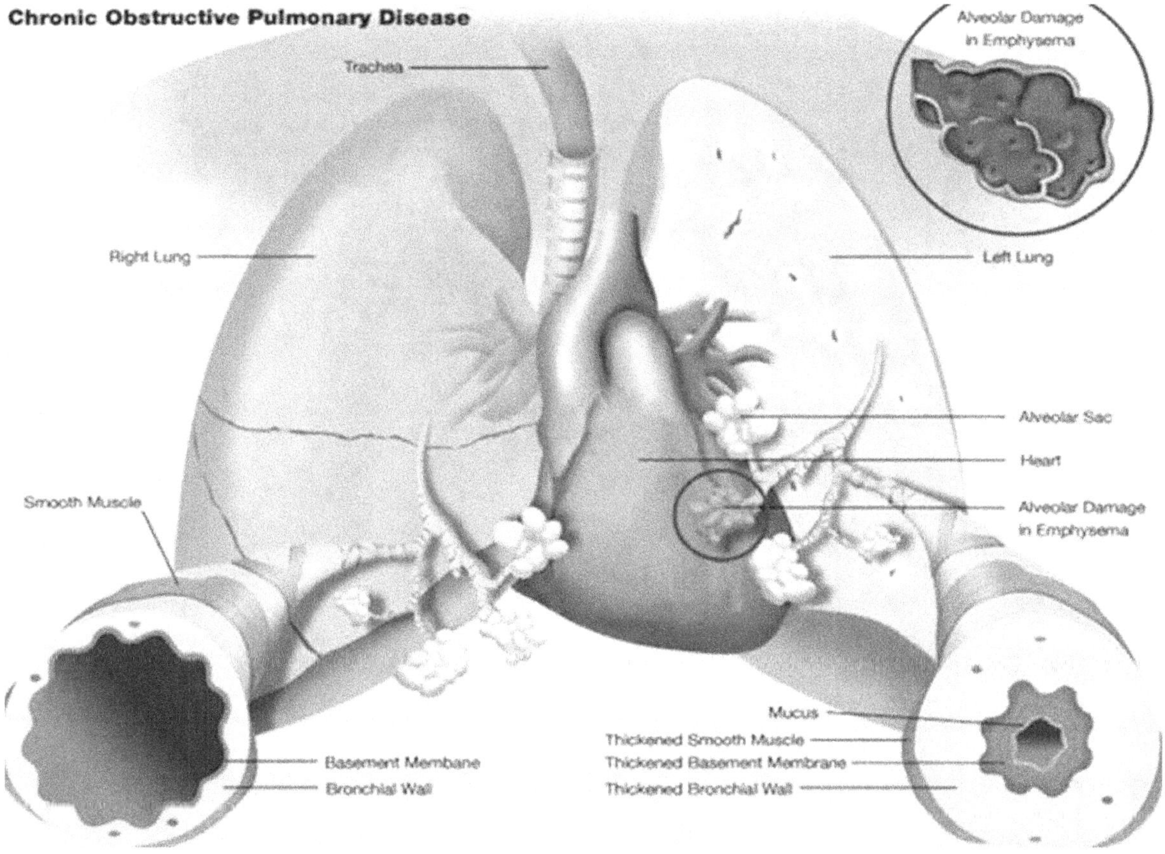

Chronic Obstructive Pulmonary Disease

COPDs reduce the capacity for your airflow during respiration. In western or allopathic medicine, bronchitis and emphysema are irreversible. They consider Bronchial asthma as an intermittent condition caused by restriction of airways and they offer relief with bronchodilator medications.

Your body is an AWESOME vehicle, designed specifically by GOD….. You are virtually indestructible and created to withstand and last. That's why when someone dies their body doesn't magically disappear. In fact, it takes years for your body to return back into the material from which it was created … this means that you could still have been in your body – LIVING!!

If you create the proper conditions in Self, then your body will do what it is created to do = Heal Self!!!!

Your body can regenerate and re-grow more than just your hair, skin and nails ….. You are created of Cells…. Your Cells divide and reproduce …. If you create the environment, then your cells will reproduce into Health and Life!

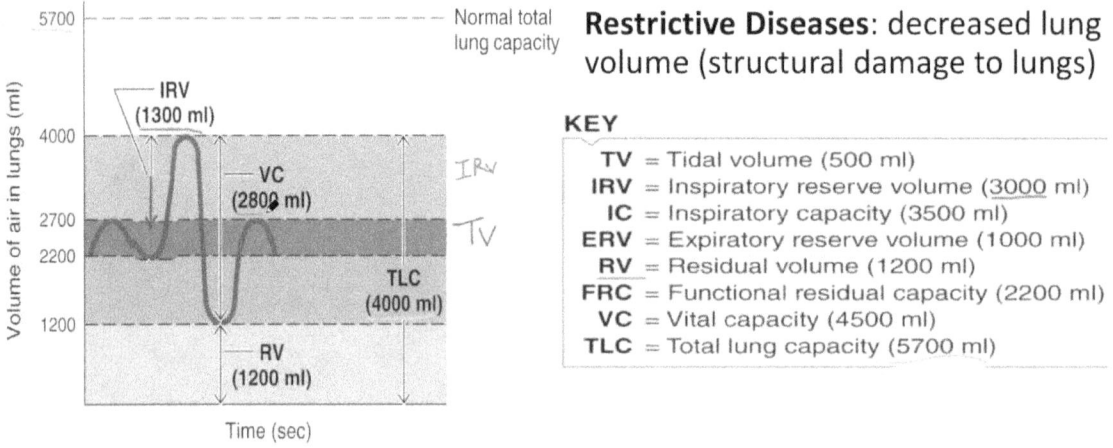

(b) Spirogram in restrictive lung disease

Understanding Restrictive Lung Diseases

Restrictive lung diseases have many causes, including diseases of the rib cage and spine such as kyphoscoliosis and pectus excavatum (sunken chest).

Other causes include pulmonary edema, pulmonary embolism, exposure to toxic substances (coal workers' pneumoconiosis, silicosis, asbestosis), chemotherapy, and radiation therapy. Often, these inflame your interstitium and fibrotic tissue begins to develop.

There are various types of neuromuscular diseases (spinal cord injury, amyotrophic lateral sclerosis or Lou Gehrig's disease, Guillain-Barré syndrome, tetanus, and myasthenia gravis) that can also cause restrictive lung disease.

Obesity and pregnancy can restrict lung expansion because of the abdomen pushing up into your thoracic cavity.

In general, those with restrictive lung diseases have reduced residual volume (RV), inspiratory reserve volume (IRV), expiratory reserve volume (ERV), forced vital capacity (FVC), and maximal tidal volume (TV).

Their Breathing has become more difficult because their respiratory muscles must work harder to inflate their lungs.

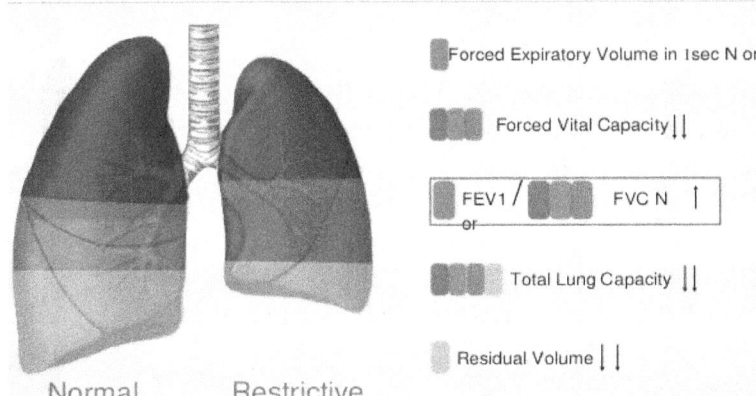

Restrictive lung diseases have numerous causes, but they all are essentially characterized by the reduced capacity to expand the lungs.

Smaller lung volumes are typically seen in people with these diseases which significantly inhibits their ability to Breathe.

Life is based on the ability to Breathe …. Which is the only difference between a Living body and a dead one = the ability to Breathe!

Evidence for Exercise

Pulmonary rehabilitation programs are often found alongside cardiac rehabilitation programs in many hospitals. Most pulmonary rehabilitation programs focus on people with COPD, although people with other types of pulmonary disease may also benefit from exercise. Support for pulmonary rehabilitation programs is limited by the fact that patients typically show little or no improvement in VO2max, tests of lung function, and mortality rates. As a result, many insurance providers are reluctant to pay for pulmonary rehabilitation because they view it as medical management rather than a way to restore the patient to normal function (as much as possible).

However, most pulmonary rehabilitation patients do improve in functional outcomes, including symptom-limited GXT, symptoms of dyspnea, quality of life, and frequency of hospitalization.

Pulmonary rehabilitation should be viewed as a desirable part of the patient's medical treatment. The overall goals are to improve the patient's general health, to optimize oxygen saturation, to make ADLs more easily accomplished, and to improve self-efficacy.

Patients with lung diseases can and do benefit from a pulmonary rehabilitation program. Although patients usually demonstrate little improvement in VO2max and pulmonary function tests, they do improve in their ability to carry out tasks and in other measures of quality of life.

Testing and Evaluation

Exercise tests are often administered to assess the patient's ability to exercise. The test may be a standard GXT on a treadmill or cycle ergometer or a simple 6 or 12 min walk test on a flat surface. In a pulmonary patient, exercise capacity is limited more by the lungs than the cardiovascular system. As a result, these patients typically experience **hypoxemia** (low arterial oxygen content) and **dyspnea** (shortness of breath).

A **pulse oximeter** is used to assess the percent saturation of hemoglobin in the arterial blood (S_aO_2) of pulmonary patients. This noninvasive device shines a light beam through the finger or earlobe. The absorption characteristics of oxygenated and deoxygenated hemoglobin in the red or infrared region are used to assess the arterial oxygen saturation.

Values for S_aO_2 below 90% indicate that the client needs supplemental oxygen to increase the driving force for diffusion of oxygen into the lungs. Frequently, a dyspnea rating scale is used to evaluate symptoms during exercise testing. Cardiovascular, pulmonary, metabolic, and power output measurements are obtained and used to evaluate the severity of disability.

In restrictive lung diseases, lung volumes are often reduced because the ability to expand the lungs is compromised. Exercise testing of patients with lung diseases, with appropriate monitoring of signs (hypoxemia) and symptoms (dyspnea) to assess the severity of the patient's condition, is beneficial.

Since exercise is recommended for increasing the health and life quality of pulmonary patients, the fitness professional should know how to prescribe exercise for this population.

The goal of a typical pulmonary rehabilitation program is your self-care, healing and increase in your Life-Span so that you can Successfully Enjoy your Abundant Life.

Aerobic training is usually accomplished with rhythmic, dynamic exercise that uses large muscle groups. Recommended modes are walking, cycling, and swimming.

The exercise modes should be enjoyable and improve the ability to perform normal daily activities.

As with healthy individuals and other clinical populations, the frequency is typically 3 to 5 days $\cdot$ wk^{-1}, with each session lasting at least 30 min. However, assigning appropriate exercise intensities poses a particular problem because Pulmonary patients usually cannot achieve the same peak HRs as healthy individuals of the same age. T

Various methods can be used to estimate the appropriate exercise intensity for pulmonary patients. Generally, the method of assigning exercise intensity varies with the level of the disability.

In patients with mild or moderate impairment, setting the intensity just below the ventilatory threshold or the point where the person became noticeably dyspneic is appropriate. Intermittent exercise, interspersed with rest, may be all that the client can tolerate. If the impairment is severe, supplemental oxygen will be needed to maintain S_aO_2 above 90%.

Individuals with emphysema should be instructed in pursed-lip breathing, which involves pressing the lips together and exhaling through a small opening in the center of the mouth. This slows the rate of respiration and prevents collapse of small airways, resulting in better oxygenation. In some instances, a resistive breathing device may be recommended to train the respiratory muscles at rest.

Upper-body exercise is recommended for pulmonary patients. This exercise can be achieved using exercise equipment that require both arm and leg muscles to operate like the rowing as mentioned in the Move YourSelf Activities Chapter.

Additionally, your resistance training can be accomplished with dumbbells, machines, or elastic bands. Increasing arm strength and endurance improves your ability to perform functional activities and decreases local muscle fatigue.

Flexibility training (e.g., stretching, tai chi) and balance training may also be incorporated to improve your functional ability, which allows you to maintain and sustain your ability to Move YourSelf!

Your Pulmonary System is the basis or foundation for your Life.

Your ability to Heal, increase your Health and Manifest your Power is built on your Pulmonary System.

You need your Pulmonary system to operate Efficiently, Effectively and at its Maximum Health in order for you to Successfully Enjoy your Abundant Life!

Move Something!

Health Benefits of Running

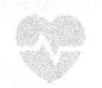

IMPROVED CARDIOVASCULAR HEALTH
Reduces the risk of heart attack and prevents high blood pressure.

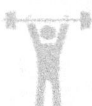

IMPROVED MENTAL HEALTH
Neurochemicals released while running can reduce symptoms of depression and anxiety. Running also reduces stress hormone levels.

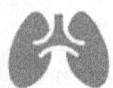

IMPROVED RESPIRATORY HEALTH
Lessens the effects of asthma and increases aerobic capacity.

IMPROVED PHYSICAL STRENGTH
Running improves physical strength in the lower body muscles. (Runners should, however, maintain a strength training program for the upper body muscles.)

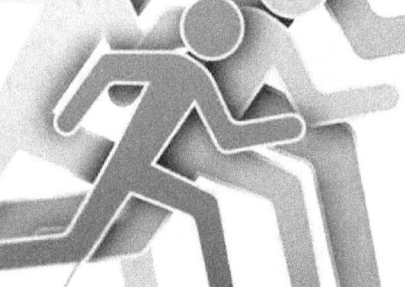

IMPROVED JOINT HEALTH
Increases strength and stability in the tendons and ligaments, thereby, preventing injuries to the hips, knees and ankles. Running also increases bone mass and helps prevent age-related bone loss.

WEIGHT MANAGEMENT
Running promotes weight loss (and tightens the skin as the weight comes off!). Losing extra body weight greatly decreases the risk of heart attack, diabetes and other chronic illnesses.

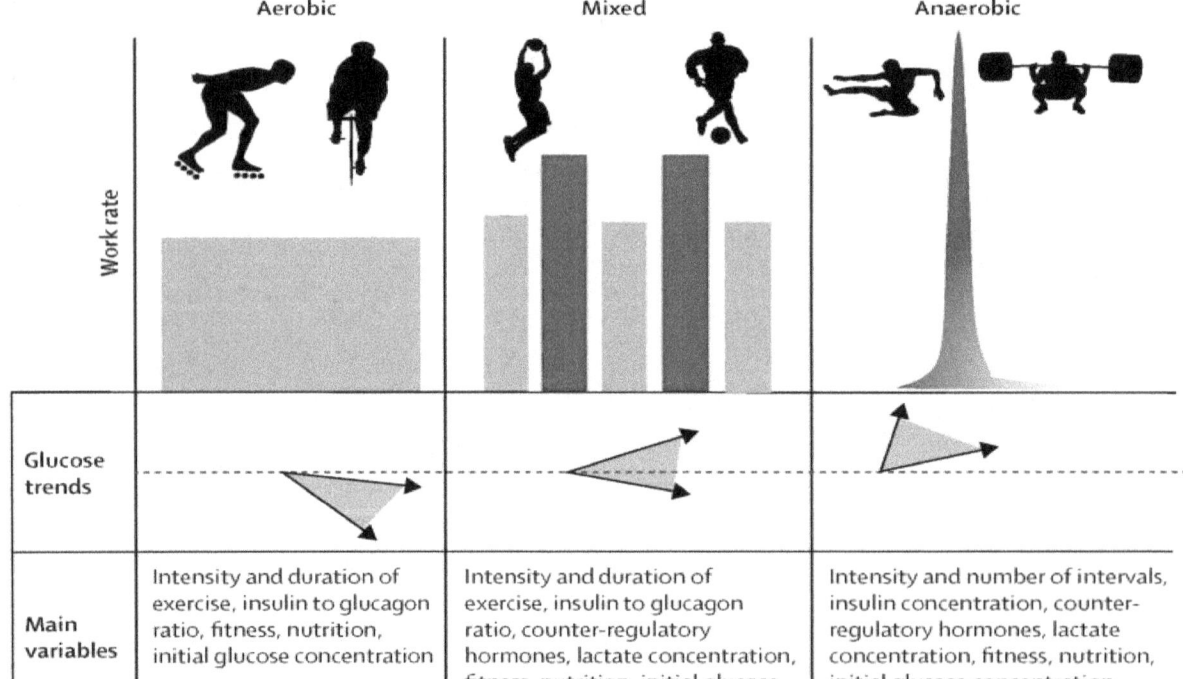

	Aerobic	Mixed	Anaerobic
Main variables	Intensity and duration of exercise, insulin to glucagon ratio, fitness, nutrition, initial glucose concentration	Intensity and duration of exercise, insulin to glucagon ratio, counter-regulatory hormones, lactate concentration, fitness, nutrition, initial glucose concentration	Intensity and number of intervals, insulin concentration, counter-regulatory hormones, lactate concentration, fitness, nutrition, initial glucose concentration

Supreme Health & Fitness! — *Health & Wellness Series ... Vol 3!*

Components of Physical Fitness

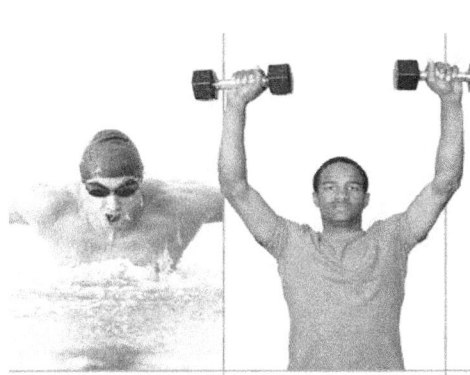
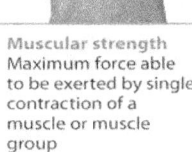
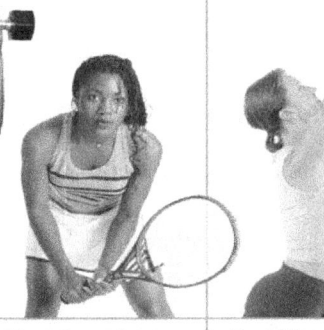
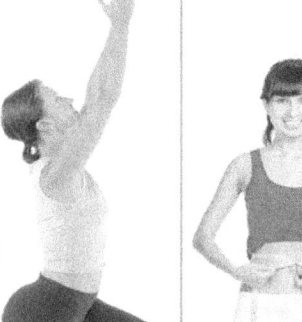
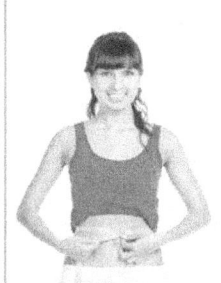

Cardiorespiratory fitness
Ability to sustain aerobic whole-body activity for a prolonged period of time

Muscular strength
Maximum force able to be exerted by single contraction of a muscle or muscle group

Muscular endurance
Ability to perform muscle contractions repeatedly without fatiguing

Flexibility
Ability to move joints freely through their full range of motion

Body composition
The relative proportions of fat mass and fat-free mass in the body

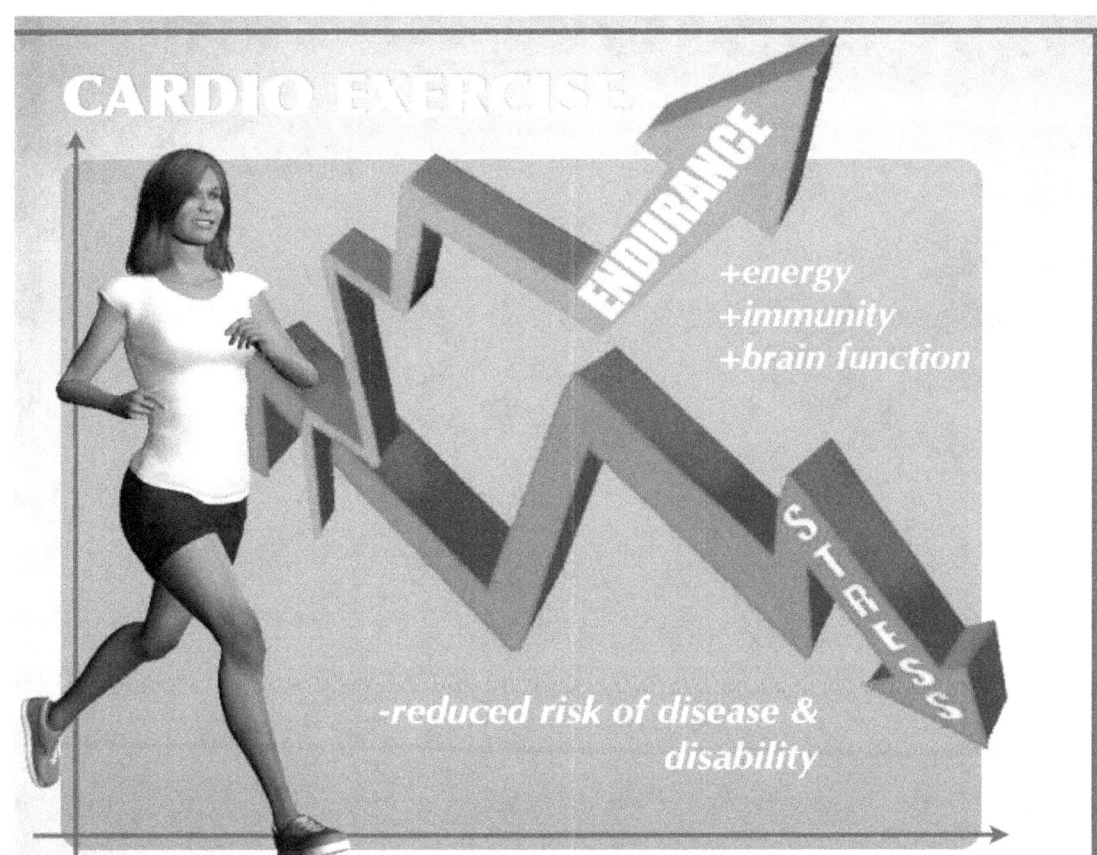

anatomy

How Muscles Function

Muscles are usually attached to bones by tendons, which can be short, long, flat, or like thin strings

When muscles contract they get shorter and thicker, pulling the tendon attached to the bone causing movement

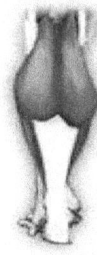

The achilles tendon attaching to the purple calf muscles is flat, thin, and long

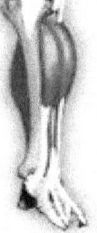

The tendons moving from the green peroneal muscles to the feet are thin cables that articulate the toes

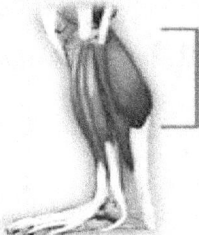

Relaxed calf muscles

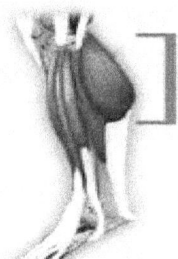

Contracted calf muscles

Muscles can only pull, and as weird as this sounds, when we do "push ups" no muscle is actually pushing. For every muscle group that performs an action there is a group that will perform the opposite action. Muscles working in these contrasting motions are what allow us to do such complex movements

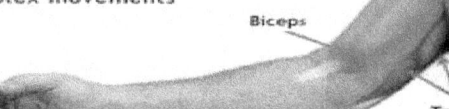

Biceps

Triceps

The biceps and triceps are two muscles that work in contrast to each other. When the arm is in this position resting on the table, both the biceps and triceps are relaxed

To lift the lower arm up the biceps have contracted. Muscles always move the bones below, so in this case the biceps lay on top of the humerus but pulls the radius and ulna up

To slam the fist down on the table, the triceps must contract which pulls on the elbow causing the the lower arm back down with force

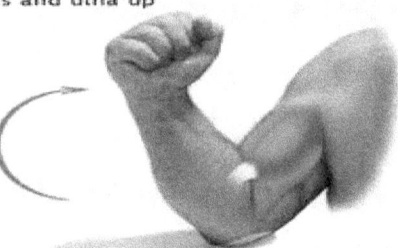

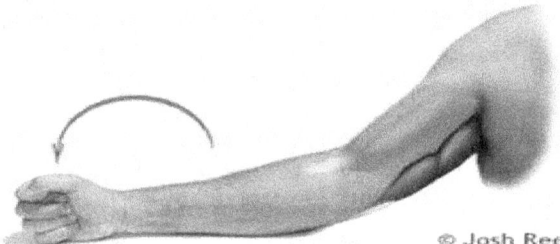

© Josh Reed

CIRCULATORY SYSTEM

- **Blood pools in the lower body "because of" gravity causing a pressure gradient**

- **70% of blood below heart level**

- **Blood Pressure normally higher in lower body than in the upper body**

- **Without the pull of gravity, the blood can no longer pool in the lower legs and feet**

- **Instead the blood collects in the head and thorax region of the body**

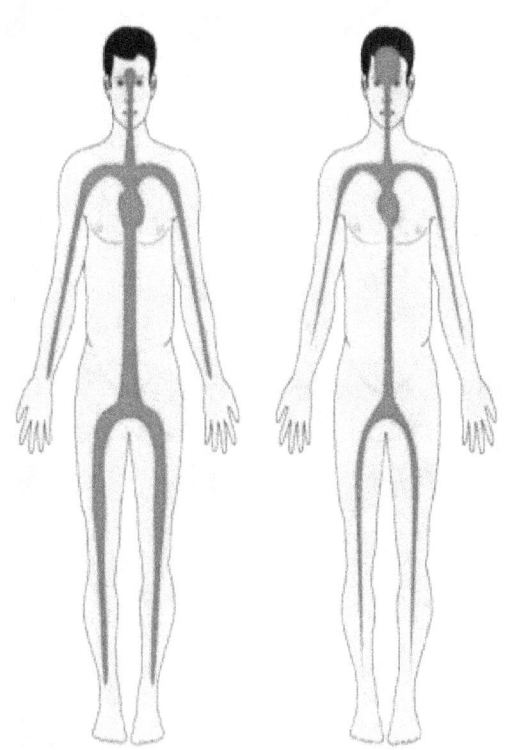

The IMPORTANCE of Moving Your Self..... Your MoveMent Regulates and Maintains Your Life Blood Circulation.

Your Circulatory Systems main function is to disperse the Breath Of Life throughout your Body – to EVERY CELL IN YOUR BODY!

Biomechanics

- Examines the internal and external forces acting on the human body and the effects produced by these forces

- Aids in technique analysis and the development of innovative equipment designs

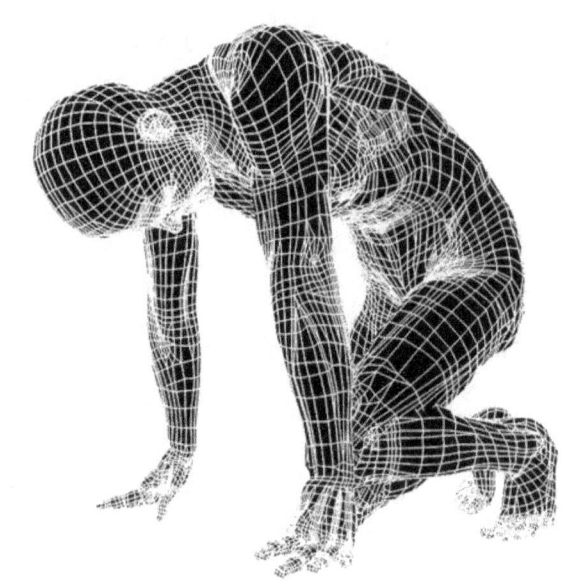

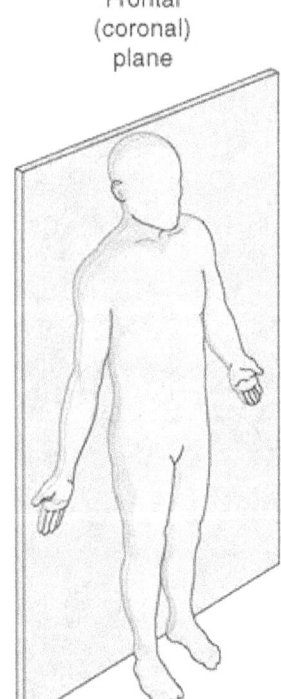

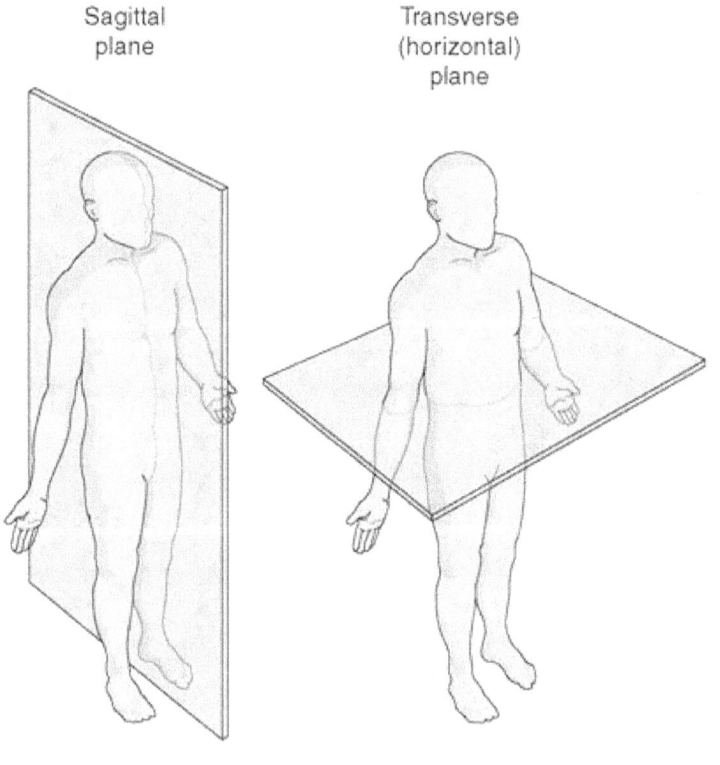

Frontal (coronal) plane

Sagittal plane

Transverse (horizontal) plane

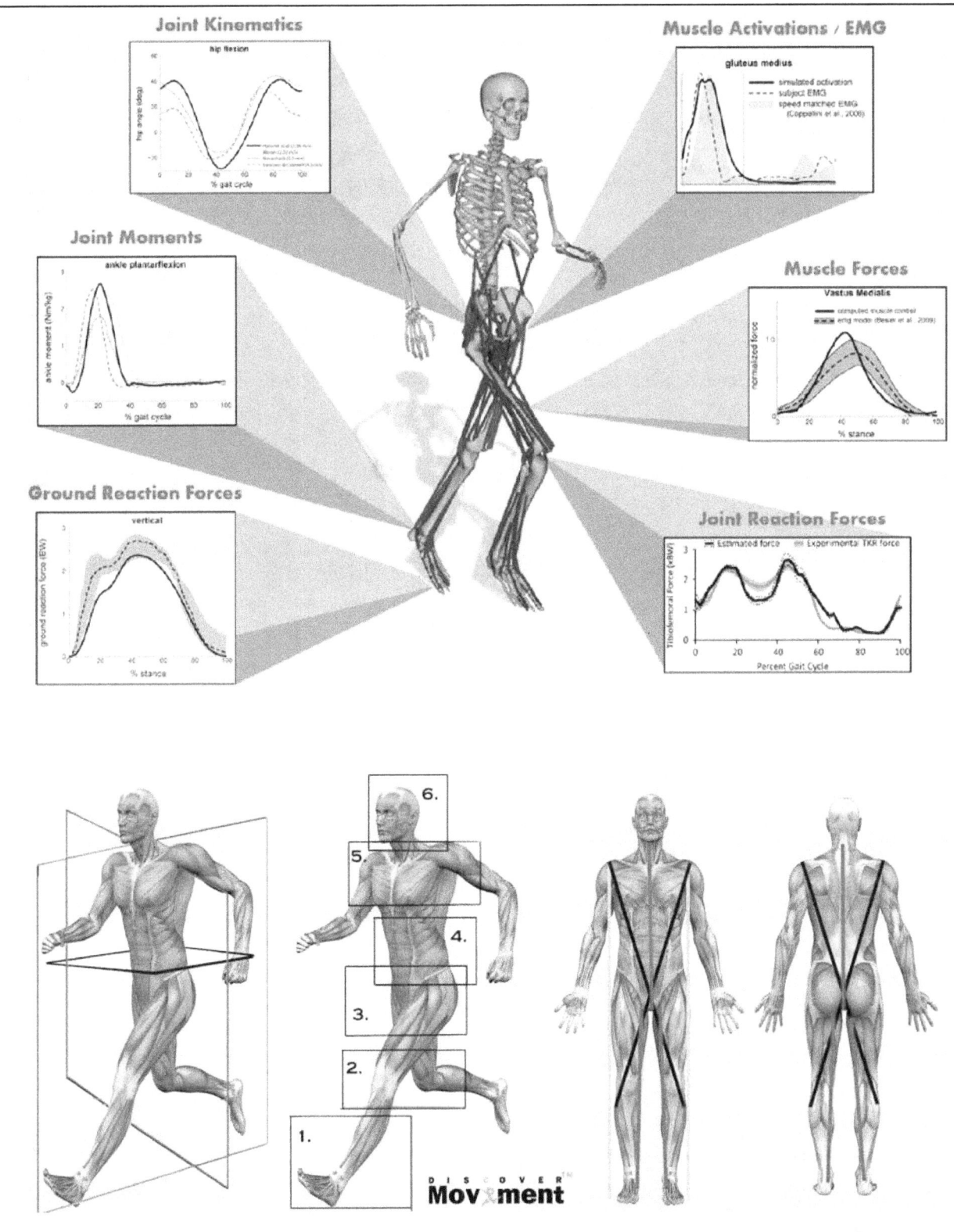

Move Something!

Chapter Twenty-One

Biomechanics – Moving YourSelf

*****

The foundation of Healing, Health and Power is KNOWLEDGE OF YOURSELF!

You must know your Anatomical structure and function which increases your ability of Control and Command over Your Body.

Think about your body as you woke up this morning. You stretched your muscles and noticed the first sensations from nerves in your eyes, ears, and skin. As you lay in bed, summoning the energy to get up you may have noticed your heart beating. You took a few deep breaths, swung your legs to the ground, and headed to the shower. After you dressed, enjoyed a hearty breakfast, and made a final trip to the bathroom, you were ready to begin the day. In that short hour before leaving home you engaged in all the essential activities of life (with the probable exception of reproduction).

Bio = Life …. Mechanics = Working Parts.

Bio-mechanics is the study of how the joints of your body move and the forces that contribute to or hinder those movements.

Understanding some key principles of biomechanics is necessary to fully understand your movement and how to Successfully keep YourSelf IN perpetual MOTION … the Motion of Life!

A Body IN Motion STAYS IN Motion until a stronger Force STOPS it … that Force is YOUR DEATH … By understanding the Bio-Mechanics of your Motion = you can CONTROL Your Motion … and You CAN Successfully Move YourSelf into the Enjoyment of Your Abundant Life!

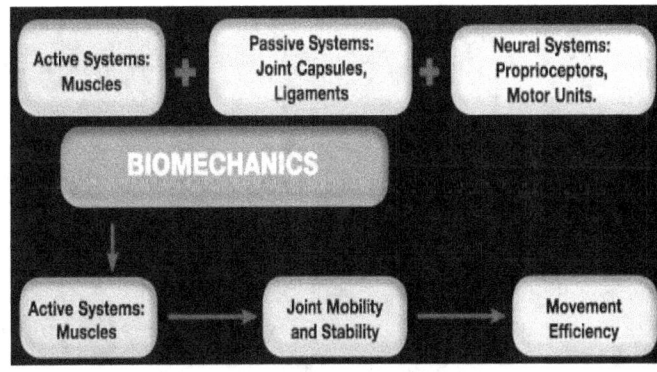

Some of the main concepts are described below.

The 3 major roles of your muscles are:

1. To **cause** your body movement to be GREATER (**concentric** action) regardless of your opposing force.
2. To **decelerate** or **control** the speed of your body movement (**eccentric** action), even if the movement was caused by another force (whether Stronger or Greater),
3. To **prevent** movement (**isometric** action).

*These 3 roles or functions are how you **Protect** yourself, **Defend** yourself and become **VICTORIOUS** over **ALL** opposition .... Including **YOUR DEATH!***

Other muscle functions include counteracting an undesirable action caused by the concentric action of another muscle and guiding movements caused by another muscle.

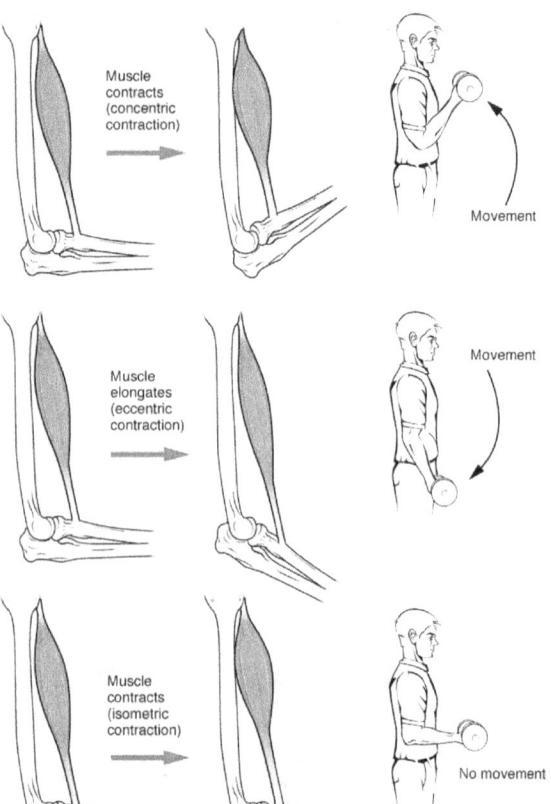

Understanding the Roles of Your Muscles

Your Skeletal muscles can act in several ways and have a variety of effects on your joint movement. They can cause movement via concentric action or decelerate movement caused by another force via eccentric action. Muscles may also act isometrically to stabilize or prevent undesirable movement.

For example, during a push-up, gravity tends to cause your lumbar spine to hyperextend. Isometric action of your trunk muscles prevents this sagging and stabilizes your lumbar region in a neutral position.

Another function of your muscle is to counteract an undesirable action caused by the concentric action of another muscle. The concentric action of many of your muscles causes more than one movement at the same joint or causes movement at more than one of your joint.

If only one of those movements is intended, another muscle must act to prevent the undesirable movement.

For example, concentric action of fibers in your upper trapezius both elevates and adducts your scapula. If only adduction is desired, fibers in your lower trapezius, which cause depression and adduction, neutralize the undesirable scapula elevation. In this example, different fibers of the same large trapezius muscle neutralize the unwanted action.

Muscles can also guide movements caused by other muscles. During activities against a great resistance, such as lifting free weights, additional muscles help maintain balance and proper direction of your movement. After the force of a prime mover has initiated a ballistic movement, other muscles guide your movement in the proper direction.

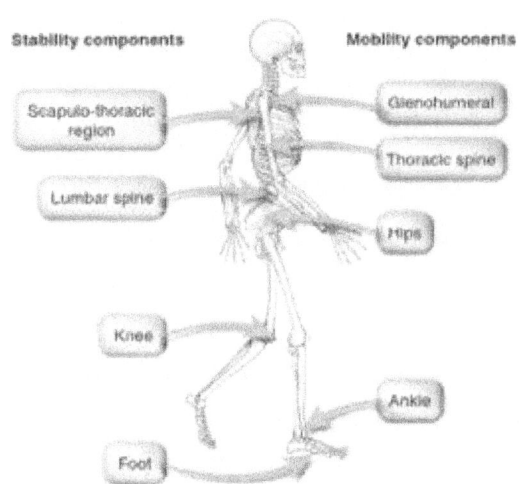

The knowledge of your Muscle movement should really underscore the Importance of Moving Yourself!

Your body is literally created to Move and Maintain your Motion of Life!

You MUST Move YourSelf MORE THAN YOU SIT STILL!

A **muscle group** includes all of the muscles that cause the same movement at the same joint. The group is named for the joint where the movement takes place and for the movement commonly caused by the concentric action of those muscles.

A muscle group includes all the muscles that act concentrically to cause a specific movement at a given joint.

Flexibility – ability to achieve a specific range of motion across one joint. Example: supine straight leg raise (hamstring flexibility).

Mobility – ability to achieve a specific range of motion across 2 or more joints simultaneously. Example: squat (ankles, knees, hips, thoracic spine)

Stability – ability to maintain a position against external forces. Example: Plank hold against gravity

Motor Control – the coordination between stability and mobility while performing functional movements. Example: Single leg squat.

Achieving Your Stability

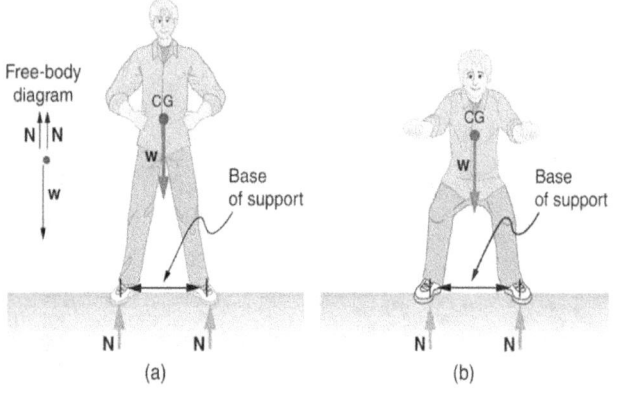

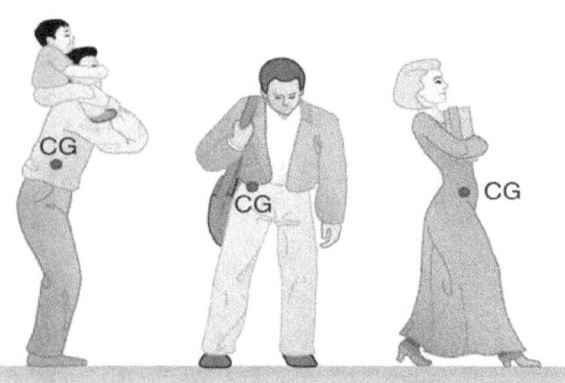

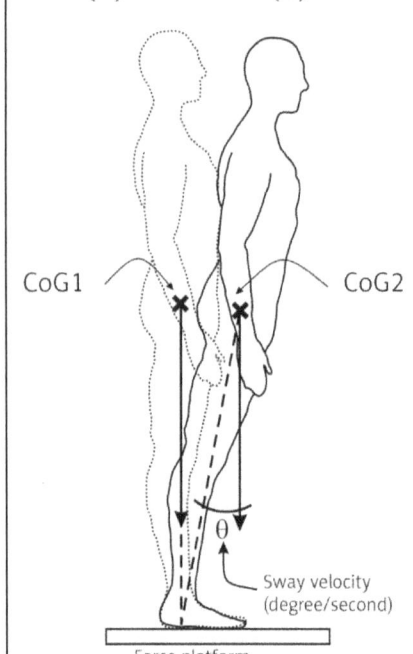

Stability is a feature of your whole body and is influenced by the position of all parts of your body. It is your ability to maintain a **stable** and **balanced** position following a disruption - such as being pushed by someone.

This science illustrates just how Awesome your body is ... that it is created to maintain its Stability and Balance in response to a disruption of your force from an external source. This means that you ARE STRONGER than anything you could ever go up against .... EVEN YOUR DEATH!

In order to maintain your balance, your center of gravity must fall within the area of your base of support. In the simple case of standing on two feet with arms at the sides, there is a roughly rectangular base of support from the toes of each foot to the heels of each foot. With your weight evenly distributed on both feet, the center of gravity will be in the middle of the base of support.

Changing your foot position will change the shape and area of your base of support.

Changing the position of your body or holding an object will alter the location of your center of gravity within your base of support.

Your Stability is proportional to the distance from your center of gravity to the edge of your base of support in the direction that an external force could or would propel you.

With the feet apart, if you lean so that your line of gravity falls directly over one foot and a pushing force is applied in the same direction of your lean, there is less stability than if your feet were together but with the line of gravity along the edge of your foot closer to the applied force.

A wide base of support in the anticipated direction of perturbation typically provides greater stability.

A lower body position and the accompanying lower center of gravity also contribute to a more stable position.

This means that you can Control and Command your body to BE Stronger than ANY External force that could come against you. This means that the ONLY thing that can STOP You IS YOU!

An object IN Motion STAYS IN MOTION until a STRONG Enough Force can Compel it to STOP ... Your DEATH is that Force in Your Life .... You are created with the Ability to produce a STRONGER Force than Death and Push it out of your Path!

You can maintain the Stable position of your Life!

Your Stability is also directly proportional to your body weight. With all other factors being equal, a heavy person is more stable than a lighter one.

Your Stability may also be increased by moving your feet apart to widen your base of support and by flexing your knees and hips to lower your center of gravity.

During standing exercises that require balance, your stability can also be aided by holding or pushing against a nearby object such as a wall or chair.

Many exercises can be executed from a sitting position, which increases your base of support and lowers your center of gravity.

To help maintain stability against a potentially upsetting force, your weight should be shifted **toward** that force.

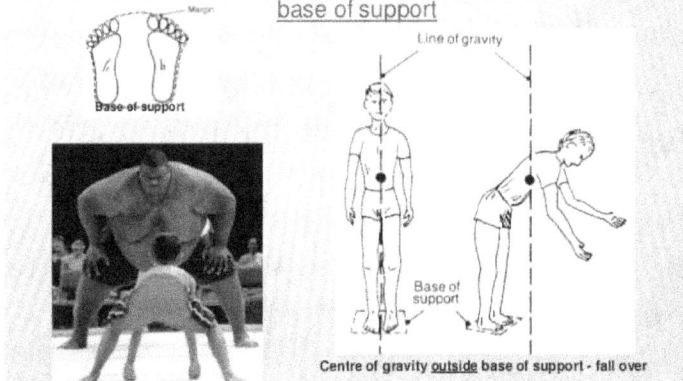

FACE YOUR OPPOSITION HEAD-ON!

Shift your Weight of Life TOWARD your Death and MOVE IT OUT YOUR WAY!!!!

Your Stability in Action

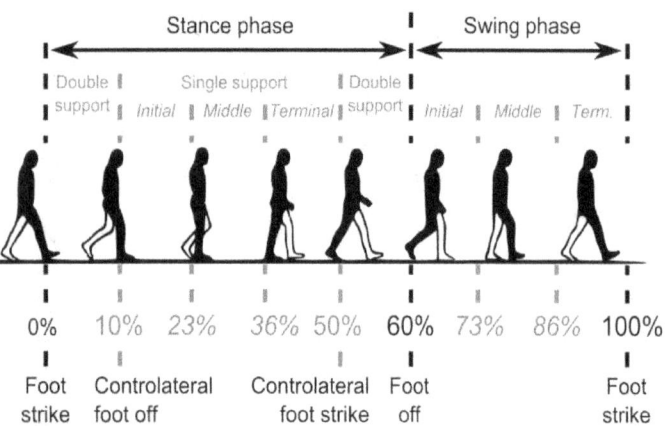

Just before the act of walking begins, a position close to instability is attained by shifting your center of gravity in the direction of your intended movement, which is closer to the anterior limits of your base of support.

During the act of walking, as the line of gravity moves outside your base of support, a new base of support is established when your other foot makes contact and your stability is restored.

In basketball, a guard who takes a charge from a forward will fall quicker and easier if she is in an unstable position—standing erect with feet closer together and weight on the heels at the moment of the collision.

Stability is directly proportional to the distance of your center of gravity from the edge of your base of support. It is inversely proportional to the height of your center of gravity above the base of support and it is directly proportional to the weight of your body.

For greater stability during standing, your knees should be flexed, your feet spread apart in the direction of an oncoming force and your body weight shifted toward the force.

Your Torque (Moment of Force)

Muscular Torques

As the forearm is flexed and extended, the moment arm changes.

The moment arm is biggest when the elbow is at 90 degrees, and gets smaller as it is flexed and extended away from this position.

A similar situation exists for most of our muscles and the joints they cross.

Explains why our muscles are apparently stronger in some joint positions than others

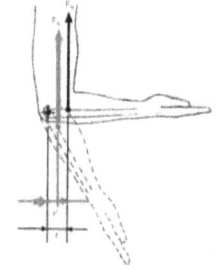

A force is any push or pull that is applied to a person or object. In your body, when a force is applied at a distance from one of your joints it produces a **torque (T),** which will typically cause your joint to rotate = Motion.

Torque is the product of the magnitude of the **force** (F) and the **force arm (FA),** which is the perpendicular distance from the axis of rotation to the direction of application of that force. Torque can be expressed as follows:

$$T = F \times FA$$

$$T_R = R \times RA$$

When two opposing forces act to produce rotation in opposite directions, one of the forces is typically designated as the **resistance force (R),** and its force arm is called the **resistance arm (RA),** producing a **resistance torque (TR)**.

In considering torque produced by your muscle to cause movement against gravity or some other external force, *F* and *FA* are designated for your muscle and *R* and *RA* are designated for gravity or other opposing forces.

Your body is created to produce the opposite amount of Force that Gravity has on your body to keep you Upright and In-Motion so that you can Successfully Enjoy Your Abundant Life!

Death is considered a Resistance Force to your Motion of Life ...

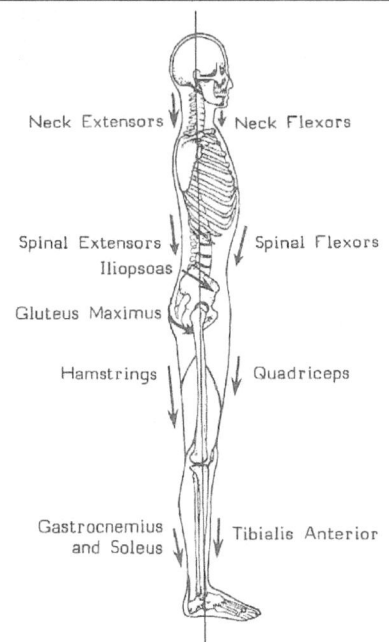

Figure 4.1. The major antigravity muscles that maintain the erect position.

So, by Moving YourSelf for at least 60 minutes a day, you can Build Up your Muscles and Body to be STRONG enough to Successfully Carry and Move you into the Enjoyment of Your Abundant LIFE!

Applying Torque to Muscle Action

Your Muscle action is a force. The force arm is the perpendicular distance from the axis of rotation of your joint to the direction of the force from its point of application (where your muscle attaches to your bone being moved).

Note that the force arm is not always parallel to the bone. This shortens the force arm, so the same muscle force produces less torque at that joint angle, or more muscle force is required to generate the same torque. This is why a dumbbell biceps curl feels harder at the start of the flexion movement compared with the middle of the flexion movement.

Skeletal Muscle Function

Torque produced by a muscle (T_m) at the joint center of rotation is the product of muscle force (F_m) and muscle moment arm ($d_\perp$).

$$T_m = F_m \times d_\perp$$

Torque Resulting From Other Forces

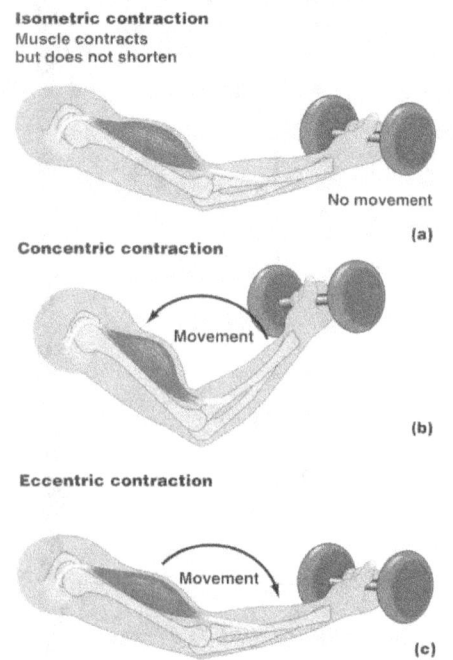

The force of gravity directed vertically downward is treated as a **resistance force**. The resistance produced by gravity acting on a body part is the **weight** of the object. The resistance arm is the perpendicular distance from the axis of rotation to the point of the object that represents its center of gravity.

The torque produced is the product of the **resistance** and the **resistance arm**. This torque can be increased by adding mass to increase both the magnitude of force (total weight of forearm and hand plus the added mass) and the length of the resistance arm if the mass is added farther from the axis of rotation.

The MORE weight or resistance that you encounter – your body has the ability to produce a GREATER Torque to allow you to Successfully withstand and/or overcome that particular weight or resistance.

The weight or resistance can be in the form of a barbell, your own thoughts or even your death. By constantly Moving YourSelf for at least 60 minutes a day, you condition your body to create perpetual Torque to produce perpetual Motion!

For muscle contraction to move a bone, the muscle force generated must produce a torque greater than the opposing or resistance torque.

In this case, the muscle action is concentric and the joint moves in the direction of the muscle torque. If the resistance torque is greater than the muscle torque, the muscle acts eccentrically and lengthens under tension. In this case, the joint moves in the opposite direction of the muscle torque (in the direction of the resistance torque). When the muscular torque equals the resistance torque, no movement occurs and the muscle acts isometrically.

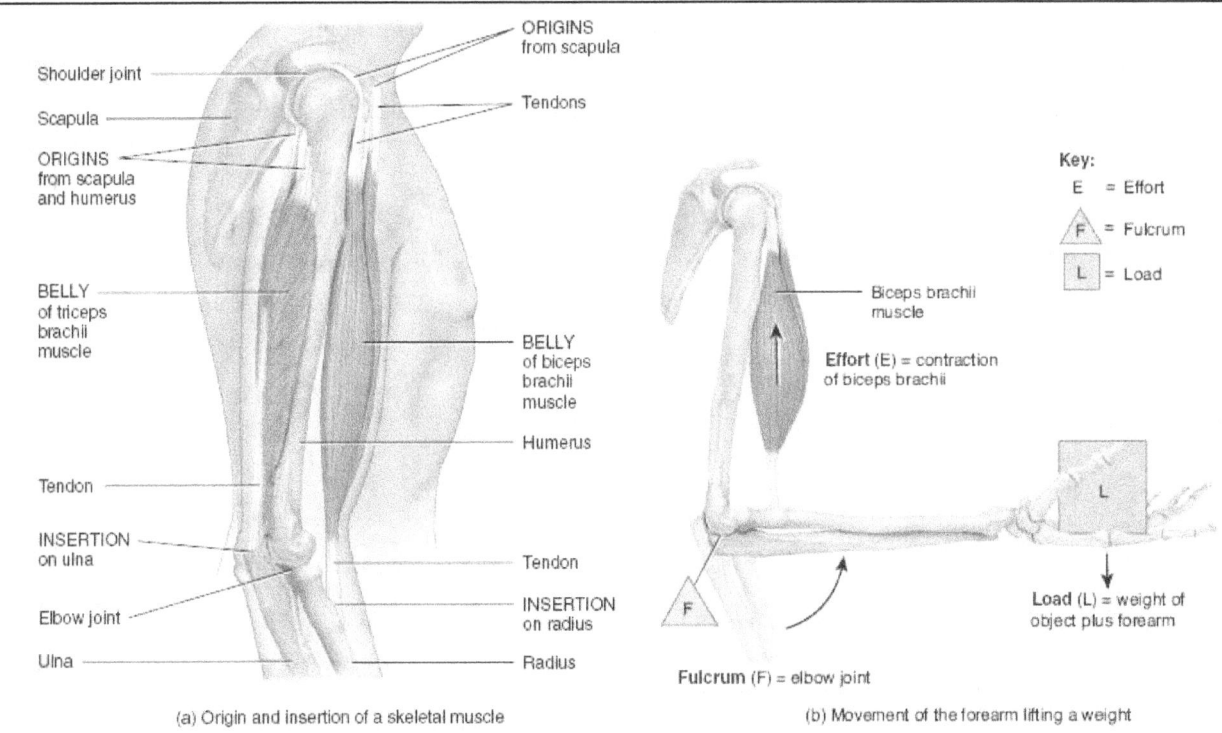

(a) Origin and insertion of a skeletal muscle

(b) Movement of the forearm lifting a weight

Applying Torque to Exercising

Knowledge of torque can be used to modify exercises for individuals. The amount of muscle force required by the exercise can be tailored to a person's needs by altering the amount of resistance, the resistance arm, or both in order to change the resistance torque.

For an example, resistance torque can be increased by adding external weight so that greater muscle force is required to overcome it. The resistance torque also can be changed by altering the position of the body parts.

The Greater the resistance torque = the Greater the Muscle Force = THE STRONGER YOU BECOME!

During an abdominal crunch, the position of the arms determines the length of the resistance arm and, therefore, the amount of resistance torque against which the abdominal muscles have to work to flex the trunk and lift the shoulders off the floor.

The arms may be held at the sides of the body to bring the upper-body mass closer to the axis of rotation and reduce the required muscle force.

To increase the challenge of this exercise, the arms can be raised with the hands on the back of the head. The resistance arm can be increased by holding the arms straight out overhead, which increases the resistance torque and therefore increases the muscle force required to perform the exercise.

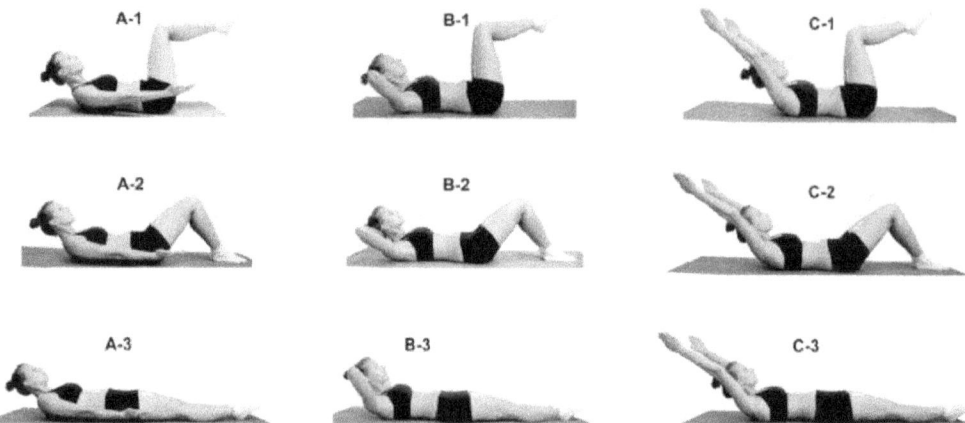

The torque that resists limb movements can be altered by modifying the amount of the resistance force and by changing the length of the resistance arm.

Rotational Inertia (Moment of Inertia)

Rotational inertia, or the resistance to change in the rotation of a body segment around a joint axis, depends on the mass of the segment and its distribution around the joint. A lower limb, for example, has more rotational inertia than an upper limb not only because it is heavier but also because its mass is concentrated a greater distance away from its axis of rotation.

The rotational inertia of body segments before or during movement depends on the mass of the segments, which cannot be changed, and on the distribution of the mass around the joints, which can be manipulated.

For example, an upper limb with the elbow extended has a greater rotational inertia than with the elbow flexed. Similarly, a lower limb with an extended knee has more rotational inertia than with the knee flexed.

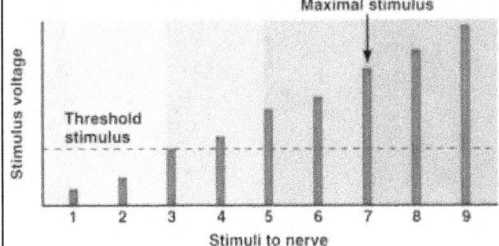

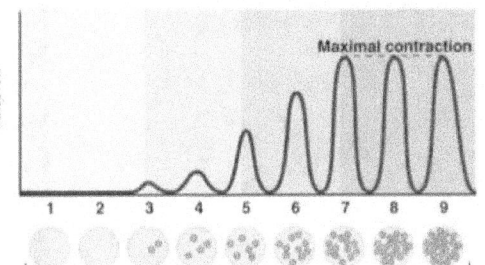

Understanding Forces of Movement

Joint movement is caused primarily by either the shortening of a muscle or the action of gravity, although other forces, such as another person pushing or pulling on a body part, may cause joint movement.

Whether a muscle contraction causes movement depends on the combined effect of the force developed and the amount of resistance from other forces.

Understanding Resist or Prevent Forces of Movement

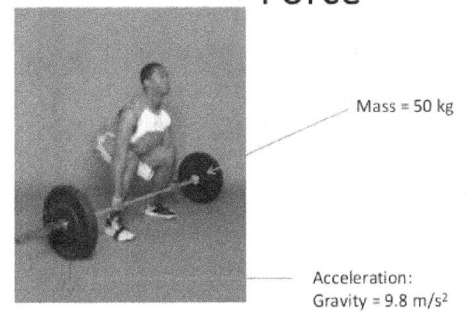

Force

Mass = 50 kg

Acceleration: Gravity = 9.8 m/s^2

Force = Mass x Acceleration
The force of this barbell = 50 kg x 9.8 m/s^2

The same forces that can cause movement may also resist or prevent movement. Joint movement caused by gravity can be resisted or decelerated by eccentric muscle action.

Gravity always resists movement occurring in a direction away from the earth.

Other forces that can resist movement include internal soft-tissue restriction by ligaments and tendons. Outside your body, exercise bands, hydraulic or air-pressure devices on resistance training equipment and the drag provided by air and water against your body moving through them can resist movement.

Strength = Maximal Force Produced
At a specific velocity

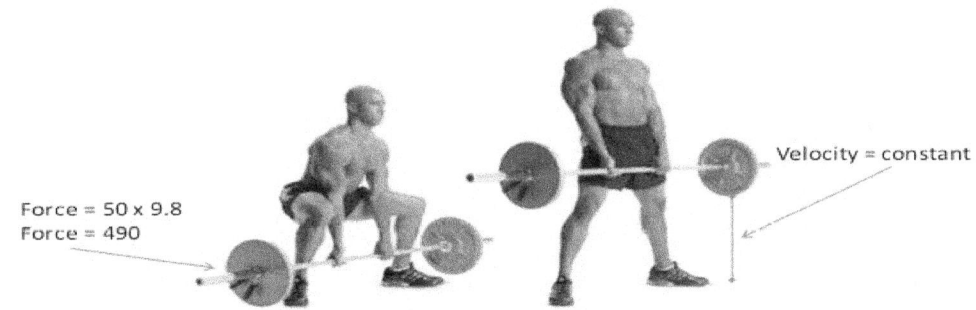

Force = 50 x 9.8
Force = 490

Velocity = constant

Because the acceleration of gravity does not change on earth, then only way to change the force is by increasing the mass

A motor neuron and the muscle fibers it innervates.

Fine control
- small motor units contain as few as 20 muscle fibers per nerve fiber
- eye muscles
  - Allow for greater dexterity because of a lower neuron to muscle fiber ratio.

Strength control
- gastrocnemius muscle has 1000 fibers per nerve fiber
  - One motor neuron controls many muscle fibers which allows for strength production.

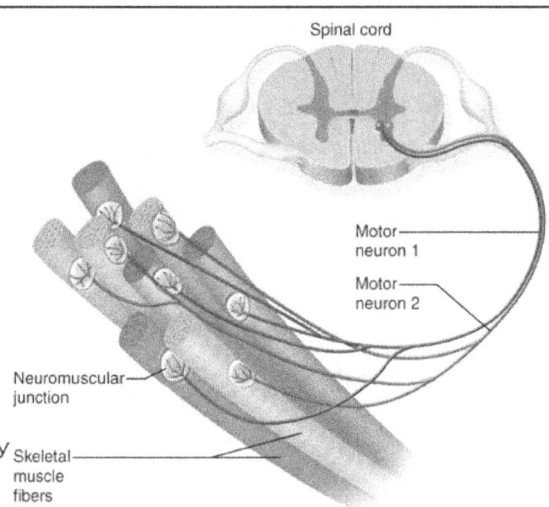

Your Muscle Action

Each muscle fiber is innervated, or receives stimuli, by a branch of your motor neuron. A **motor unit** consists of a single motor neuron, its branches, and all the muscle fibers that it innervates. With a sufficiently strong stimulus, each muscle fiber within that motor unit responds maximally; muscular tension increases as a result of the stimulation of more motor units (**recruitment**) or an increased rate of stimulation (**summation**).

Your need to Heal and become Healthy and Powerful can be your Strong Stimulus.

Your wany to Successfully Enjoy your Abundant Life can become your Strong Stimulus.

This means that you can use your Brain to formulate the necessary Thought to produce your determined Strong Stimulus to stimulate ALL of your muscles to Move YourSelf INTO Your Healing, Health and the Enjoyment of your Abundant Life!

Role of the nervous system in muscle contraction

- Specialized neurons that trigger muscle contraction are known as MOTOR NEURONS
  - As the axon of a motor neuron approaches the muscle it branches out into dozens of smaller fibers — allows one nerve to stimulate MANY different muscle fibers

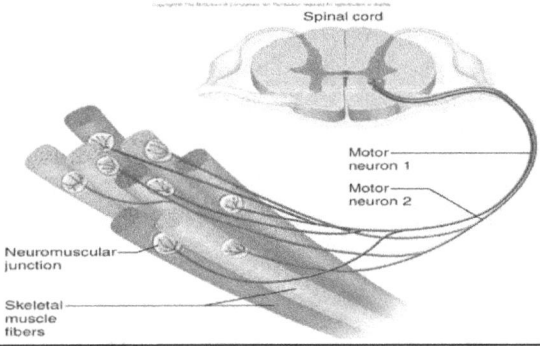

- This arrangement helps coordinate the timing of the contractions of the 1000s of muscle fibers found in a muscle

- Although each nerve fiber can stimulate 100s of muscle fibers, one muscle fiber can only be stimulated by ONE nerve fiber — prevents the muscle fiber from getting "mixed signals"

A muscle whose primary purpose is a strength or power movement (e.g., the gastrocnemius) rather than a delicate movement (e.g., the finger muscles) has a large number of muscle fibers and many muscle fibers per motor unit.

When a muscle develops tension, it tends to shorten toward the middle, pulling on all of its bony attachments.

Whether the attached bones move as a result of that muscle action depends on the amount of muscle force and the resistance to that movement from other forces.

The three major muscle actions are **concentric**, **eccentric**, and **isometric**.

Muscular Power

- Power = Velocity of muscular force development x amplitude of muscular force development
    - Velocity is how fast the fiber contracts
    - Amplitude is how much tension it produces

Motor Units

average motor unit — 200 muscle fibers for each motor unit

small motor units - fine degree of control
- 3-6 muscle fibers per neuron
- eye and hand muscles

large motor units — more strength than control
- many muscle fibers per motor unit
- powerful contractions — gastrocnemius — 1000 muscle fibers per neuron

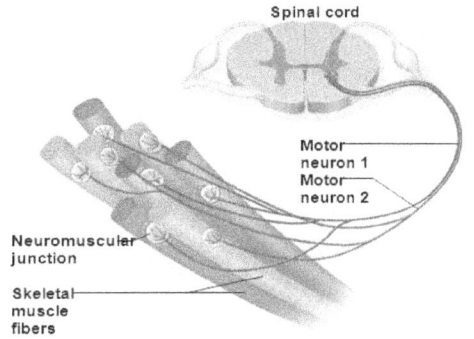

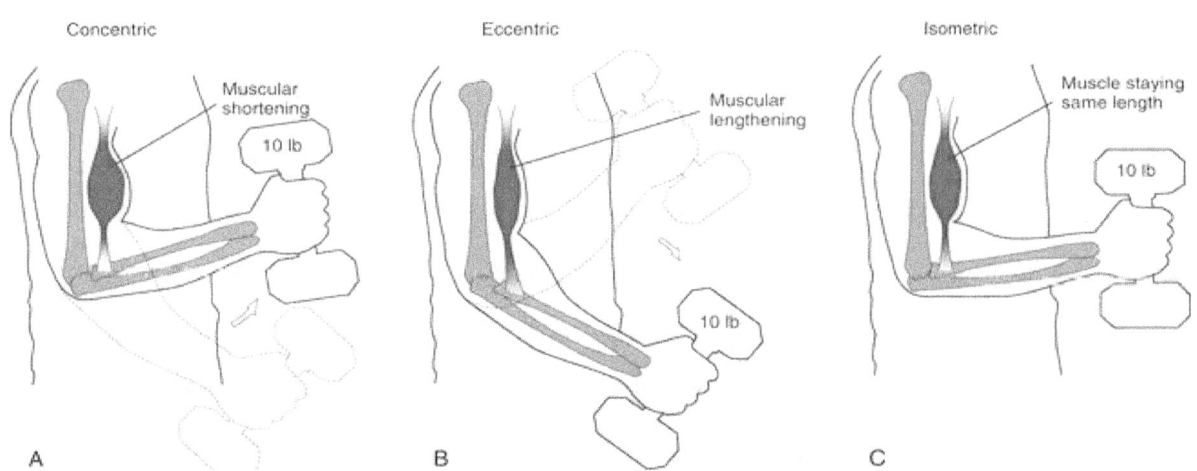

A — Concentric

B — Eccentric

C — Isometric

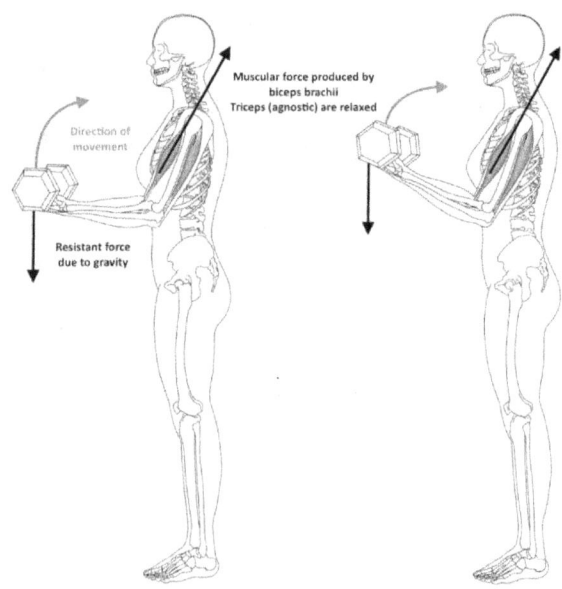

Understanding Concentric Action

A concentric action is also necessary for your rapid movement, regardless of the direction of other forces. When an external force could cause the desired movement without any muscular action but would be too slow, your concentric actions produce the desired speed.

This shortening action pulls the points of attachment on each bone closer to each other, causing movement at the joint. The muscles responsible for the flexion act with sufficient force to shorten, which pulls the forearm toward the humerus. Although the pull is on all the bones of attachment, usually only the bone farthest from the trunk (i.e., more distal) moves during a concentric action.

To exercise muscles by using gravity as the resisting force, the movements must be done in the direction opposite the pull of gravity (i.e., away from the Earth).

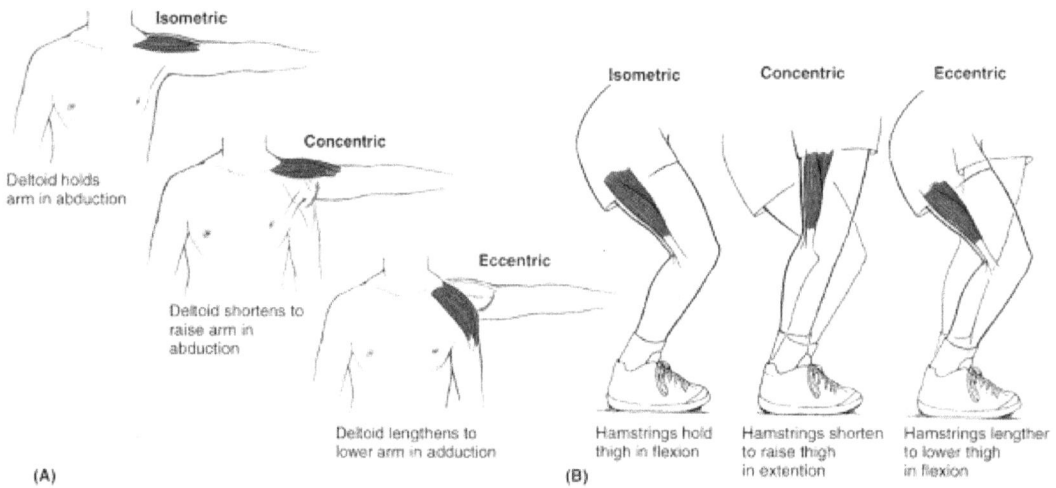

Stand up from a semi-squat position, your body must extend at the hip joints and knee joints, but gravity resists that extension. Your muscles must develop sufficient force to overcome the force of gravity as your muscle shortens in a concentric action, pulling on your bones to cause extension.

Resistance training with free weights uses gravity as the resistance.

A muscle that is very effective in causing a certain joint movement is a prime mover, or **agonist.** Assistant movers are muscles that are not as effective for the same movement.

During a concentric action, muscles that act opposite to the muscles causing the concentric action, the **antagonist** muscles, are mostly passive and lengthen as the agonists shorten.

For an example, for your elbow to flex against gravity, your muscles responsible for your elbow flexion act concentrically, while the antagonists, or your muscles responsible for elbow extension, relax and lengthen passively.

Antagonist

- The role played by a muscle acting
  - to control movement of a body segment against some other non-muscle force
  - to slow or stop a movement

- Force development during eccentric action
  - Check ballistic movements
- Relaxation during concentric action

Understanding Eccentric Action

Your **eccentric action** occurs when your muscle generates tension that is not great enough to cause your movement but instead slows the speed of your movement in the opposite direction caused by another force.

Your muscle exerts force, but its length increases while it is under tension. Shoulder abduction requires concentric action, but gravity will adduct the upper limb back to the side of the body.

To adduct your upper limb more slowly than gravity does, the same muscles that acted concentrically to abduct your upper limb now act eccentrically to control the speed of upper limb.

Eccentric actions may also occur when the maximum effort of your muscle is not great enough to overcome the opposing force.

Movement due to the opposing force will still occur despite the maximally activated muscle, which is lengthening under tension.

Eccentric contraction – working against gravity

- Sitting Down

- Hip – Flexion
- Agonist – Gluteals

- Knee – Flexion
- Agonist – Quadriceps

- Ankle – Dorsiflexion
- Agonist – Gastrocnemius

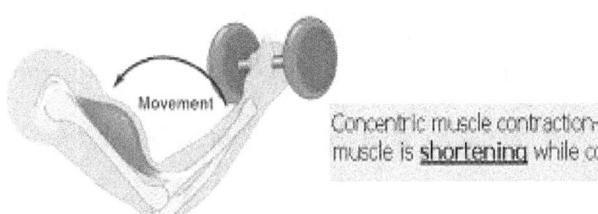
Concentric muscle contraction—The bicep muscle is **shortening** while contracting.

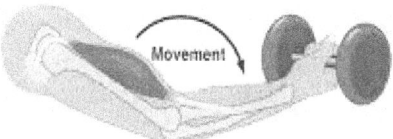
Eccentric muscle contraction—The bicep muscle is **lengthening** while contracting.

An example of this may occur when a person with the elbow joint flexed to 90° is handed a heavy weight. The exerciser tries to flex the elbow joint or even maintain the 90° position but lacks the strength to do so. The elbow joint extends despite the efforts to flex it.

Muscles that are antagonists to the eccentrically acting muscles will passively shorten during the movement.

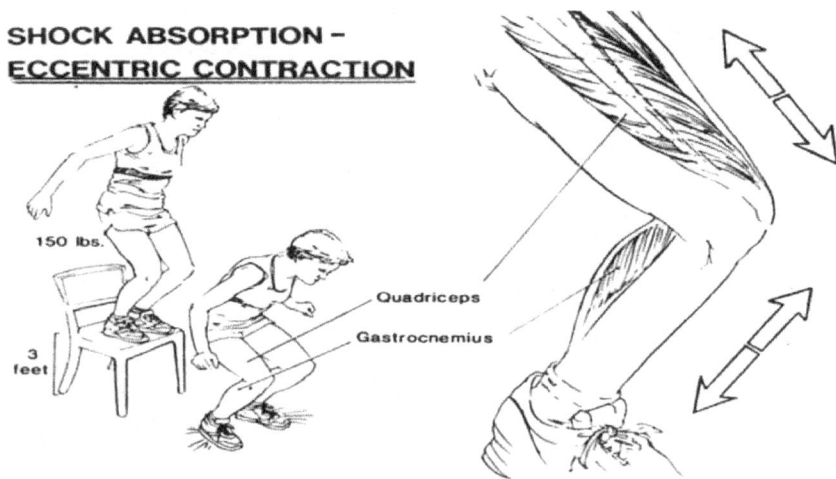

Figure 2. Eccentric contraction of the quadriceps and gastro-soleus muscle groups effectively dissipates the force of impact following a jump from a height.

Understanding Your Ballistic Movements and Muscle Action

Your **ballistic movement** is a fast movement that occurs when resistance is minimal, as in throwing a ball, and requires a burst of your concentric action to initiate it.

Once your movement has begun, these initial muscles relax because any further action would cause your movement to slow.

You have other muscles that actively guide your movement in the appropriate direction. At the end of your movement, eccentric action of muscles that are the antagonist to the initial muscles decelerates and stops the movement. For an example, one of the most important movements in throwing is internal rotation of the shoulder joint. The muscles responsible for internal rotation act **quickly** and **concentrically** to begin the throwing motion. After the ball is released, the muscles responsible for external rotation act eccentrically to **slow** and **stop** the movement during the follow-through.

The reverse is true for the windup, or preparation for the actual throw.

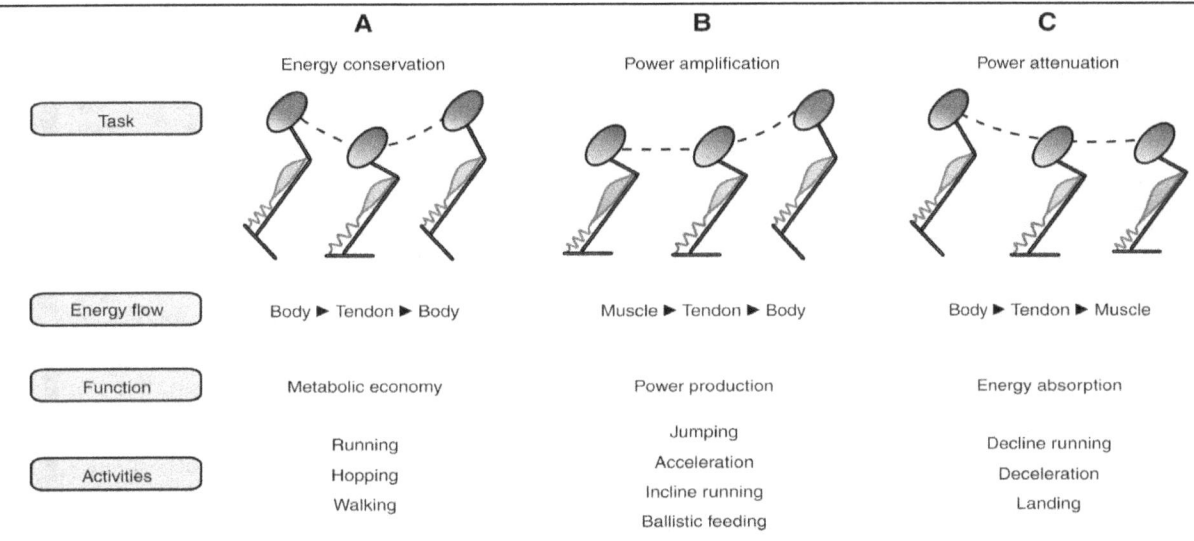

Understanding Isometric Action

During an **isometric action,** or static action, your muscle exerts a force that is equal in magnitude to an opposing force.

The muscle length does not change and the joint position is maintained: The contractile part of your muscle shortens, but the elastic connective tissue lengthens proportionately, so there is no overall change in the entire muscle length.

Holding your upper limb in an abducted position or maintaining a semi-squat position requires isometric action, producing just enough muscle force to counteract the pull of gravity and result in no movement.

The effort involved in trying to move an immovable object (e.g., pushing against a wall) is another example of an isometric action; although the amount of muscular force can be maximal, the joint does not move.

The posterior pelvic tilt desired during some exercises is maintained by isometric action of your anterior trunk muscles after they have acted concentrically to tilt your pelvis backward.

ISOMETRIC

Exercise in which one contacts muscles but does not move body parts

Examples:
- Planks
- Wall sits
- Side planks
- Push up holds
- Dead hang
- Split squats

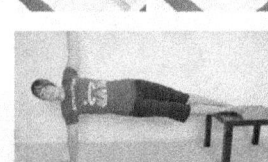

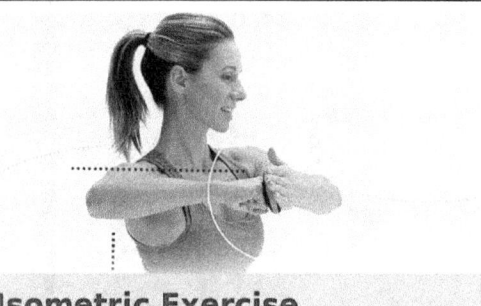

Isometric Exercise

Isometric exercise has been practiced for over 5,000 years and is the **foundation of both yoga and pilates**.

Isometrics is **static muscle exercise** in which you engage your muscles against each other or against a static object making it easy to exercise anywhere.

Scientific research has proven that isometric exercise is one of the **fastest and most efficient ways to build strength, burn fat and tone your body**.

During all resistance exercises that involve your arms or legs, your trunk muscles should act isometrically to stabilize your trunk and help prevent injury.

KEY Knowledge

During **concentric** muscle action, your muscle shortens and the joint moves in the direction your muscle is pulling = Your Body Moves where You Command.

During **eccentric** muscle action, your muscle lengthens and the joint moves in the opposite direction than your muscle is pulling.

During the action of **isometric** muscle contraction there is no change in the length and the joint does not move.

These exercises are practice of Control and Command of Self ... to increase your ability to Move YourSelf into your Healing!

Isotonic contraction		Isometric contraction
Concentric	**Eccentric**	
• Concentric contraction in the biceps brachii during the **upward phase** of exercise	• Eccentric contraction in the biceps brachii during the **downward phase** of exercise	• Isometric contraction occurs in the biceps brachii when the muscle is **holding the weight still**
• Biceps brachii produces tension and **shortens**	• Biceps brachii produces tension and **lengthens**	• Biceps brachii develops tension and **stays the same length**
• It pulls the **forearm upwards to cause flexion** of the elbow	• It **slows the lowering of the forearm and controls extension of the elbow**	• It **stops flexion and extension of the elbow**

Tips for Exercising Muscle Groups and Common Exercise Mistakes

Many errors that occur during exercise and movement activities result from a lack of knowledge of musculoskeletal anatomy rather than a lack of muscular strength or coordination. Applying basic knowledge allows exercisers to perform better and more safely. This section offers tips for each major muscle group.

Your Shoulder Girdle & Shoulder Joint

Movement can be enhanced and more of your muscles become involved if your shoulder girdle movements are deliberately incorporated with shoulder joint movements. These muscles can be optimally involved in the following exercises and movements:

• Forward reaching. Glenohumeral joint flexion can be accompanied by scapular elevation and upward rotation if you reach your fingertips as far forward as possible.

• Push-up. At the completion of a push-up, your scapulae can be protracted to raise your chest a bit more off the floor.

• Overhead reaching. Normally, some scapular elevation is involved when your upper limb is overhead. A conscious effort to reach as high as possible will involve your scapula elevators more. Conversely, a deliberate attempt to keep your shoulders down and your neck long requires concentric action by your scapula depressors.

• Sideward reaching. During horizontal abduction at your shoulder joint, your upper limb can be moved farther back with scapular retraction.

Your Elbow & Radioulnar Joints

Flexion against resistance requires concentric action of your flexor muscles at the elbow joint. The degree to which these muscles are strengthened, however, is affected by **supination** and **pronation** actions. Your biceps brachii attaches to the radius, and this bone rotates when your forearm pronates, stretching out your biceps and reducing its contribution to your elbow flexion. Thus, elbow flexion with the radioulnar joint in a pronated position (a reverse curl) is a weaker movement than a traditional curl with the forearm in a supinated position. A reverse curl puts more emphasis on the brachialis at the expense of your biceps.

Triceps push-downs, in which elbow extension occurs with your radioulnar joints in the pronated position, require your wrist flexors to stabilize your wrist joint, whereas triceps pull-downs (supinated position) utilize your wrist extensors, which are usually much weaker than your flexors. If you want to concentrate on building your elbow extensors – try performing triceps push-downs.

Your Wrist Joint

During wrist flexion and extension curls, your wrist muscles are affected by the position of your radioulnar joints. Gravity acts as resistance for wrist flexion when your radioulnar joints are in the supinated position and as resistance for extension when your radioulnar joints are in the pronated position.

Your Vertebral Column and Lumbosacral Joints

In general, neither neck hyperextension nor hyperflexion is desirable action or position. The same pairs of muscles that act concentrically to cause flexion and extension can be strengthened or stretched, one side at a time, by cervical lateral flexion and rotation. You should tilt or turn your head from side to side rather than bend your neck forward or backward.

Although hyperextension may not be contraindicated for the young, it teaches bad habits and is best avoided.

Many exercises require appropriate positioning of your lumbosacral joint and lumbar vertebrae and actions by your trunk muscles for either movement or stabilization.

When performing an abdominal curl-up or crunch, you should begin with a backward pelvic tilt that is maintained throughout the curl-up and return movement. If the backward pelvic tilt cannot be maintained or you feel tightness or an ache in your lumbar area, **you should STOP!** If the problem is inadequate strength to maintain the backward tilt, then you should modify to one where you have the sufficient abdominal strength to perform correctly.

A full curl-up, in which you come up to a sitting position, requires hip flexion by your hip flexor muscles during the last stages of the exercise. Initially, the abdominal muscles concentrically tilt the pelvis backward and then flex the vertebral column. Once flexion is achieved, these muscles act isometrically to keep your pelvis tilted backward and your trunk in a flexed position. During a full curl-up, you can feel a sticking point that occurs when your trunk flexion is complete and your hip flexors begin to bring your trunk to an upright position.

Doing partial curl-ups or crunches helps eliminate the role of your hip flexors and maintain focus solely on strengthening your abdominal muscles.

The leg lift is also considered an abdominal exercise, but unfortunately, it is often not taught correctly. From a supine position on the floor, your legs are lifted and held up by the concentric and then isometric action of your hip flexors. Some of your hip flexors also pull your lumbosacral joint into a forward-tilted position. Your abdominal muscles must prevent that forward tilt and maintain a flattened lumbar spine and posterior pelvic tilt. The backward pelvic tilt should precede the hip flexion, and, as in the case of the curl-up, if the proper tilt cannot be maintained, the exercise should not be done in that fashion.

The pelvis also tends to tilt forward during overhead upper-limb movements from a standing position. This can be prevented by keeping your arms in front of your ears and flexing your knees slightly.

When weights are lifted from a supine position, as in the bench press, there is a tendency to hyperextend your lumbar spine and tilt your pelvis forward. Although this tendency can allow you to lift a somewhat heavier weight, it does not increase the work of your upper limb and chest muscles, and it puts your lower back into a compromising position. Bench presses are best done with your hips and knees in a flexed position and your feet on the bench or a bench extension to maintain a posterior pelvic tilt. Upright presses are best done seated with your back supported.

Your Hip Joint

A common error during side-lying leg raises for the hip abductors is the attempt to move the foot as high as possible. Because the ROM for true abduction is limited (about 45°), you will externally rotate the top limb, which turns your foot out and allows it to go higher. However, this rotation changes the muscle involvement more to your hip flexors. To exercise your primary abductor muscles, your limb should not be rotated and your toes should face forward, not upward.

In backward lower-limb movements for strengthening the gluteus muscles, hip extension is limited primarily by the tightness of your hip ligaments. Your limb can appear to be more extended if it is accompanied by a forward pelvic tilt. You should be cautioned to keep your pelvis in its neutral position in order to focus on your gluteal muscles, even though some apparent hip extension is lost.

Your Knee Joint

Hyperflexion can strain and stretch your knee ligaments and put pressure on your menisci. Therefore, a maximum squat depth to a 90° angle at your knee joint is recommended. During any lunging movements or forward–back stride positions in which your front knee is flexed, your knee should be over or in back of your foot and not in front.

Any knee position that puts a twisting pressure on your knee joint should also be avoided. The hurdler position, with one limb out to the back and side with a flexed knee, should be avoided; instead, both legs should be out in front.

A common exercise position is standing with feet your shoulder-width apart. You should have your feet turned slightly outward (7°-10°). The appropriate toe-out position is one that positions your kneecaps facing forward. During any squatting or standing movement, your knee should be in line directly above your foot (not moving to the outside or inside of your foot) to avoid straining your lateral and medial knee ligaments and to develop good lower-extremity positioning habits.

Performing the exercise in front of a mirror is recommended to enable you to monitor the position of your knee relative to your foot.

Your Ankle Joint

If the squat exercise is performed with your heels of your feet resting on a low block, your soleus muscles are exercised more than they would be if your feet were flat. This position with your heels up shortens your gastrocnemius muscles even more (they are already shortened by your flexed knee), limiting their ability to generate force.

Your soleus muscles, which do not cross your knees, aren't shortened to the same extent. To increase the force production of your gastrocnemius muscles, the squat could be done with the balls of your feet on the block.

Your Subtalar Joint

Your subtalar joint plays a role in adapting to uneven surfaces. A way of exercising your invertors and evertors is to walk across, instead of up and down, a ramp or hill.

KEY Knowledge

During exercises involving your vertebral column and lumbosacral joints, you should remember to achieve a posterior (backward) pelvic tilt before initiating the exercise and should maintain the tilt throughout the exercise to protect your lumbar spine.

For exercises involving your knee, you should remember to keep your knee in line above your foot when observing themselves in a mirror. Your knee should also stay behind or above your foot when observed from the side.

Defining Power

- Power is intimately tied to Work
    - Power is work per unit time

- Work refers to the force exerted on an object and the distance the object moves in the direction in which the force is exerted
    - Work = Force x Distance

- Power is how much work was performed in a given time
    - Power = Work/Time

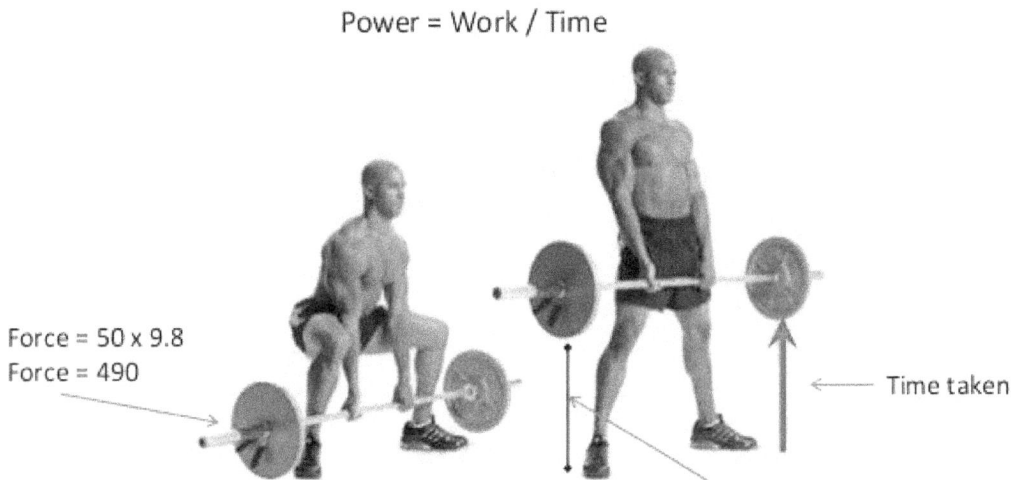

Power = Work / Time

Force = 50 x 9.8
Force = 490

Time taken

Distance = .75 m

Work = Force x Distance = 490 x .75 = 367.5
In a deadlift, work does not change for a given weight.
Thus, the time taken to do the work will determine power.

Calculate the difference in power when the movement takes 3 sec vs. 2 sec

- Strength is intimately related to maximal force production
- Force = mass x acceleration
  - Often times people forget about the acceleration component of force
  - Acceleration = over coming gravity
- Acceleration is a change in velocity per unit time
  - Velocity is the rate of change in position
- The best definition of strength is
  - The maximal force that a muscle can generate at a specified velocity

- Force is an influence which causes an object to undergo a change acceleration
  - Force = Mass x Acceleration
- Strength is the maximal force a muscle can generate at a specified velocity
  - Strength = force x velocity
- Power is the work done in a given amount of time
  - Work = force x distance
  - Power = work/time

Neural Factors Related to Muscular Strength & Power

- The 2 neural control factors that are intimately involved with displaying strength and power are
  - Recruitment
  - Rate Coding

Neural Factors Related to Muscular Strength & Power

- In general, muscular force is greater when
  - 1. More motor units are involved with the contraction
  - 2. The motor units are greater in size (fast twitch motor units, which are the most difficult to recruit)
  - 3. The rate of neural firing increases in speed and efficiency
    - Rate coding – how well a message goes from your brain and down your spinal cord to eventually reach and signal the individual muscle motor units to fire

Move Something!

Chapter Twenty-One

Biomechanics – Life Movement & Motion

*****

Your Skeletal Anatomy

Most of the 200 distinct bones in your skeleton are involved in your movement. Their high mineral component gives them rigidity, while their protein component reduces their brittleness.

The two types of bone tissue are **cortical** and **trabecular** bone. Cortical, or compact, bone is the dense, hard outer layer of a bone.

Trabecular bone, also known as spongy or cancellous bone, has a lattice-like structure to provide greater internal strength along the lines of stress within a bone but with less overall weight than solid bone.

Your Bones are living tissue and are constantly being remodeled in adaptation to the loading demands placed on them.

Your Bones are divided into four classifications according to their shape: **long**, **short**, **flat**, and **irregular**.

Your Bones are designed to hold your God-Body TOGETHER so that you can Successfully Enjoy Your Abundant Life!

Your Bones are designed to MOVE!

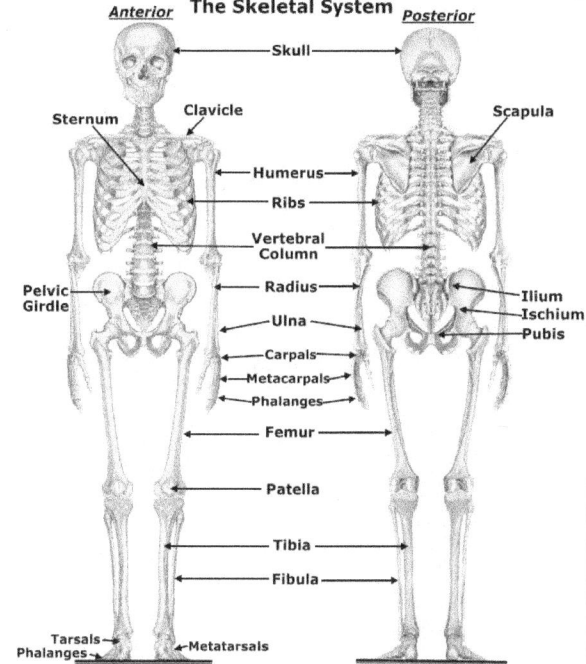

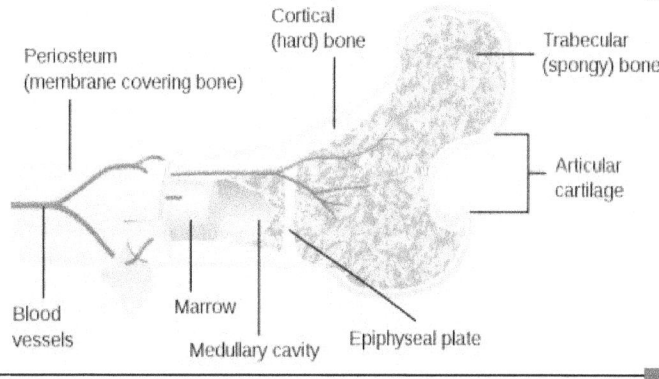

Your Long Bones

Your long bones are found in your limbs and digits and serve primarily as levers for your movement. Each of your long bones has several distinct features.

Your **diaphysis,** or shaft, is made up of thick, compact bone surrounding the hollow medullary cavity. It is characteristic of long bones that the shaft is longer than it is wide.

Your **epiphyses,** or expanded ends, are composed of spongy bone with a thin outer layer of compact bone.

Your **articular cartilage** is a thin layer of hyaline cartilage covering the articulating surfaces (the surfaces of a bone that come into contact with another bone to form a joint) that provides a smooth, low-friction surface and helps absorb shock.

Your **periosteum** is a fibrous membrane covering the entire bone (except where the articular cartilage is present) to serve as an attachment site for muscles. Examples of long bones include your femur in your thigh, your ulna in your forearm, and your phalanges in your digits.

Classification of Bones by Shape

- **Long bones**
    - Longer than they are wide
    - All limb bones except the patella, wrist, and ankle bone are long bones.
- **Short bones**
    - Cube-shaped bones (in wrist and ankle)
    - Sesamoid bones (within tendons → patella)

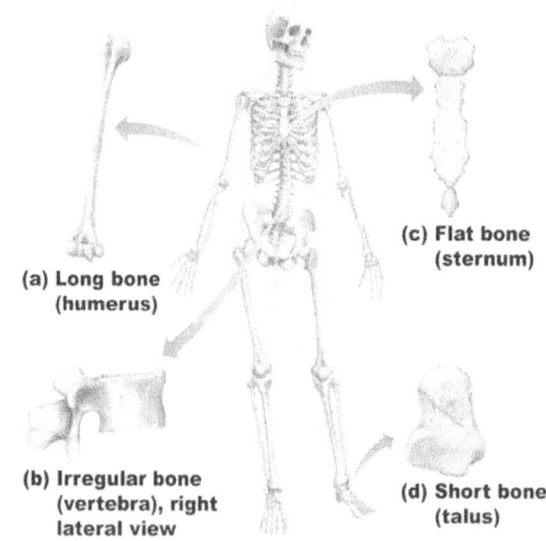

(a) Long bone (humerus)
(b) Irregular bone (vertebra), right lateral view
(c) Flat bone (sternum)
(d) Short bone (talus)

Your Short, Flat and Irregular Bones

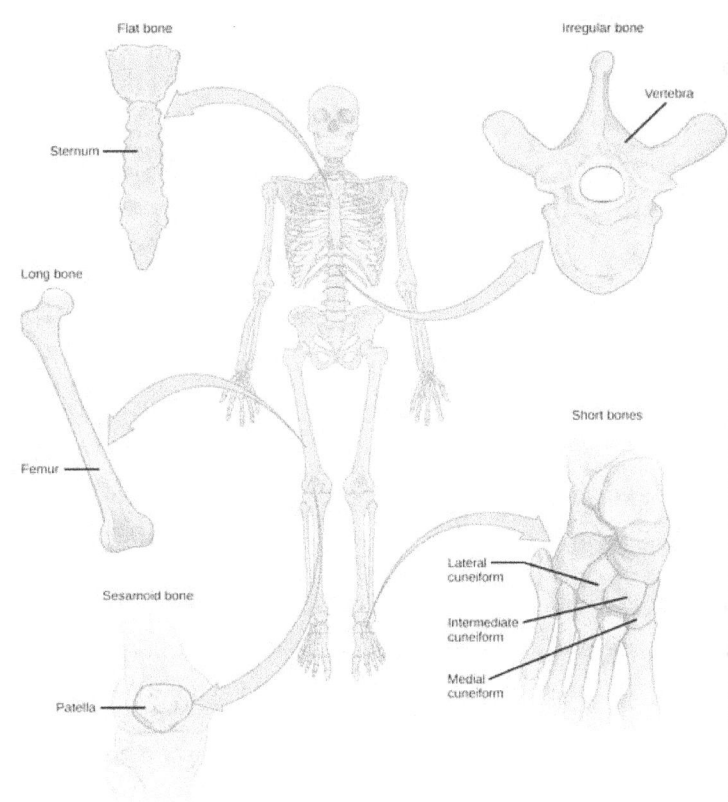

In addition to long bones, your skeleton is made up of **short** bones, **flat** bones, and **irregularly** shaped bones. Your **tarsals** (in your ankle) and **carpals** (in your wrist) are your short bones, and they are approximately as wide as they are long. Their composition (internal trabecular bone covered with a thin outside layer of cortical bone) provides light weight and strength. Their roughly cubic shape decreases the potential for movement between adjacent bones.

Your flat bones, such as your **ribs**, **ilia** (wings of your pelvis), and **scapulae** (shoulder blades), serve primarily as broad sites for your muscle attachments and, in the case of your ribs and ilia, to enclose cavities and protect your internal organs. These bones have a broad, flattened structure. They are composed of trabecular bone covered with a thin layer of cortical bone.

Your **ischium** (inferior part of your pelvis), **pubis** (anterior part of your pelvis) and **vertebrae** are irregularly shaped bones that protect internal parts and support your body in addition to being sites for your muscle attachments.

An additional category of bone, sesamoid, is reserved for those few bones in your body that are embedded within a tendon. The role of these bones is to modify the way a tendon crosses a joint. Your **patella** (kneecap) is a sesamoid bone embedded in the quadriceps tendon at your knee.

Your Planes & Axes of Movement

Anatomical terminology enables the accurate description of position and movement of the human body.

To describe joint movements, reference is made to rotation about one or more of three axes and to movement in one of three cardinal planes.

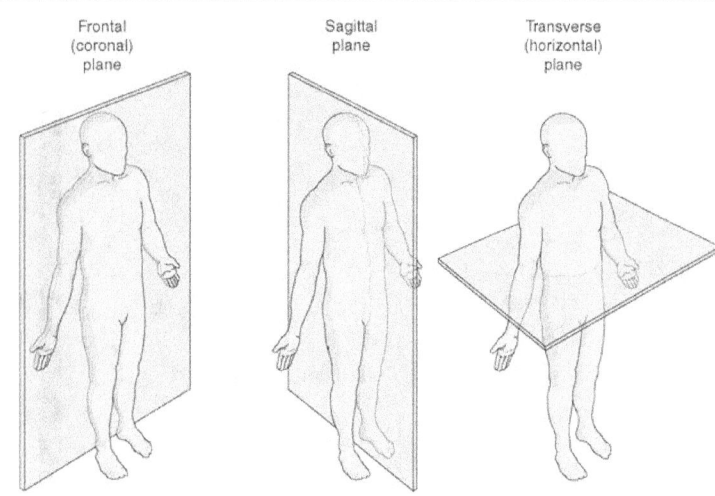

These planes are perpendicular to each other and represent a side view (**sagittal** plane), front or back view (**frontal** or **coronal** plane), and top view, looking down from above (**transverse** plane).

Movement observed in each plane is a rotation about an axis that is perpendicular to the plane. The reference position for describing movement is the anatomical position (standing erect, arms hanging at sides, palms facing forward, feet shoulder-width apart).

Your mediolateral axis is perpendicular to your sagittal plane and joint rotations about this axis are **flexion** and **extension**.

Your **anteroposterior** axis is perpendicular to your frontal plane and joint rotations about this axis are abduction and adduction. Your longitudinal or vertical axis is perpendicular to your transverse plane, and rotations about this axis are **internal** and **external rotation.**

Your Joint rotations are described according to how your distal segment (body part just below the joint) moves relative to your proximal segment (body part just above the joint).

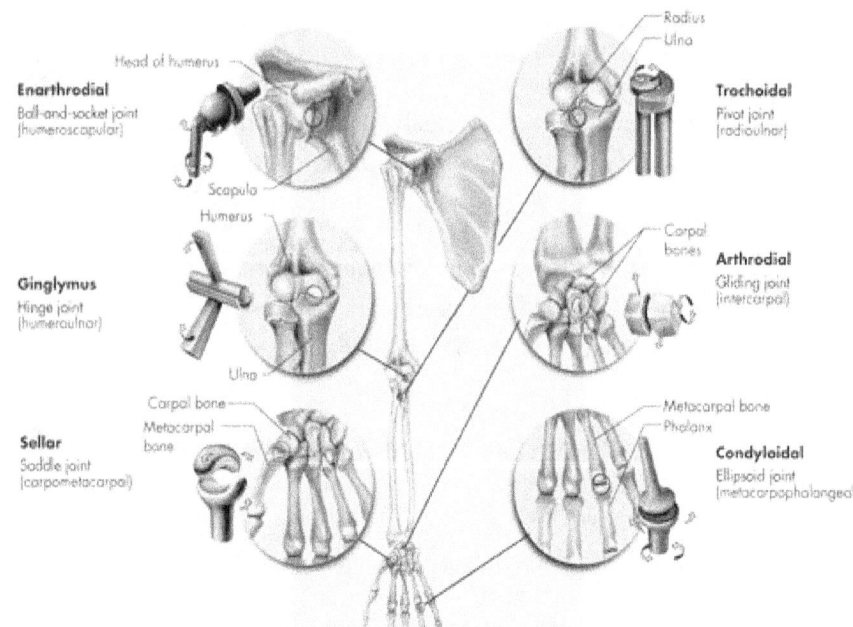

Joints, which are the places where two or more of your bones meet, or articulate, are often classified according to the amount of movement that can take place at those sites.

Your **Ligaments,** which are tough, fibrous bands of connective tissue, connect your bones to each other across all joints.

Your Joints are classified as **synarthrodial**, **amphiarthrodial**, or **synovial** based on how much they can move. **Synarthrodial joints** are immovable joints. Your bones merge into each other and are bound together by fibrous tissue that is continuous with your periosteum. Your **sutures**, or lines of junction, of the cranial (skull) bones are prime examples of this type of joint.

Amphiarthrodial Joints

Your Amphiarthrodial joints, or cartilaginous joints, allow only slight movement between bones. Usually a fibrocartilage disc separates your bones and movement can occur only by deformation of the disc.

Examples of these joints are your **tibiofibular** and **sacroiliac** joints and the joints between the bodies of your vertebrae in your spine.

Symphysis

- Joint separated by a fibrocartilage pad that allows very slight movement between the bones
- Examples - The symphysis pubis and intervertebral discs

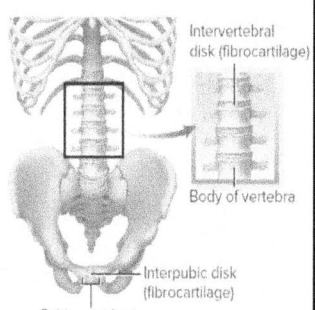

Diarthrodial Joints

Your Diarthrodial joints, more commonly known as **synovial** joints, are freely movable joints that allow greater movement direction and range; most of the joint movements during physical activity occur at these joints.

Your synovial joints are the most common type and include most joints of the extremities.

Strong and inelastic ligaments, along with connective and muscle tissue crossing the joint, maintain their stability.

- known as synovial joints
- freely movable
- composed of sleevelike *joint capsule*
- secretes synovial fluid to lubricate *joint cavity*

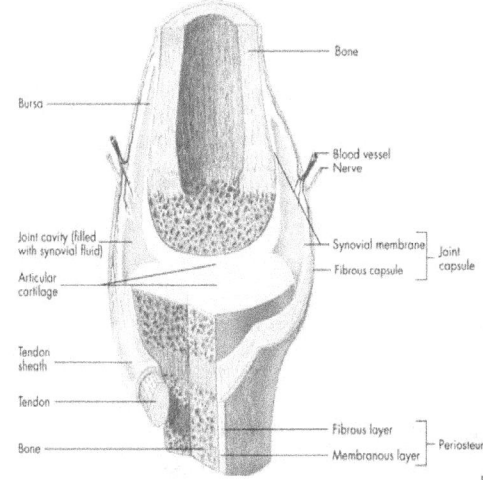

Your synovial joints have several distinguishing characteristics. The articulating surfaces of the bones are covered by articular cartilage, a type of hyaline cartilage that reduces friction and contributes to shock absorption between the bones. Each joint is completely enclosed by an **articular capsule,** whose thickness varies from thin and loose to thick and tight.

Your **synovial membrane** lines the inner surface of the capsule. It secretes synovial fluid into the **joint cavity,** the space enclosed by your articular capsule. Synovial fluid bathes your joint to nourish the articular cartilage and reduce friction when bones move. Normally, the joint cavity is small and, therefore, contains little synovial fluid, but an injury to the joint can increase the secretion of synovial fluid and cause swelling.

Functional Classification of Synovial Joints

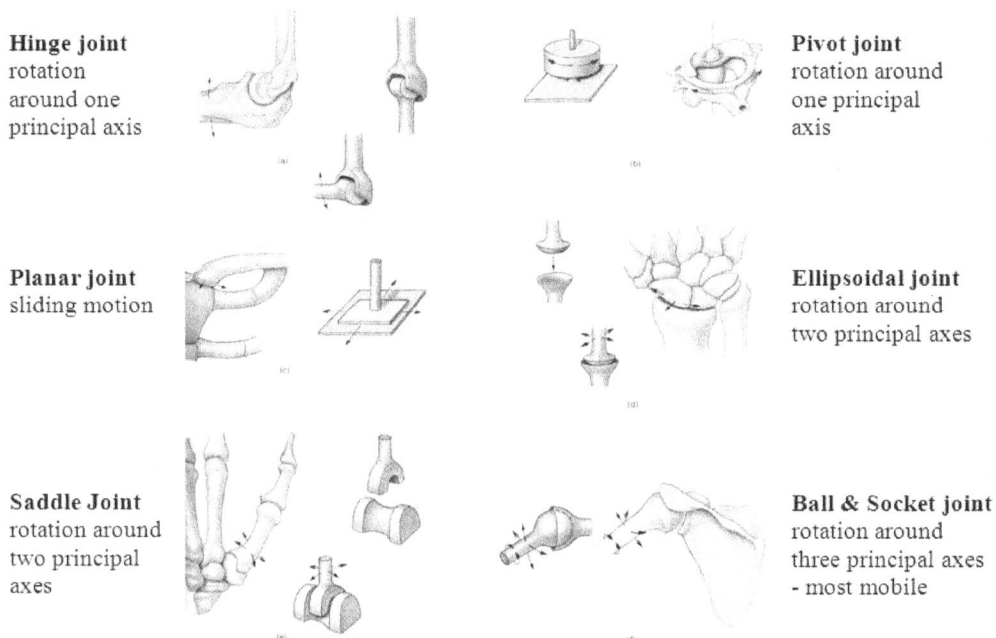

Hinge joint — rotation around one principal axis

Pivot joint — rotation around one principal axis

Planar joint — sliding motion

Ellipsoidal joint — rotation around two principal axes

Saddle Joint — rotation around two principal axes

Ball & Socket joint — rotation around three principal axes - most mobile

Some synovial joints, such as your **sternoclavicular** and **knee** joints, also have a partial or complete fibrocartilage disc between your bones to aid shock absorption and, in the case of your knee, to give greater stability to the joint.

The partial, C-shaped discs between your femur and your tibia at your knee are called **menisci.** To reduce friction or rubbing as tendons move during muscle contraction, your tendons often are surrounded by tendon sheaths—cylindrical, tunnel-like sacs lined with synovial membrane.

For example, the two proximal tendons of your biceps brachii pass through these tunnels in the bicipital groove of your humerus. **Bursae,** or sacs of synovial fluid that lie between your muscles, tendons, and bones, also reduce friction between the tissues and act as shock absorbers.

Many bursae are found around the shoulder, elbow, hip, and knee. Bursitis, or the inflammation of a bursa, can result from repeated friction or mechanical irritation. The moveable joints in your body are diarthrodial (synovial) joints. The bony surfaces are covered in smooth articular cartilage and your joint cavity is filled with synovial fluid, which lubricates the joint,

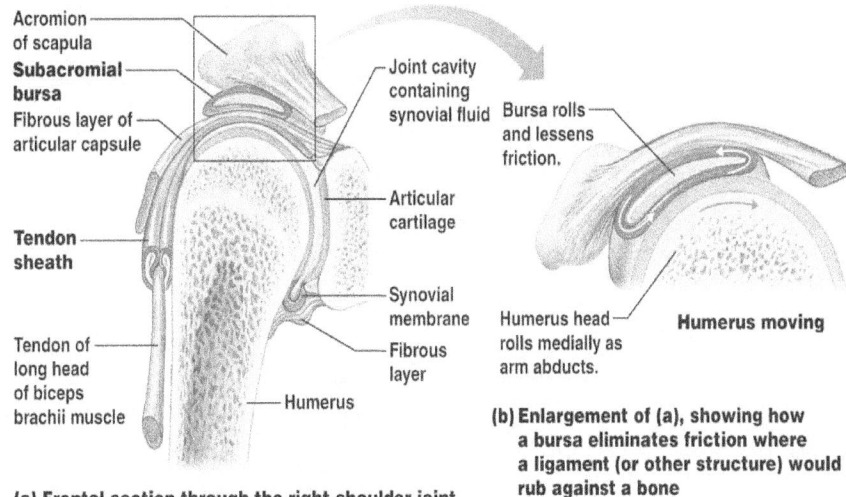

(a) Frontal section through the right shoulder joint

(b) Enlargement of (a), showing how a bursa eliminates friction where a ligament (or other structure) would rub against a bone

Your joints are the hinges to ensure your movement. Your dietary choices have a direct impact on the health and condition of your joints.

The level and amount of your activities determines the physical ability of your joints to Successfully Move You into the Enjoyment of Your Abundant Life!

Determining Factors - Your Direction and Range of Motion

The primary movement at a joint is rotation about one or more axes. Some joints may exhibit a small amount of sliding (translation) between the bones. The limits to direction and the **range of motion** (ROM) at a joint are determined primarily by the shape of the bones at their articulating ends. Depending on the bone shape, joints may rotate about one, two, or three axes. Ball-and-socket joints, which are found at the hip and shoulder, allow a wide range of movement in all directions as the ball rotates within the socket.

Hinge joints, such as the elbow and ankle joints, have only one axis of rotation due to the structure of the interlocking bones.

Other types of joints include ellipsoidal joints, such as the wrist, and saddle joints, such as the sternoclavicular joint, whose shapes permit rotation about two axes. Pivot joints, such as the proximal radioulnar joint, permit rotation about one axis only, the longitudinal axis. Gliding joints, such as between the tarsal bones in the foot, have minimal sliding movement between the bones.

The length of the ligaments and to a lesser extent their **elasticity,** or ability to stretch passively and return to their normal length, also limit ROM. For example, the iliofemoral ligament at the anterior hip joint is a strong but short ligament that prohibits much hip extension.

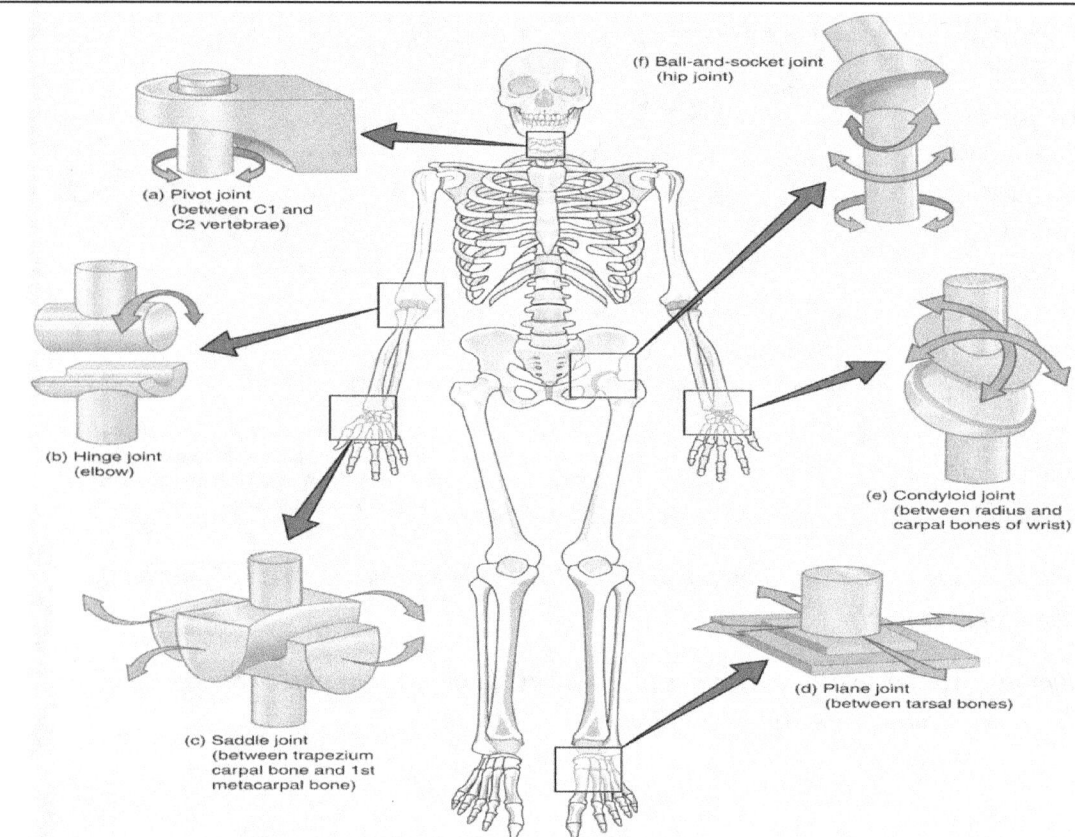

The limits to range and direction of motion at a joint are determined by the shape of the articulating bones and the length of ligaments crossing the joint.

Your Specific Joint Movements

Specific terminology is used to describe the direction of movement at the various joints. This ensures that movements are described accurately and can be immediately understood. The anatomical position serves as a point of reference. Terminology generally relates to movements within planes and about axes.

Flexion and **extension** are movements in the sagittal plane about a mediolateral axis. Flexion is moving the distal segment forward and upward from the anatomical position to bring two body segments closer together. Extension is the return from flexion, moving the segment in the opposite direction.

Abduction and **adduction** are movements in the frontal plane about an anteroposterior axis. Abduction is moving the distal segment out to the side and away from the body from the anatomical position, whereas adduction is the return toward the anatomical position from abduction, moving the segment in the opposite direction. Internal and external rotation are movements in the transverse plane about a longitudinal axis.

Joint range of motion is measured from anatomical neutral, normal standing postion. These ranges are general guidelines and individuals vary. For example, women tend to be more flexible than men and may have a greater overall range of motion. Comparing range of motion between sides of the body is one of the best ways to distinguish normal and limited range of motion.

Neck
Flexion: 90°
Touch chin to sternum.
Extension: 55°
Look upwards.
Lateral flexion: 35°
Bring ear to shoulder.
Rotation: 70°
Turn head to the left or right.

Hip
Flexion: 130°
Flex knee and bring thigh close to abdomen.
Extension: 30°
Move thigh backward without moving the pelvis.
Abduction: 45°
Move thigh laterally away from midline.
Adduction: 20°
Bring thigh forward and across midline.
Internal rotation: 40°
Flex knee & swing lower leg away from midline.
External rotation: 45°
Flex knee & swing lower leg toward midline.

Ankle
Plantarflexion: 50°
Bend ankle so toes point down
Dorsiflexion: 20°
Bend ankle so toes point up.
Supination/Inversion: 30°
Turn foot so the sole faces in.
Pronation/Eversion: 15°
Turn foot so the sole faces out.

Shoulder
Abduction: 180°
Raise arm away from body, above head.
Adduction: 45°
Bring arm toward and across midline.
Horizontal extension: 45°
Swing arm horizontally backward.
Horizontal flexion: 130°
Swing arm horizontally forward.
Extension: 50°
Raise arm backward.
Forward flexion: 180°
Raise arm forward over head.

Lumbar Spine
Flexion: 75°
Bend forward at the waist.
Extension: 30°
Bend backward at the waist.
Sidebending: 35°
Bend to the side at the waist.

Elbow
Flexion: 150°
Bend arm bringing wrist to shoulder.
Extension: 180°
Straighten arm from flexion.
Supination: 90°
Turn lower arm so palm faces up.
Pronation: 90°
Turn lower arm so palm faces down.

Knee
Flexion: 130°
Bring heel toward hamstring.
Extension: 0°
Straighten out knee as much as possible.
Internal rotation: 10°
Twist lower leg toward midline.

Wrist
Flexion: 80°
Bend wrist, palm toward palmar forearm.
Extension: 70°
Bend wrist, palm toward dorsal forearm.
Radial deviation: 20°
Bend wrist toward radius.
Ulnar deviation: 45°
Bend wrist toward ulna.

Internal rotation is turning a segment toward the midline of the body from the anatomical position.

External rotation is the return toward the anatomical position, turning the segment in the opposite direction.

Your Shoulder Girdle

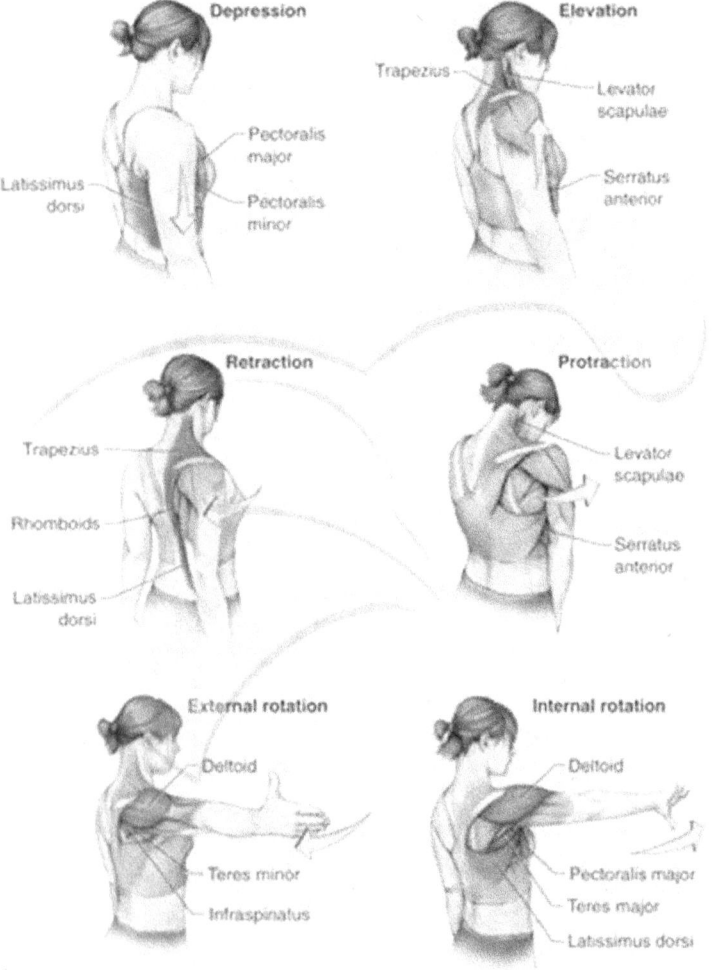

The primary articulation between your scapula (shoulder blade) and your thoracic cage (ribs) is not a traditional joint because there is no direct contact between your bones, which have several muscles between them.

However, there is a large ROM of the scapula on the thoracic cage that has its own terminology.

Your **Vertical** movements are *elevation* (upward movement) and *depression* (downward movement).

Your **Horizontal** movements are *protraction* or *abduction* (out to the side) and *retraction* or *adduction* (in toward the spine).

Your **Rotational** movements are *upward* and *downward rotation*.

The Movements of your shoulder girdle combine with the movements of your shoulder joint to provide the large ROM found at your shoulder.

Your shoulder girdle also includes your **sternoclavicular** joint, between your sternum (breastbone) and **clavicle** (collarbone) and your **acromioclavicular** joint, between your scapula and clavicle. These joints move when your scapulothoracic joint moves.

Your Shoulder Joint

Your glenohumeral joint is a ball-and-socket joint, so it can move in all directions—flexion, extension, abduction, adduction, internal and external rotation as well as circumduction (tips of the fingers trace a circle in the sagittal plane).

Horizontal adduction and horizontal abduction are additional movements of your upper limb toward and away from your midline when it is positioned in the transverse plane (parallel to the ground).

The relationship between your scapulothoracic and shoulder joints is called *scapulohumeral rhythm*.

Your glenohumeral joint alone cannot reach the full ROM seen at the shoulder because it is restricted by the bone structure at the joint.

However, the glenoid fossa that makes up part of your glenohumeral joint is part of your scapula, so if your scapula also moves, greater ROM can occur and be achieved.

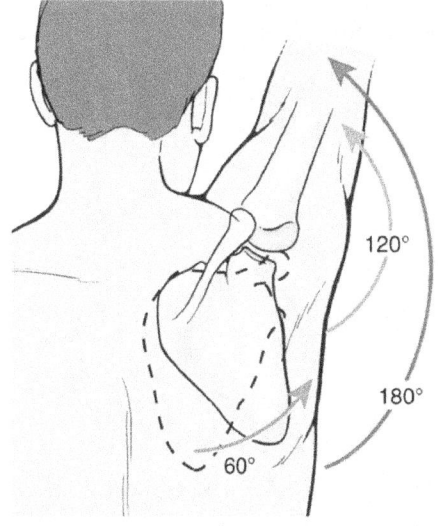

(C) Scapulo-humeral rhythm. The scapula and humerus move in 1:2 ratio. When the arm is abducted 180 degrees, 60 degrees occurs by rotation of the scapula, and 120 degrees by rotation of the humerus at the shoulder joint.

Your Elbow Joint

Your elbow joint is the articulation between your humerus and your two forearm bones, your **radius** and **ulna**.

Your ulnohumeral joint is your primary joint and as a hinge joint, it limits movements to flexion and extension.

Your radiohumeral joint is also part of your elbow joint, but it does not provide much bony stability.

The ability of some individuals to hyperextend the elbow joint is due to differences in the shape of their articulating surfaces.

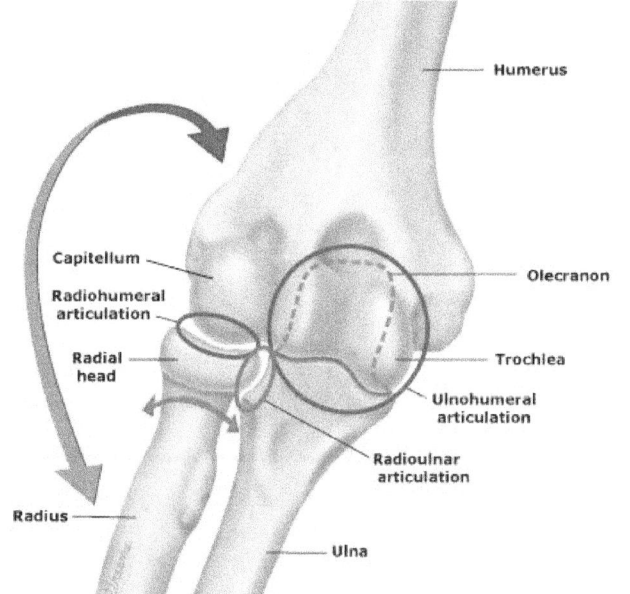

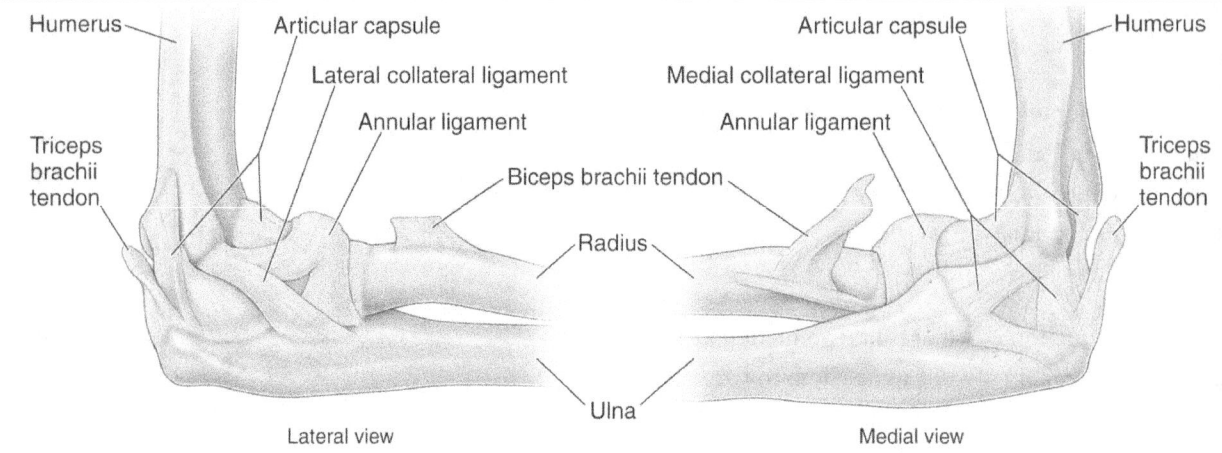

Lateral view / Medial view

Your Radioulnar Joints

Your **radius** and **ulna** articulate with each other both **proximally** and **distally** in your forearm.

Your joint movements are **pronation** and **supination**. Although the wrist is not involved in these movements, the position of your radioulnar joints can be identified by the direction your palms face. When the arms hang down alongside your trunk, your palms face forward in the supinated position and toward your back in the pronated position.

In the supinated position, both your radius and ulna are parallel with each other; in the pronated position, your radius lies across and on top of your ulna.

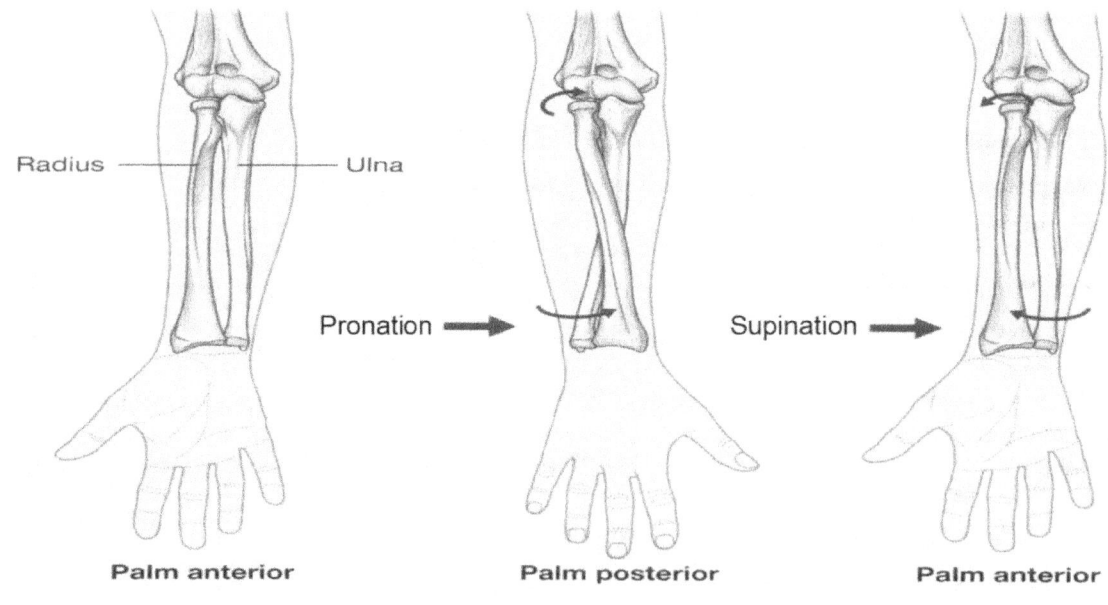

Your Wrist Joint

Your wrist joint consists of your **radiocarpal** and **ulnocarpal** articulations between your forearm bones and your carpal bones of your wrist.

Your Movements at your wrist include joint **flexion**, **extension**, **abduction** (radial flexion), and **adduction** (ulnar flexion).

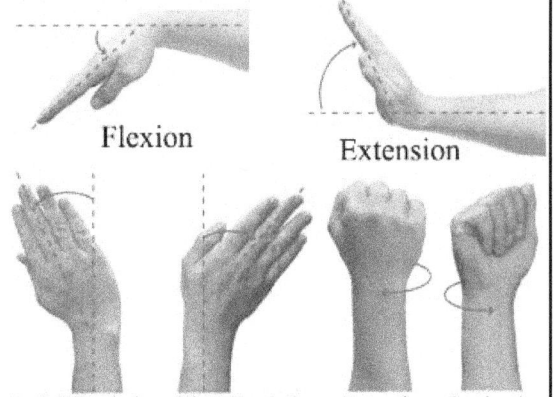

Flexion | Extension
Radial Deviation | Ulnar Deviation | Pronation | Supination

Your Metacarpophalangeal and Interphalangeal Joints

Your metacarpophalangeal joints are the knuckles of your hand. The second through the fifth joints move in **flexion** and **extension** as well as **abduction** and **adduction** of your fingers. Your metacarpophalangeal joint of your thumb allows only **flexion** and **extension**.

The ability of your opposable thumb to touch the tips of all your other digits comes from movement at your carpometacarpal joint.

Your interphalangeal joints of your fingers and thumb are hinge joints that flex and extend.

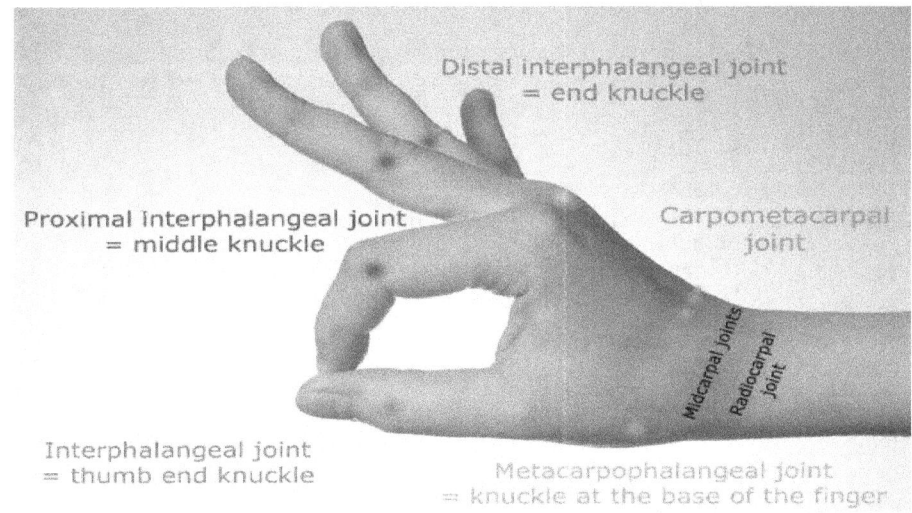

Your Vertebral Column

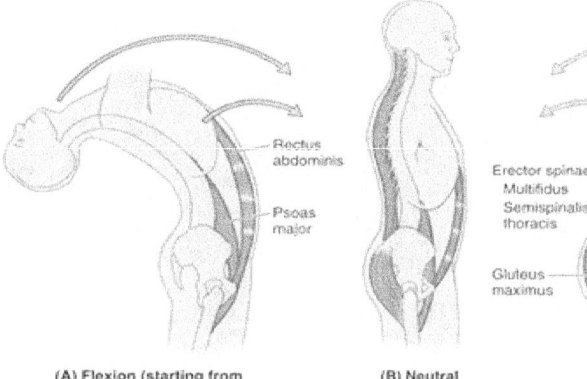
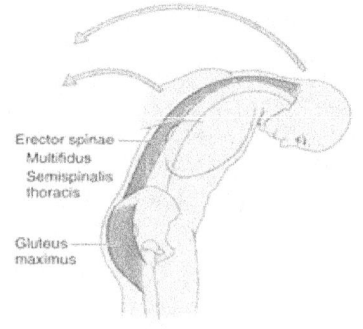

Your vertebral column contains 24 individual vertebrae and your sacrum.

Although movement between adjacent vertebrae is just a few degrees, when combined over the whole vertebral column, the ROM of your trunk is substantial.

Your Movements of your trunk occur in all three planes: **flexion** and **extension**, **lateral flexion** to the left and right, and **rotation** to the left and right.

Your Lumbosacral Joint

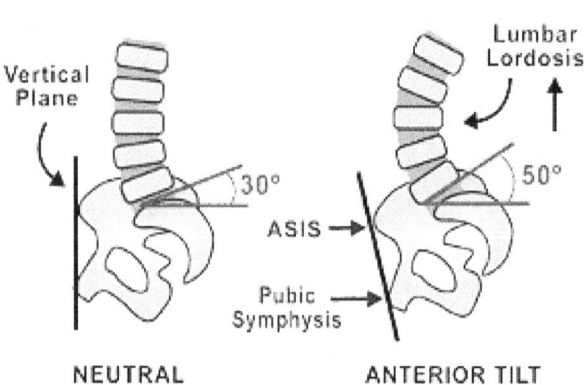

Your pelvis tilts mainly at the joint formed by your fifth lumbar vertebra and your sacrum. A reference for the direction of pelvic tilt is a line between your anterior and posterior superior iliac spines in your sagittal plane.

When your pelvis tilts anteriorly, the angle between the horizontal and the line between your iliac spines increases.

With your posterior pelvic tilt, the angle of the line between your iliac spines becomes closer to the horizontal.

Your Anterior pelvic tilt is accompanied by extension of your lumbar spine, whereas a backward tilt results in a flattening out of your lumbar spine.

Your Hip Joint

Your hip joint is a ball-and-socket joint similar to your shoulder (glenohumeral joint), but the bony socket at your hip is much deeper compared with your shoulder.

The deep socket makes your hip more stable than your shoulder, but at the expense of total ROM.

For example, extension is less at your hip than at your shoulder.

Your Movements at your hip joint are **flexion**, **extension**, **abduction**, **adduction**, **internal rotation**, **external rotation** and **circumduction** (a movement combining flexion, extension, abduction and adduction that results in your foot moving in a circular motion).

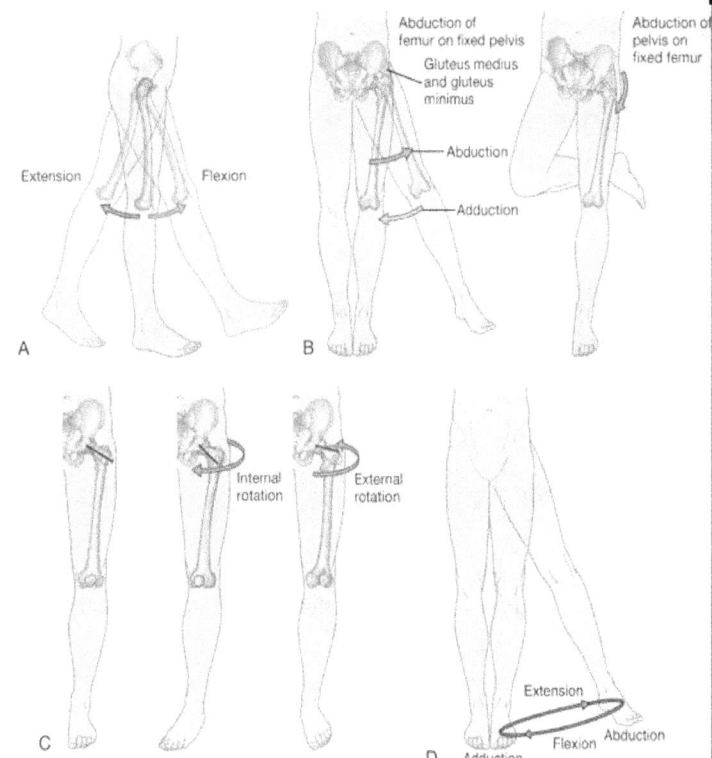

Your Knee Joint

The tibiofemoral joint is your primary knee joint. Your knee does not have good bony stability in flexion due to the flattened surface of your tibial plateau; therefore, it relies on your ligaments to provide your stability, which, unfortunately, makes it vulnerable to injury.

Flexion and **extension** are the major movements at the knee. When the knee is in a flexed position, limited **rotation**, **abduction**, and **adduction** are possible.

Joint Motions
- abduction/adduction
- dorsiflexion/plantarflexion
- flexion/extension/hyperextension

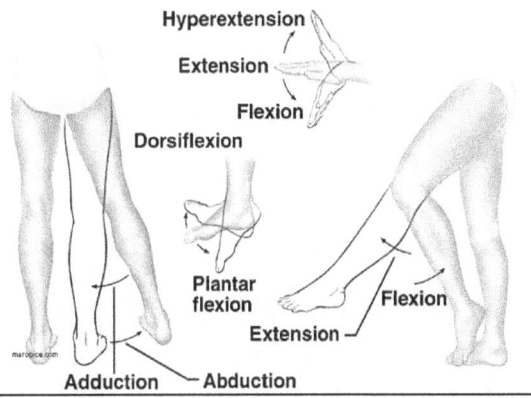

Ankle Joints

- Talocrural Joint
- Type: Hinge
- Movements:
  - Plantarflexion
  - Dorsiflexion

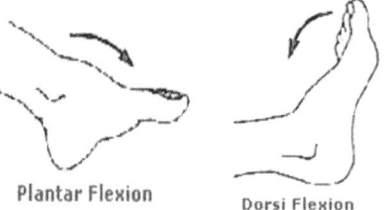

- Subtalar Joint
- Type: Gliding
- Movements:
  - Inversion
  - Eversion

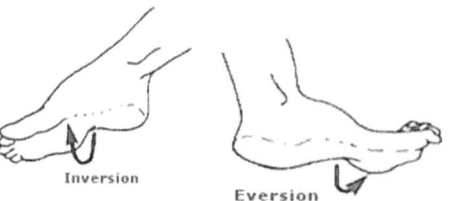

Your Ankle Joint

Also called your **talocrural joint**, your ankle joint is limited to movement in one plane only. **Plantar flexion** is pointing your foot downward and **dorsiflexion** is pulling the foot up toward the shin.

Your Subtalar Joint

Your subtalar joint contributes to pronation and supination movements of your foot. In the frontal plane, these movements are **eversion** and **inversion**.

In combination with other foot joints, your subtalar joint lowers your medial longitudinal arch (pronation) via a combination of **eversion**, **dorsiflexion**, and **abduction**.

The opposite movement is supination, and it raises the arch via a combination of **inversion**, **plantar flexion**, and **adduction**.

Your Skeletal Muscle

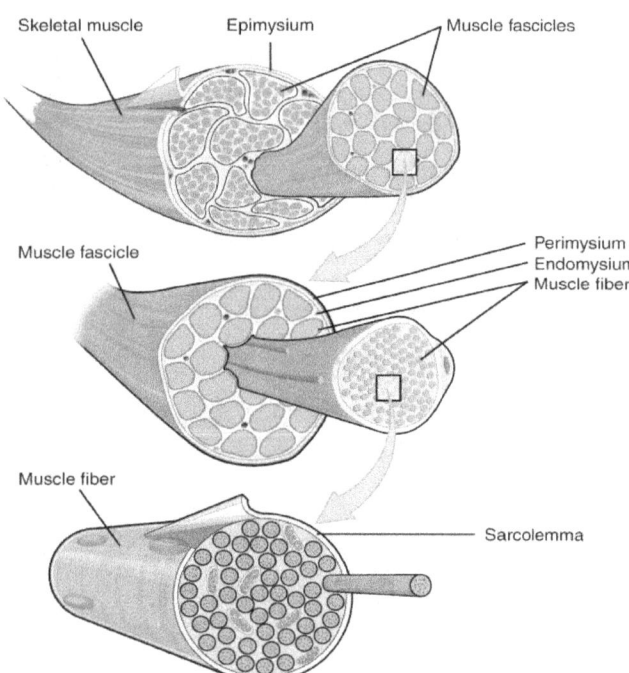

Your Skeletal, or also called voluntary, muscles consist of thousands of **muscle fibers** (e.g., your brachioradialis has approximately 130,000 fibers; your gastrocnemius has more than 1 million) and **connective tissue**.

Each fiber is enclosed by the **endomysium**, a type of connective tissue.

The **fascicles,** or bundles of fibers grouped together, are surrounded by your **perimysium,** and the entire muscle is enclosed by your **epimysium.**

The **tendon** is the passive part of your muscle and is made up of elastic connective tissue.

Each muscle attaches to bone at the periosteum or alternatively to deep, thick fascial tissue via tendons and the perimysium and epimysium connective tissues.

The **size** and **shape** of your tendons depend on the functions and shape of your muscles that they are attached to.

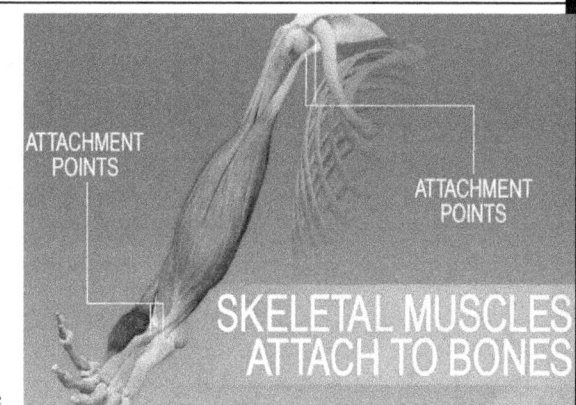

Some tendons can be easily seen and palpated just under the surface of the skin, such as the hamstring muscle tendons at the sides of the posterior aspect of the knee and the Achilles tendon inserting into the posterior heel.

Other muscles, such as your supraspinatus and infraspinatus (muscles of the rotator cuff in your shoulder), are attached directly to your bone with no observable tendon.

Broad and flat tendons, such as your proximal tendinous sheath of the latissimus dorsi, are **aponeuroses.**

Other muscles lie underneath the surface muscles.

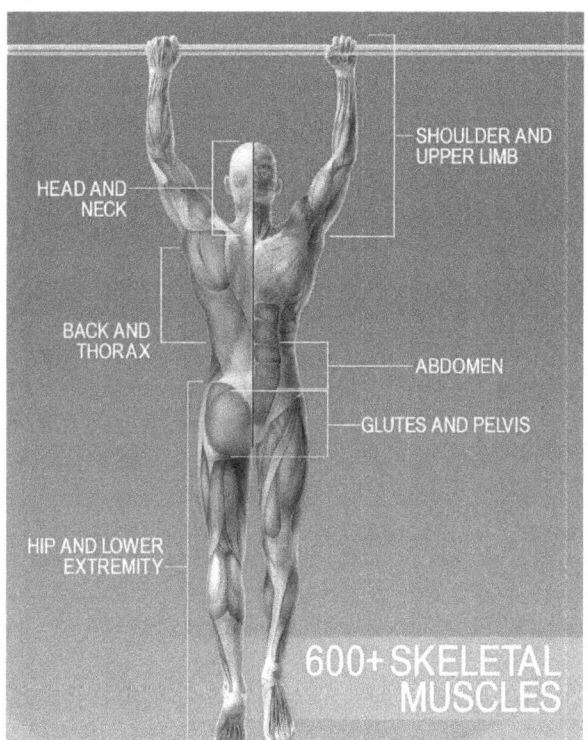

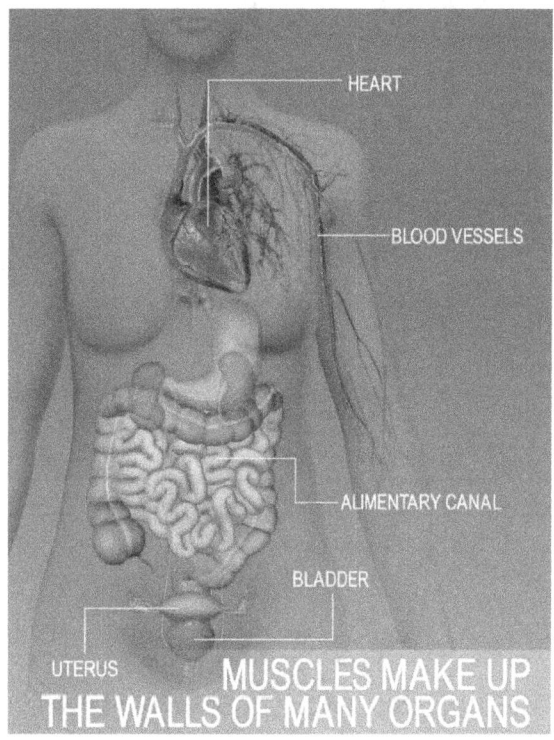

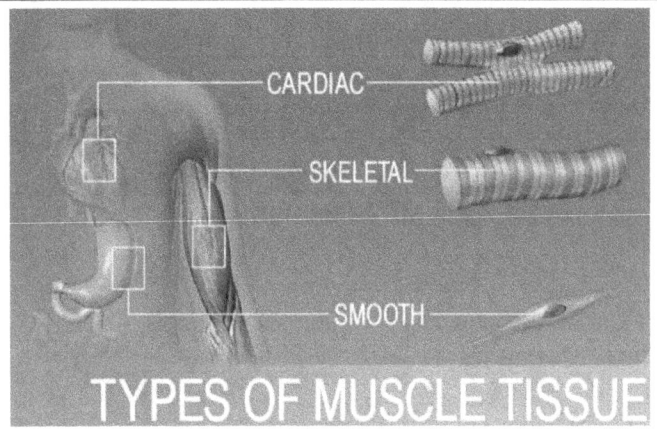
TYPES OF MUSCLE TISSUE

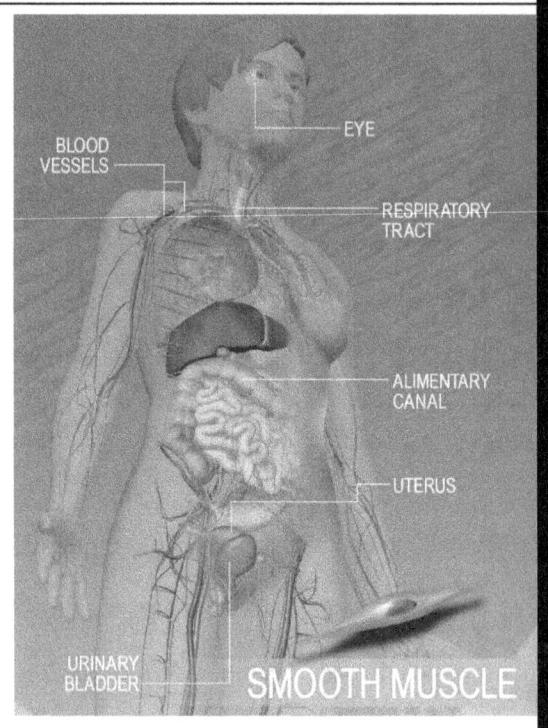
SMOOTH MUSCLE

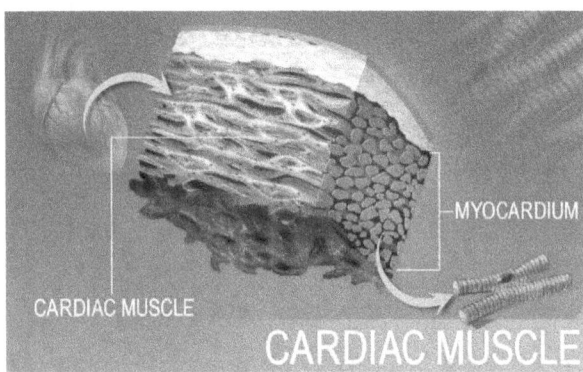
CARDIAC MUSCLE

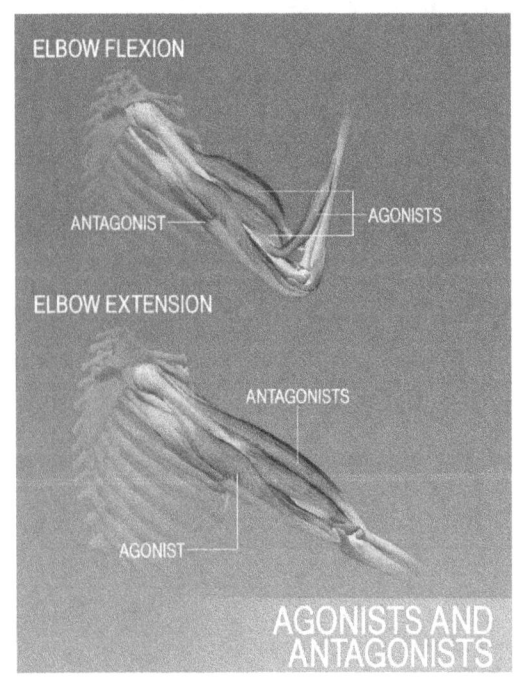
AGONISTS AND ANTAGONISTS

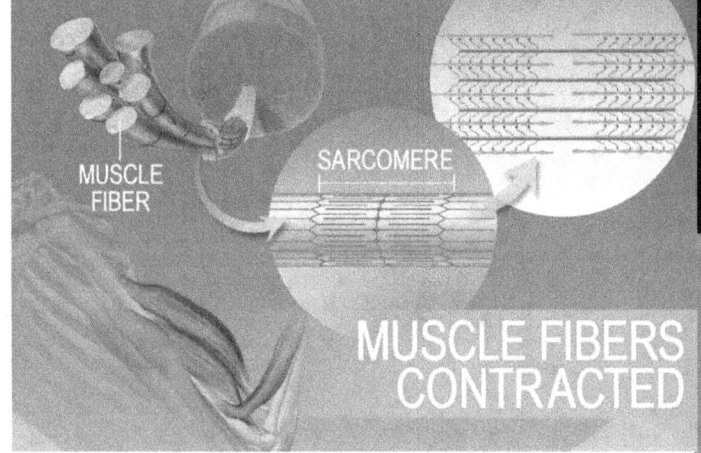
MUSCLE FIBERS CONTRACTED

Muscular System Response to Long Term Exercise

- Increased number of **Mitochondria** and **Myoglobin** stores
  - Myoglobin is a site for oxygen storage in the muscle
  - Mitochondria produce energy as glucose combines with O_2 to produce ATP
- Increased **Muscle Strength**
- This is a response to muscles being used more than they are used to – they are overloaded. Overloading can be done by increasing resistance (weight).

Skeletal System

- Regular exercise slows the rate of skeletal ageing. Active people have **greater bone mass** than sedentary people.
- Strength training and weight-bearing exercises help increase bone mass e.g. Netball, tennis, basketball, walking
- Increases in **calcium** and **collagen** in the bones add the strength. This reduces the risk of osteoporosis.

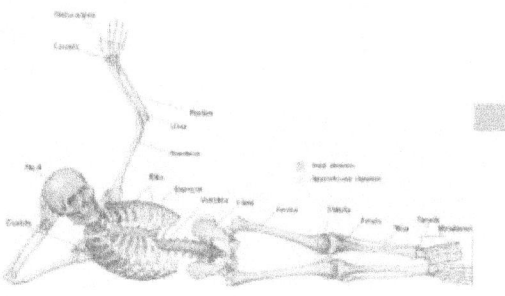

•Increased Production of synovial fluid
Secretion of synovial fluid allows movement in the joints. Regular exercise reduces the thickness of the fluid allowing a greater range of movement in the joint

Human Strength and Power

- Biomechanical Factors in Human Strength
  - Muscle Length
    - **At resting length:** actin and myosin filaments lie next to each other; maximal number of potential cross-bridge sites are available; the muscle can generate the greatest force.
    - **When stretched:** a smaller proportion of the actin and myosin filaments lie next to each other; fewer potential cross-bridge sites are available; the muscle cannot generate as much force.
    - **When contracted:** the actin filaments overlap; the number of cross-bridge sites is reduced; there is decreased force generation capability.

Strength-to-Mass Ratio

- Strength-to-mass ratio of larger athletes is often less than smaller athletes
  - Greater muscle volume relative to CSA
    - CSA is a 2 dimensional phenomenon
    - Volume is a 3 dimensional phenomenon
- Hypertrophy
  - Volume increases in greater proportion compared to CSA
- Thus, when body size increases, body mass increases more rapidly than does muscular strength

Body Size

- The reason that smaller athletes are stronger than larger athletes pound for pound is because of the fact that smaller athletes can have equal cross-sectional area of muscles as larger athletes, but the smaller athletes have less muscular volume

- So what?
- If an athlete increases muscle mass by 15% and force production by 10%
  - Reduction in ability to accelerate his/her body
- More strength focus in taller athletes

Strength-to-Mass Ratio

- Strength-to-Mass ratio is intimately related to cross-sectional area and muscular volume

- Most athletics involved moving the body through space

- The strength-to-mass ratio directly reflects the athlete's ability to accelerate his or her body

Move Something!

The Cool Down

Creating Your Change

*****

Unfortunately, translating the desire to change a health-related behavior into action can be a challenge for most people. They may wish to be more active or to eat a healthier diet but may not have the knowledge, skills, or motivation to make the necessary behavior modifications and stick to them. To help people adopt and maintain a healthier lifestyle, the fitness professional should understand basic principles of behavior change and develop the skills to put those principles into practice.

Even a little physical activity performed on a regular basis may reduce the risk of heart disease. The more exercise people do, the more benefit in reducing risk.

Key findings of the study by Harvard School of Public Health researchers found:

- •As little as 2.5 hours of moderate-intensity physical activity per week (150 minutes) can lower a person's overall risk of heart disease by 14%.

- •The risk of developing coronary heart disease gets progressively lower the more physical activity a person does. While 150 minutes is beneficial, 300 minutes weekly will achieve even better results.

- **Now**, if you utilize my calculations and increase your level of exercise to at least 60 Minutes a day … just 420 Minutes a week ….. You Can Heal, Restore, Repair and Gain the Power you need to Successfully Enjoy Your Abundant Life!

This study corroborates federal guidelines—even a little bit of exercise is good, but more is better. Researchers noticed a significant gender difference that showed that exercise had a greater effect in reducing heart disease risk in women than in men.

For clients who are sedentary, the first step in programming is establishing a regular routine of physical activity. In most cases, this means a structured walking program (or equivalent if orthopedic limitations exist) that focuses on the routine of activity.

The program might begin with a short (10 min) bout of activity to realize success and provide a reference point for later modifications.

Remember, if a client has been inactive for many years, taking a few weeks to get into the habit of physical activity is not unreasonable.

Easy 3 Step Phase to Get ACTIVE!

Phase 1: Regular Walking

The first phase for sedentary individuals is to gradually increase the amount of moderate-intensity physical activity in their regular routine. Walking is the most popular activity. The major goal is to increase the amount of physical activity that can be done comfortably, so no emphasis on intensity is necessary at this point. People in this phase start with the distance they can easily walk without pain or fatigue and then gradually increase the distance and pace until they can complete about 30 minutes of moderate-intensity activity (e.g., 2 mi at 4 mi $\cdot$ hr-1, or 3.2 km at 6.4 km $\cdot$ hr-1) each day. People with orthopedic limitations can substitute a weight-supported activity such as cycling, rowing, or swimming for walking.

Even though some may not be able to achieve this initial goal of 30 minutes, a regular pattern of light physical activity still provides health-related benefits and is better than being sedentary.

Phase 2: Recommended Work Levels for a Change in Fitness

Once phase 1 is accomplished, participants are taught about recommended levels of work for fitness changes. There are some people that may not be interested in moving beyond a walking program that they can do most days of the week. For Health and Wellness, this is not an issue, especially since the health-related benefits of physical activity can be realized with a walking program.

For those who want to move on to more vigorous activities, a work–relief interval training program is introduced— light jogging is the work, and walking is the relief. The participant walks, jogs a few steps, then walks, and so forth. Gradually, light jogging covers more distance than walking, until the person can lightly jog continuously for 20 to 30 minutes at the THR.

People interested in cycling and swimming (see later in this chapter) also can use interval training. People interested in group classes should transition from the walking program to the lower-intensity version of the class, if one is available.

If a lower-intensity version is not available, you should communicate with the instructor to get pointers on how to transition into the class.

Phase 3: Variety of Fitness Activities

Once the base of physical activity has been established and the transition to regular vigorous-intensity physical activity has occurred, you will be able to participate in a wider range of physical activities.

Phase 3 is quite individualized and is based on the person's interests.

The purpose is to promote continued activity by having people participate in an activity they naturally enjoy. Some people prefer to continue to stretch, walk, and jog; some prefer to exercise alone; and others enjoy working out with other people.

Some people like cooperative and relatively low-level competitive activities, and others like the thrill of competition. Some enjoy a variety of movement forms, while others enjoy repeating similar activities.

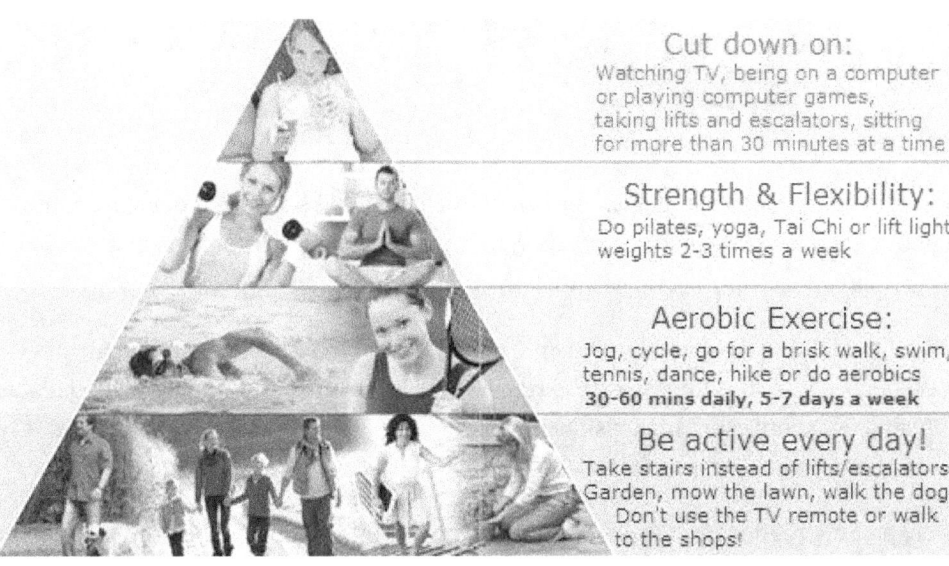

Behavior Change

Behavior modification theory is based on the assumption that behavior is learned and can be changed by modifying the antecedents (stimuli, cues) and consequences (rewards, punishments). A cue could be a flyer listing the benefits of walking during lunch, and a reward could be a certificate presented to the aerobics participant with the best attendance.

Your 'cue' for your behavior change should be to improve your Health condition!

Your 'cue' should be that you want to Improve the Quality of your Life!

Your 'cue' should be that you want to Enjoy Your Abundant Life!

People may start exercising to lose weight but later train for a road race because they enjoy a sense of accomplishment from running.

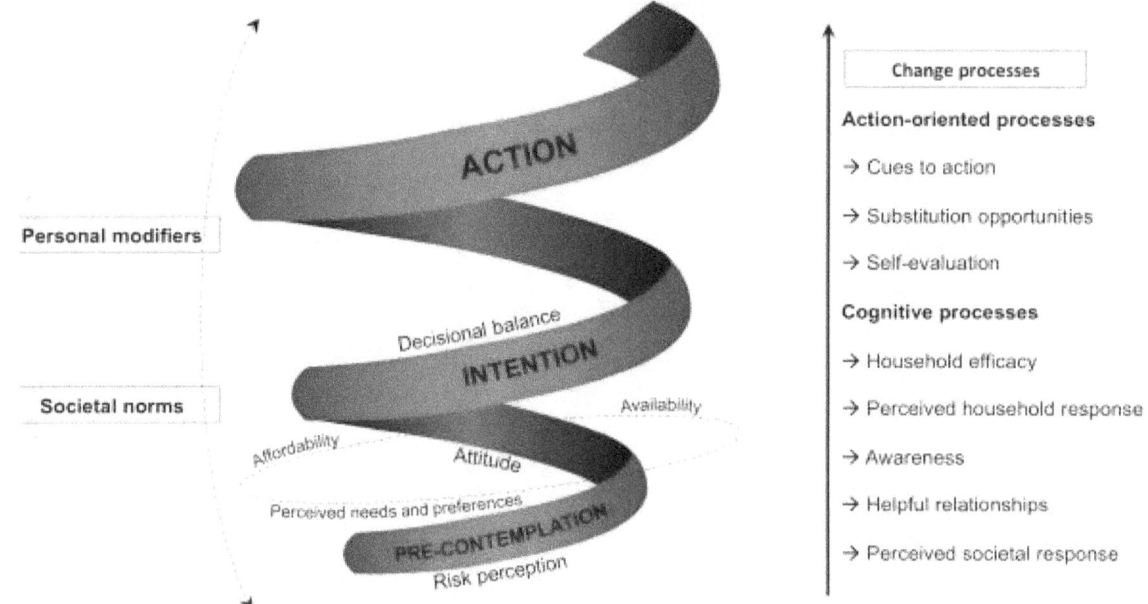

Although there are several effective strategies for behavior change that have been developed, most theories of behavior treat change as an all-or-none event. In other words, participants go from being sedentary to being regularly active in response to an intervention.

The transtheoretical model was developed in the 80's and presents change as a dynamic process whereby attitudes, decisions, and actions evolve through stages over time. Although the model was developed to explain how people stop high-risk behaviors, I have adapted, utilized and applied it with measurable success for promoting exercise.

The rest of this chapter highlights the stages of change and ways this model can be used to help you think about, decide to begin and continue an active lifestyle.

Stages of Change

1. **Precontemplation**: In this stage, you are not necessarily seriously thinking about changing an unhealthy behavior in the next 6 months, but you may be aware that you NEED to make a change or you are denying the need to change.

2. **Contemplation**: This is the level where you are seriously thinking about changing an unhealthy behavior within the next 6 mo.

3. ***Preparation***: This is a transitional stage in which you intend to take action within the next month. Some plans have been made, and you are striving to determine what to do next.

4. ***Action***: This stage is the 6 months following your overt modification of an unhealthy behavior. Your amount of Motivation and investment in your behavior change is sufficient in this stage, but it is the busiest and least stable stage and has the highest risk of relapse.

5. ***Maintenance***: Maintenance begins after you have successfully adhered to your new healthy behavior for a minimum of 6 months. Research shows that the longer you stay in maintenance, the lower the risk of relapse.

Stage of change	Description
Precontemplation	The individual has no intention to take action within the next 6 months and is generally unaware or under-aware of the problem.
Contemplation	The individual intends to take action within the next 6 months. He or she is aware that a problem exists but has not yet made a commitment to take action
Preparation	The individual intends to take action within the next 30 days and has taken some behavioural steps in this direction
Action	The individual changes his or her overt behaviour for less than 6 months
Maintenance	The individual changes his or her overt behaviour for more than 6 months and works to prevent relapse and consolidate the gains attained

Attitudes, Beliefs and Behavioral Skills to Influence Behavior Change

The "**how**" of behavior change in the transtheoretical model includes your **attitude**, your **beliefs**, your **behavioral skills** that are expected to change as you progresses through the stages.

These change elements are **self-efficacy**, **decisional balance**, and **processes of change**.

• ***Self-efficacy*** is confidence in your ability to engage in a positive behavior or abstain from an undesired behavior. Expectation of success is important in making your decision to change and in maintaining your new Healthy behavior. Types of self-efficacy include confidence to accomplish the elements of a task, which is important when beginning your new behavior and confidence to overcome personal and environmental barriers (coping, barrier self-efficacy), which is important for adhering to your new Healthy behavior.

• ***Decisional balance*** refers to evaluating and monitoring potential gains (pros, benefits) and losses (cons) arising from any decision. Perceived gains increase and perceived losses decrease in respect to the target behavior as you moves through the stages of change.

Transtheoretical Model of Behavior Change *(continued)*

Attitudes, beliefs, and behavioral skills that influence behavior change
- Self-efficacy (belief in capability to engage in a specific behavior successfully)
- Decisional balance (evaluating the pros and cons of the target behavior)
- Processes of change (strategies used to change behavior)
  - Experiential/cognitive
  - Behavioral

- **Processes of change** are strategies used to change your behavior. Experiential or cognitive processes are strategies that involve your thoughts, attitudes, and awareness.

Behavioral processes involve taking specific actions directed toward yourself or the environment.

For an example, seeking out information about the best exercise for losing weight is a cognitive process and creating reminders to register for a water aerobics class is a behavioral process.

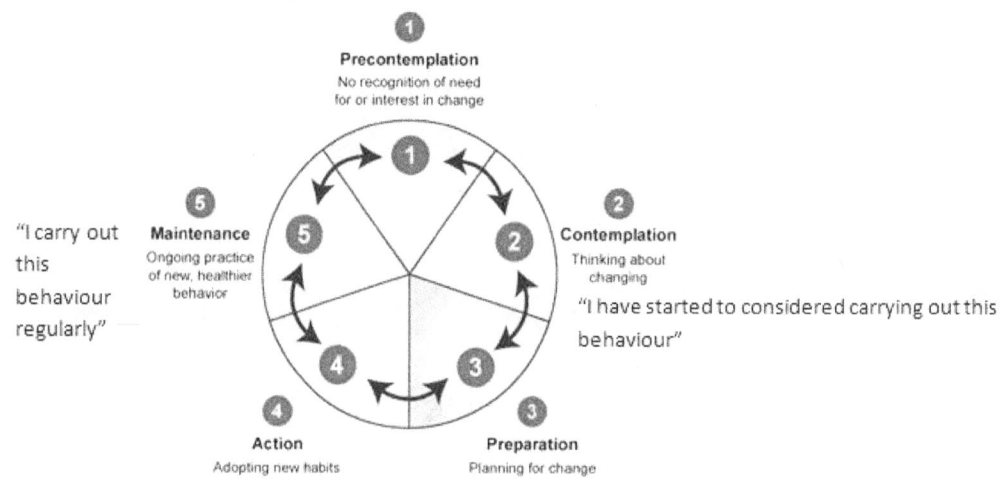

Applying the Transtheoretical Model to Exercise

I am applying the transtheoretical model is applied to exercise by matching or targeting the appropriate intervention strategy according to your physical activity history and readiness for change.

For an example, if you were in the precontemplation stage the goal would be to get you to begin thinking about changing their level of physical activity. I would discuss information from with you of any fitness test(s) or health risk appraisal followed by education about personal benefits of physical activity and we would develop an appropriate strategy for you.

The goal ultimate goal in this contemplation stage would be to motivate you and help you to prepare to take action.

If you were in the preparation stage then you would be performing some exercise but would realize that it is not enough and I would be there to help you to set up a personalized exercise program.

I would educate you and bring to your awareness the many Excellent and Awesome benefits of exercise.

This particular stage also represent there still being barriers that must be resolved. Whereas if you were in the contemplation stage you may not be ready to set goals, but if you are in the preparation stage then you are ready to set goals and get a personalized exercise prescription.

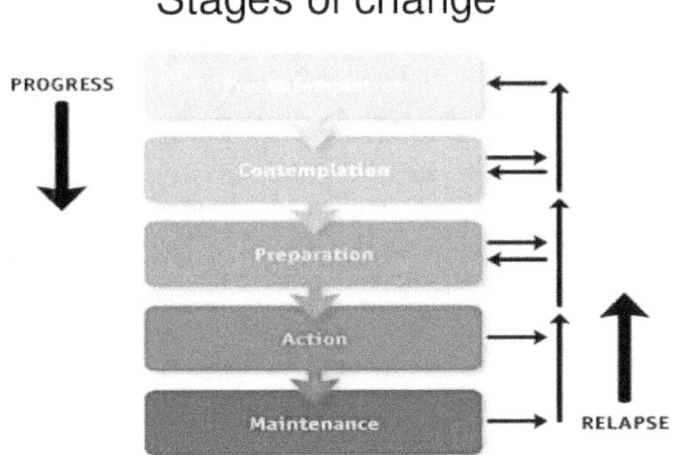

In the action stage, you are participating in regular activity, but exercise has not become a habit for you yet. You would be considered to be at a high risk of relapsing into a more familiar, inactive lifestyle.

Relapse prevention, you be applied by me to help keep you on track to the maintenance stage.

Movement from the action stage to the maintenance stage follows a decrease in the risk of relapse and an increase in self-efficacy.

Helpful strategies include periodic reevaluations of goals and updates of plans for coping with life events such as travel, inclement weather, or medical events that can disrupt regular exercise.

A variety of strategies and programs can be used to motivate sedentary and low-active individuals to consider becoming more active and adopt regular exercise.

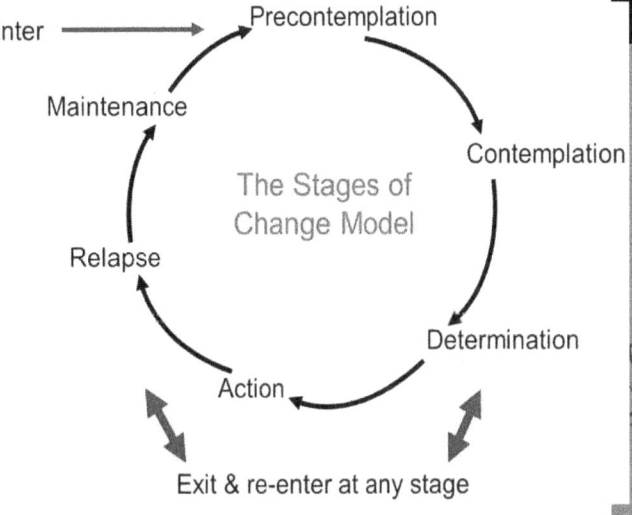

Many of these approaches are based on understanding the knowledge, attitudes, beliefs, and behavioral skills that foster adoption of a regular exercise program in the early stages of change.

I want to discuss a few specific factors related to promoting the adoption of regular exercise and a review of strategies to increase motivation.

Encouraging Exercise: Advancing Pre-contemplators and Contemplators

People in precontemplation are sedentary and have no plans to start exercising. They may be in this stage because they lack information about the long-term personal consequences of physical inactivity. They also may be demoralized from previous unsuccessful attempts to stick with an exercise program and may have low self-efficacy for exercise.

People in the precontemplation stage may feel defensive about their lifestyle because of social pressures to be physically active. They have no personally compelling reasons to change, and the costs of exercising seem to outweigh the benefits.

For me, given these attitudes and beliefs, I help to reinforce your perceptions about the benefits of exercise. I love to utilize activities to help you develop a personal value for exercise and I provide useful information about the role of exercise in a healthy lifestyle to help you to move into the next stage of your growth and development. Sedentary individuals move to the contemplation stage because of information that is convincing, personal, and timely.

Contemplators are planning to become more physically active, but they are still ambivalent about changing. They know the need for exercise but may not have be active long enough to see or feel a healthy change.

Exposure to physically active role models, enhancement of perceived benefits, and strengthening of psychosocial variables such as self-efficacy for exercise are other factors that influence exercise adoption.

The cognitive processes of change, such as increasing knowledge about the health benefits of regular exercise and being aware of how one's inactivity affects others, are critical in these early stages of your change to a Heathy LifeStyle.

Theory of Planned Behavior

FOCUS ON BELEIFS THAT AFFECT INTENTION

MODIFYING FACTORS AND ENVIRONMENT

- Demographic
- Attitudes to target Behavior
- Personality

Beliefs, Evaluation of Behavioral Outcomes (combined=ATTITUDES),

normative beliefs, Motivation (combined=SUBJECTIVE NORM)

Control beliefs, perceived power (self-efficacy) (combined=PERCEIVED CONTROL)

INTENTION  Action

Influencing Exercise Adoption: Successful Planning for the Preparation Stage

In the preparation stage you are performing some exercise, but not enough to meet health and fitness guidelines. My goal as a Health and Wellness professional would be to help you move to the action stage and regular exercise.

A thorough assessment of personal, social, and environmental factors that offer support of your current level of activity can be particularly useful. A comprehensive assessment can establish physical fitness, motivation, goals, supports, barriers, and other factors to consider when developing a specific plan for change and implementing strategies.

Behavioral strategies come into play more as you begin to move from your preparation stage. Goal setting, behavioral contracts and time management training are practical strategies to use with-in your preparation stage, and information from an assessment will help tailor an intervention to your specific needs and situation.

Exercise Adoption

- The most important factor in starting exercise program is the individual.
- A person cannot be coerced into starting to work out.
    - He or she must be ready to make a change.
- Applying the transtheoretical model of behavioral change principles will help increase the chances of success when adopting a new behavior.
- Factors that motivate individuals to start exercising may not be the same factors that keep them exercising.

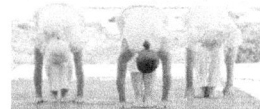

Your Personal Influences

Your individual characteristics that influence your initiation of exercise include demographics, activity history, past experiences, perception of health status, perception of access to facilities, time, enjoyment of exercise, aptitudes, beliefs, self-motivation and self-efficacy. Exercise history is an important factor in your current level of physical activity. Your past exercise experience also can influence your current and/or future expectations about exercise and self-efficacy and high exercise self-efficacy is associated with increased exercise participation.

Your Motivation is another variable influencing your exercise adoption. Your Motivation depends on your expectations for future benefits or outcomes from exercise, such as your good health, your improved appearance, improved stress management, enjoyment, and opportunities for competition.

It also varies in degree of your self-determination and your **intrinsic** motivation is the most self-determined, whereas your **extrinsic** motivation is motivation based on satisfying others or on the consequences of the behavior.

The self-determination theory describes motivation on a continuum from extrinsic to intrinsic and links motivation to seeking to meet basic human needs of competency, autonomy, and relatedness.

Self-motivation for exercise is the ability to continue an exercise program without the benefit of external reinforcement. Participants high in self-motivation are probably good at goal setting, monitoring exercise progress, and self-reinforcement and are high in intrinsic motivation. People with little self-motivation may need more external reinforcement and encouragement (e.g., group activities and social support) to adopt and adhere to exercise, but even people with high intrinsic motivation can benefit from social support.

Your Perceived behavioral control is significantly correlated with your intention to exercise. If you believe that you have more control over the exercise and have choices about when and how to exercise, you are more likely to begin a program.

Becoming Healthy can and should be your Motivation for you to Move SomeThing!

Enjoying Your Abundant Life should be Motivation for you to Move YourSelf!

Helping Individuals Change Health Behaviors

- **Knowledge**
    - A theoretical model to explain and predict behavior (transtheoretical model)
    - Factors that influence health behaviors: attitudes, beliefs, and behavioral skills
- **Skills**
    - Behavior change strategies matched to stage of motivational readiness
    - The ability to listen effectively and respond empathetically

Your Social Influences

Your Social support involves your level of comfort, your amount assistance, and information provided by individuals or groups. Practical help, such as providing problem-solving tips or a ride to the fitness facility, can result in tangible benefits to the participant, but emotional support also plays a key role.

For an example, emotional support (encouragement and expressions of care, concern, and sympathy) could be helpful when or if you should become emotionally stressed.

Other types of emotional support include esteem support (reassurance of self-worth, expressions of liking or confidence in another person), network support (expressions of connection and belonging), and even informational support (information and advice).

Exercising with a group can also meet your need for relatedness described by self-determination theory.

Social support for exercise from family, friends, and physicians is usually associated with physical activity and the success or continuation of it. Spouses appear to provide a consistent, positive influence on exercise participation; in one study, individuals who joined a fitness center with their spouse had better adherence and lower dropout rates than married individuals who joined without a spouse.

This means to get your Loved Ones (not just your spouse) to Move SomeThing with you!

You and you Family can Successfully Move YourSelves in the Enjoyment of Your Abundant Lives!

Group factors may be particularly important for older adults and people who are motivated to exercise primarily for social reinforcement.

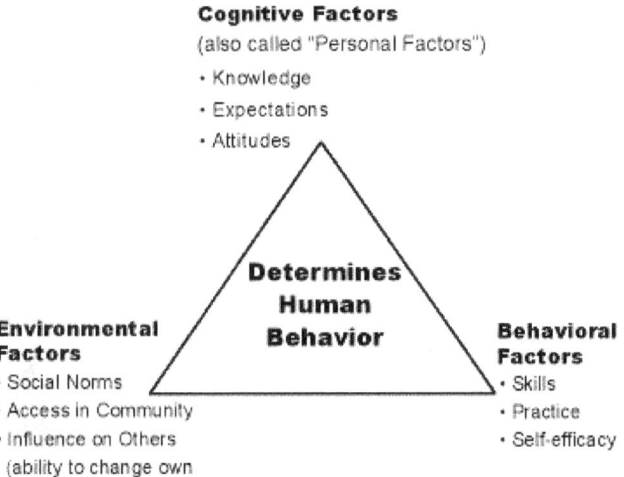

Social support definitely plays a big role in exercise adherence and most research supports that having other people involved does have a positive influence on your behavior.

Your Environmental Influences

Research has shown that social support, environmental prompts, and convenience are factors in exercise adoption.

Environments or communities that have cues for exercise – like easily accessible facilities and few real or perceived barriers, make sustaining an exercise program easier.

Where you can have or see posters, e-mails, self-sticking notes, visibly located exercise equipment and bike and walking paths are examples of some examples of environmental cues.

The convenience of exercise is influenced by the sequence, or chain, of behaviors that must be completed for the person to complete each exercise session. There is a greater potential for a break in the link if a person must leave work, drive home, gather up exercise clothes, drive to a facility, park, sign in, and change clothes to walk on a treadmill than if the person walks around the neighborhood first thing in the morning.

The primary reason most people give for not exercising is lack of time. Time can be a true determinant, a perceived determinant, an indication of poor time management, or a rationalization for the lack of motivation to be active.

This is why I eliminate all of this by promoting that you Move YourSelf WHEREVER and HOWEVER you can.

The emphasis is not on WHERE you exercise or move …. If your Home is where your 'snack food' is or where you eat your late-night snacks, then its in your home where you should Exercise and Move YourSelf into Your Health and Wellness!

Why pay someone to exercise at their facility when you can do the SAME things at home …. And get better Mental, Spiritual, Physical and Financial benefits!

Cognitive Restructuring: Reframe Negative Statements Into Positive Statements

Negative Statements

- I'm never going to get in shape.
- I'm fatter than everyone else in the class.
- I've tried to stay with exercise and each time I fail.
- It's just impossible to find time to exercise with my schedule.

Positive Statements

- Change takes time. I didn't get out of shape overnight, and I am making progress bit by bit.
- Everyone has to start somewhere. Other people have worked long and hard to get where they are.
- Every time I begin a new exercise program, I get closer to sticking with it for good.
- I can take a little time for myself to exercise every day because I deserve it. I'm the one in control.

Your Assessment

Regardless of the intervention, you having a complete comprehensive fitness and psychosocial assessments are necessary to select and carry out the appropriate strategies of behavior change for in your preparation and early action stages.

Reassessment should be conducted periodically to evaluate the effectiveness of the plan.

First, the problem must be identified and defined in behavioral terms. For an example, being overweight is not the problem but rather the result of overeating and under-exercising.

As a Health and Wellness professional I can and do also help you to formulate and decide what can be realistically changed and what cannot.

It's YOUR Body ... you have to know what it needs and/or where you want to go ..... with the underlying question or motivating factor being the answer to the question ......

HOW LONG DO YOU WANT TO LIVE?

Whatever you answer to this question is will be the determining or motivating factor in How you choice to eat and your level and amount of Exercise.

Health Belief Model

FOCUS ON INDIVIDUAL BELIEFS THAT AFFECT MOTIVATION

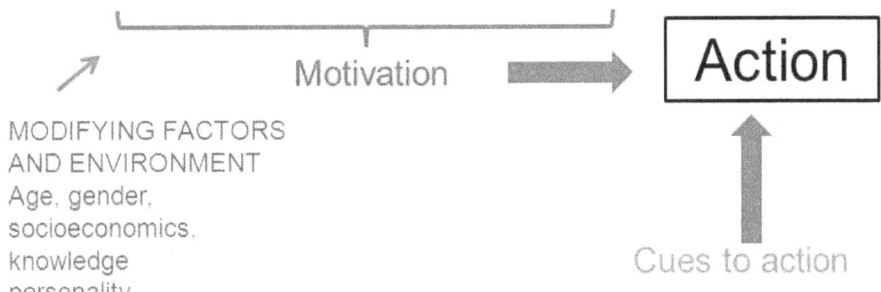

Motivational Principles from Self-Determination Theory

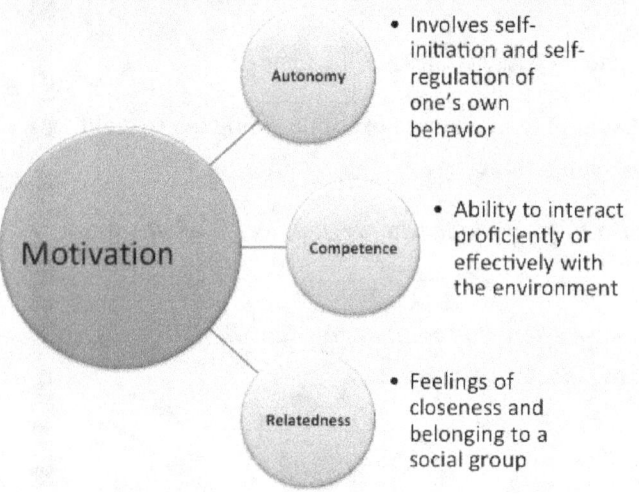

Self-determination theory is a theory of human motivation developed by Deci and Ryan in the 1980s that has been applied to promoting exercise.

According to this theory, humans are naturally inclined toward growth and development and have a set of basic psychological needs that are universal.

Motivation to engage in activities results from the fundamental needs for **competency**, **autonomy** and **relatedness**.

Satisfying these three basic psychological needs will foster intrinsic motivation and therefore enhance positive behaviors and mental health as well as the persistence of healthy behavior.

As a Health and Wellness professional I can and actually do help nurture your exercise motivation by setting up exercise tasks that help you develop your sense of mastery, making sure you have a say in your exercise program ... It's Your Body and Life. ..... I just want you to BE the BEST YOU CAN BE!

I want you to go where you want to go!

Motivational Strategies

- *Provide positive, practical behavioral feedback.*

- *Encourage group participation and group support to offer the opportunity for your social reinforcement, camaraderie and commitment.*

- *Recruit a partner and peers to support your behavioral change.*

- *Make your program enjoyable. Use upbeat, positive music.*

- *Develop a flexible routine to decrease your boredom and increase interest and enjoyment. Consider activities such as games and backpacking as alternatives.*

- *Provide periodic exercise testing to show your progress toward your goals, increase your sense of competency, and offer a Great opportunity for your positive reinforcement.*

- *Use effective strategies for your behavioral change, such as personal goal, contracts, and self-management, to foster and boost your personal control and perceived competency, which help to emphasize goals that are meaningful to you.*

- *Note and record your daily progress to be able to give yourself immediate, positive feedback. Encourage your own self-monitoring.*

- *Recognize goal achievement in notes to yourself or bulletin boards. Your Individual effort increases when your effort is or made identifiable.*

- *Set up group or individual competitions. Do a family and friends activity to promote group Health!*

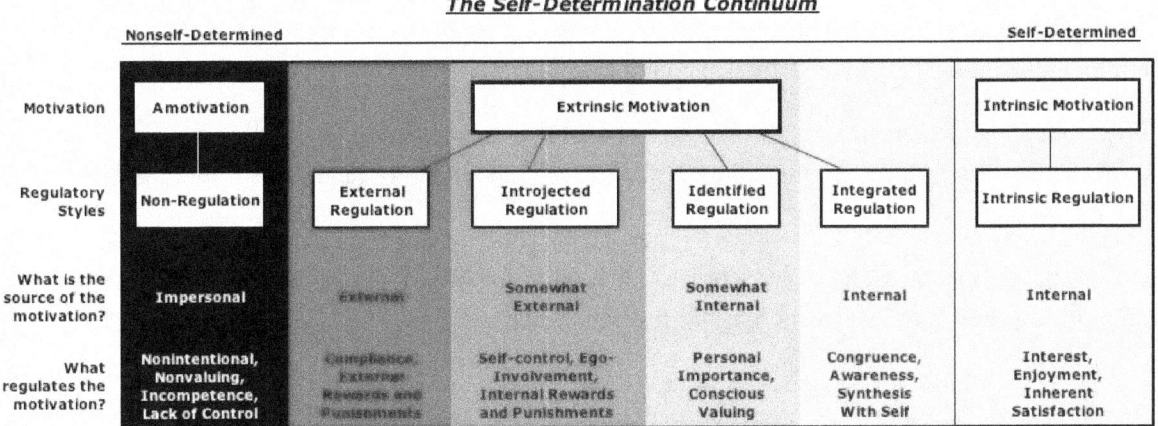

Next, examine your past attempts at behavior change. Find out what worked, what did not, and why.

This information will be useful in setting goals and identifying high-risk situations.

Because its your Body, you must be abreast and aware of everything that happens and be able to articulate the direction you want to go with your Health and Wellness!

Participants in exercise who are there because a doctor prescribed exercise may need help finding personal reasons for exercising or in the continuation of it.

This can be a sticking point for many. Don't let yourself get stuck here!

The ability for you to Successfully Enjoy Your Abundant Life should be Motivation enough to get you to Move SomeThing!

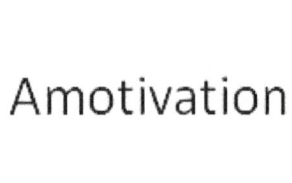

There are many reasons for beginning an exercise program (e.g., health, weight loss, anxiety reduction), but the initial motivation may not be why you continue to exercise.

Most often, people start exercise to achieve an outcome of exercise or to avoid guilt (extrinsic motivation) rather than for personal enjoyment, expression of creativity, or demonstration of mastery (intrinsic motivation).

Extrinsic motivation can be useful to get people started, but research has shown that developing intrinsic motivation for exercise is necessary for long-term maintenance.

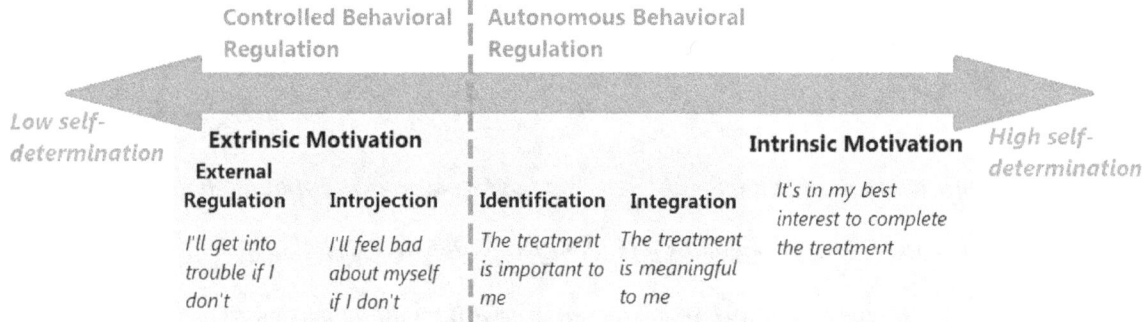

Self-Monitoring

Part of the assessment process can be accomplished by self-monitoring, in which you record information about your target behavior and also indicate any and all of your thoughts, feelings, and situations before, during and after your behavior.

You can successfully identify your internal and external cues and your resultant behavioral consequences that inhibit and/or prompt your want or ability to Move YourSelf.

Barriers and supports also become evident with self-monitoring. As a Health and Wellness professional, I can and do help you to develop successful strategies to cope with your barriers and use your supports.

Your chain of behaviors encompassing exercise can also be evaluated and weak links identified.

Immediate benefits and reinforcements tailored to individual preferences can also be established at critical links in your chain. Tablets, computer programs, calendars, graphs, and charts can be used for self-monitoring as part of the initial assessment and as a way to record progress. Fitness tracking apps are also available for smartphones and PDAs.

Goal Setting

The purpose of **goal setting** is to accomplish a specific task in a specific time frame.

Goals can be as simple and time limited as making a sandwich for lunch and as complicated and encompassing as earning an advanced degree or Healing YourSelf and Successfully Enjoying Your Abundant Life!

Goal setting provides you a plan of action that focuses and directs your activity and emphasizes a clear link between your behavior and your outcome.

Effective goal setting has several characteristics:

- Goals should be **behavioral**, **specific**, and **measurable**.

Plans are easier to make if your goal is stated in behavioral terms. For example, a goal of walking 4 days $\cdot$ wk^{-1} for 30 to 45 min is easier to implement than a goal to get in shape. Specific, measurable goals make it easier for you to monitor your progress, make adjustments and know when your goal has been accomplished.

- Goals also must be **reasonable** and **realistic**.

Your goal might be achievable, but your personal and your situational constraints can make it unrealistic. Losing 2 lb $\cdot$ wk^{-1} (0.9 kg $\cdot$ wk^{-1}) through diet and exercise is reasonable for many people, but it may be almost impossible for the working parent of three who has minimal time for exercise and cooking. Unrealistic goals set you up to fail, which can damage self-efficacy and adherence to the program for behavior change.

By using information from your assessment and self-monitoring, I can and do help you to set positive, realistic behavioral goals based on your age, sex, fitness, health, interests, exercise history, skills, and schedule. Both your short-term and long-term goals should be included.

Your Short-term goals mobilize your effort and direct your present actions, but both your short- and long-term goals lead to a more effective plan of action

Goal setting is an essential strategy for exercise behavior change and adherence, and the importance of short-term process goals for fostering intrinsic motivation and adherence.

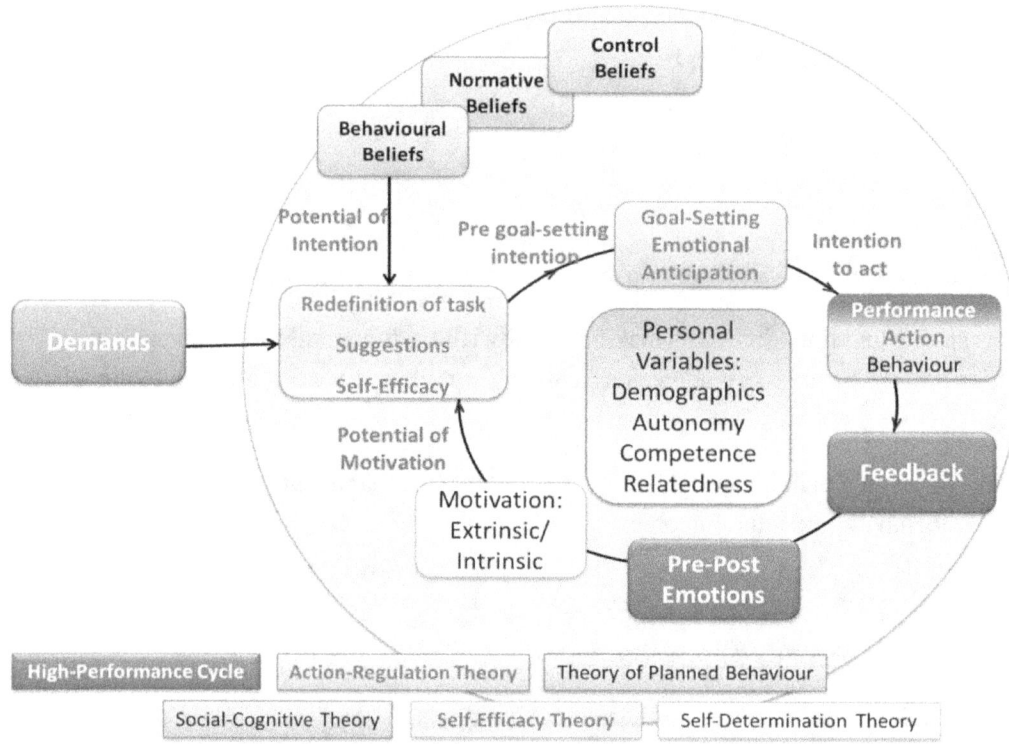

Reinforcement

Social **reinforcement** and self-reinforcement are crucial in your action phase, especially because the longer you have been inactive before starting to exercise, the longer it takes until exercise itself becomes reinforcing.

Immediate consequences of exercise can be soreness and fatigue, so external, immediate, positive rewards are necessary for beginners.

Monitoring your progress is rewarding and can involve charting miles walked after each session or asking for feedback from instructors after a difficult exercise class.

Positive reinforcement from others can enhance self-efficacy, especially when feedback comes from people who are important to the participant.

But no matter what …. The Path to your Health and Wellness …. The Journey to Your Abundant Life starts with You Move SomeThing!

Move Something!

WHAT Are YOU Moving?

YourSelf!

WHERE Are YOU Going?

Abundant LIFE!

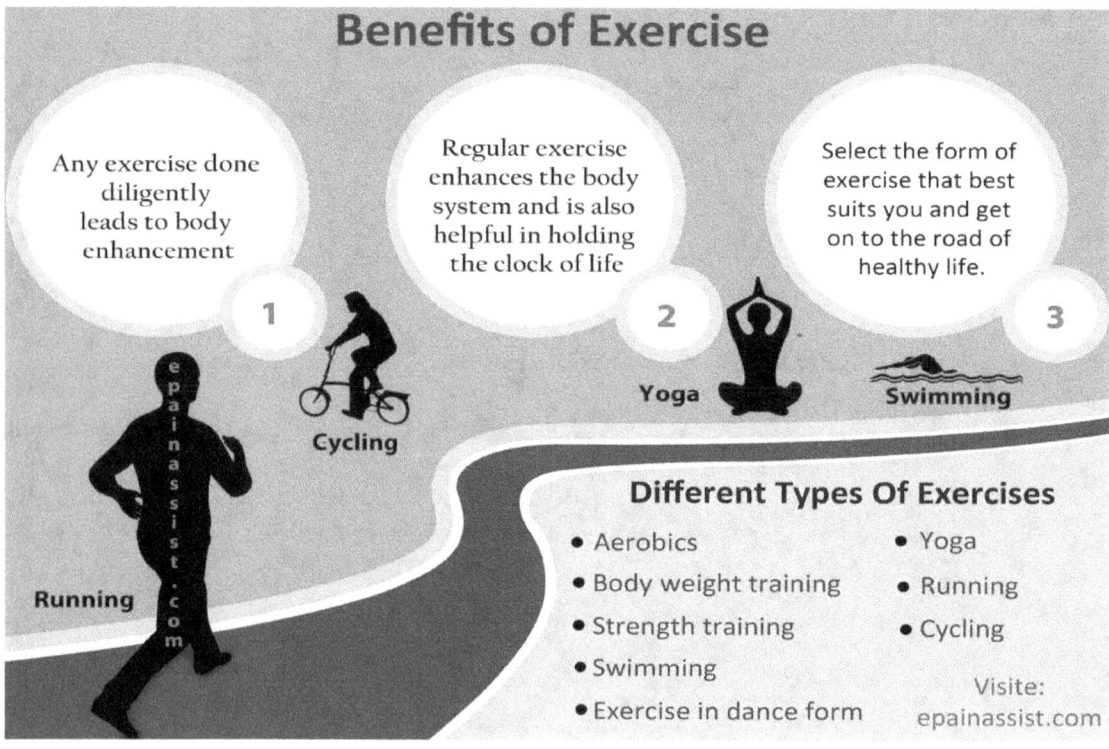

Resources

1. Carr, G.A. 2004. *Sport mechanics for coaches.* 2nd ed. Champaign, IL: Human Kinetics.
2. Floyd, R.T. 2009. *Manual of structural kinesiology.* 17th ed. Boston: McGraw-Hill Higher Education.
3. Gray, H., P.L. Williams, & L.H. Bannister, eds. 1995. *Gray's anatomy: The anatomical basis of medicine and surgery.* New York: Churchill Livingstone.
4. Hall, S. J. 2007. *Basic biomechanics.* 5th ed. Boston: McGraw-Hill.
5. Hamill, J., & K. Knutzen. 2009. *Biomechanical basis of human movement.* 3rd ed. Philadelphia: Lippincott Williams & Wilkins.
6. Hay, J.G., & J.G. Reid. 1988. *Anatomy, mechanics and human motion.* 2nd ed. Englewood Cliffs, NJ: Prentice Hall.
7. Alexander, C. 2011. *Water fitness lesson plans and choreography.* Champaign, IL: Human Kinetics.
8. Bravata, D.M., C. Smith-Spangler, V. Sundaram, A.L. Gienger, N. Lin, R. Lewis, C.D. Stave, I. Olkin, and J. R. Sirard. 2007. Using pedometers to increase physical activity and improve health - a systematic review. *JAMA.* 298:2296-2304.
9. Fenton, M. and D.R. Bassett, Jr. 2006. *Pedometer walking.* Guilford, CT: Lyons Press.
10. Franklin, B.A., N.B. Oldridge, K.G. Stoedefalke, and W.E. Loechel. 1990. *On the ball.* Carmel, IN: Benchmark Press.
11. Franklin, B.A., N.B. Oldridge, K.G. Stoedefalke, and W.E. Loechel. 2001. *The sport ball exercise handbook.* Monterey, CA: Exercise Science.
12. Franks, B.D., and E.T. Howley. 1998. *Fitness leaders' handbook.* 2nd ed. Champaign, IL: Human Kinetics.
13. Garrick, J.G., and R.K. Requa. 1988. Aerobic dance—A review. *Sports Medicine* 6:169-179.
14. Giese, M.D. 1988. Organization of an exercise session. In *Resource manual guidelines for exercise testing and prescription,* ed. S.N. Blair, P. Painter, R. Pate, 244-247. Philadelphia: Lea & Febiger.
15. Kasser, S.L. 1995. *Inclusive games: Movement fun for everyone.* Champaign, IL: Human Kinetics.

16. Londeree, B.R., and M.I. Moeschberger. 1982. Effect of age and other factors on maximal heart rate. *Research Quarterly for Exercise and Sport* 53:297-304.
17. McSwegin, P.J., and C.L. Pemberton. 1993. Exercise leadership: Key skills and characteristics. In *ACSM's resource manual for guidelines for exercise testing and prescription.* 2nd ed. Ed. J.L. Durstine, A.C. King, P.L. Painter, J.L. Roitman, L.D. Zwiren, and W.L. Kenney, 319-326. Philadelphia: Lea & Febiger.
18. New Games Foundation. 1976. *The new games book.* Garden City, NY: Dolphin Books.
19. Seaman, J. 1999. Physical activity and fitness for persons with disabilities. *PCPFS Research Digest*.
20. U.S. Department of Health and Human Services (HHS). 2008. *2008 Physcial Activity Guidelines for Americans.* www.health.gov/paguidelines/guidelines/default.aspx.
21. Williford, H.N., M. Scharff-Olson, and D.L. Blessing. 1989. The physiological effects of aerobic dance—A review. *Sports Medicine* 8:335-345.

References

4. Åstrand, P.-O. 1952. *Experimental studies of physical working capacity in relation to sex and age.* Copenhagen: Ejnar Munksgaard.
5. Åstrand, P.-O., K. Rodahl, H.A. Dahl, and S.B. Strømme. 2003. *Textbook of work physiology.* 4th ed. Champaign, IL: Human Kinetics.
6. Bassett Jr., D.R. 1994. Skeletal muscle characteristics: Relationships to cardiovascular risk factors. *Medicine and Science in Sports and Exercise* 26:957-966.
7. Bassett, D.R., and E.T. Howley. 1997. Maximal oxygen uptake: Classical versus contemporary viewpoints. *Medicine and Science in Sports and Exercise* 29:591-603.
8. Bassett, D.R., and E.T. Howley. 2000. Limiting factors for maximal oxygen uptake and determinants of endurance performance. *Medicine and Science in Sports and Exercise* 32:70-84.

9. Bouchard, C., R. Lesage, G. Lortie, J. Simoneau, P. Hamel, M. Boulay, L. Perusse, G. Theriault, and C. Leblank. 1986. Aerobic performance in brothers, dizygotic and monozygotic twins. *Medicine and Science in Sports and Exercise* 18:639-646.
10. Brooks, G.A. 1985. Anaerobic threshold: Review of the concept, and directions for future research. *Medicine and Science in Sports and Exercise* 17:22-31.
11. Brooks, G.A., T.D. Fahey, and T.P. White. 2005. *Exercise physiology: Human bioenergetics and its application.* 4th ed. New York: McGraw-Hill.
12. Claytor, R.P. 1985. *Selected cardiovascular, sympathoadrenal, and metabolic responses to one-leg exercise training.* Unpublished doctoral dissertation. University of Tennessee at Knoxville.
13. Coggan, A.R., and E.F. Coyle. 1991. Carbohydrate ingestion during prolonged exercise: Effects on metabolism and performance. *Exercise and Sport Sciences Reviews* 19:1-40.
14. Costill, D.L. 1988. Carbohydrates for exercise: Dietary demands of optimal performance. *International Journal of Sports Medicine* 9:1-18.
15. Coyle, E.F. 1988. Detraining and retention of training induced adaptations. In *Resource manual for guidelines for exercise testing and prescription,* ed. S.N. Blair, P. Painter, R.R. Pate, L.K. Smith, and C.B. Taylor, 83-89. Philadelphia: Lea & Febiger.
16. Coyle, E.F., M.K. Hemmert, and A.R. Coggan. 1986. Effects of detraining on cardiovascular responses to exercise: Role of blood volume. *Journal of Applied Physiology* 60:95-99.
17. Coyle, E.F., W.H. Martin III, S.A. Bloomfield, O.H. Lowry, and J.O. Holloszy. 1985. Effects of detraining on responses to submaximal exercise. *Journal of Applied Physiology* 59:853-859.
18. Coyle, E.F., W.H. Martin III, D.R. Sinacore, M.J. Joyner, J.M. Hagberg, and J.O. Holloszy. 1984. Time course of loss of adaptation after stopping prolonged intense endurance training. *Journal of Applied Physiology* 57:1857-1864.
19. Cureton, K.J., P.B. Sparling, B.W. Evans, S.M. Johnson, U.D. Kong, and J.W. Purvis. 1978. Effect of experimental alterations in excess weight on aerobic capacity and distance-running performance. *Medicine and Science in Sports* 10:194-199.
20. Davis, J.H. 1985. Anaerobic threshold: Review of the concept and directions for future research. *Medicine and Science in Sports and Exercise* 17:6-18.
21. Edington, D.W., and V.R. Edgerton. 1976. *The biology of physical activity.* Boston: Houghton Mifflin.
22. Ekblom, B., P.-O. Åstrand, B. Saltin, J. Stenberg, and B. Wallstrom. 1968. Effect of training on circulatory response to exercise. *Journal of Applied Physiology* 24:518-528.
23. Faulkner, J.A., D.E. Roberts, R.L. Elk, and J. Conway. 1971. Cardiovascular responses to submaximum and maximum effort cycling and running. *Journal of Applied Physiology* 30:457-461.
24. Fleck, S.J., and L.S. Dean. 1987. Resistance-training experience and the pressor response during resistance exercise. *Journal of Applied Physiology* 63:116-120.

25. Fox, E.L., R.W. Bowers, and M.L. Foss. 1998. *Fox's the physiological basis for exercise and sport.* 6th ed. Dubuque, IA: Brown.
26. Franklin, B.A. 1985. Exercise testing, training, and arm ergometry. *Sports Medicine* 2:100-119.
27. Gisolfi, C., and C.B. Wenger. 1984. Temperature regulation during exercise: Old concepts, new ideas. *Exercise and Sport Sciences Reviews* 12:339-372.
28. Hickson, R.C., H.A. Bomze, and J.O. Holloszy. 1977. Linear increase in aerobic power induced by a strenuous program of endurance exercise. *Journal of Applied Physiology: Respiratory, Environmental and Exercise Physiology* 42:372-376.
29. Hickson, R.C., H.A. Bomze, and J.O. Holloszy. 1978. Faster adjustment of O_2 uptake to the energy requirement of exercise in the trained state. *Journal of Applied Physiology: Respiratory, Environmental and Exercise Physiology* 44:877-881.
30. Hickson, R.C., C. Foster, M.L. Pollock, T.M. Galassi, and S. Rich. 1985. Reduced training intensities and loss of aerobic power, endurance, and cardiac growth. *Journal of Applied Physiology* 58:492-499.
31. Hickson, R.C., C. Kanakis Jr., J.R. Davis, A.M. Moore, and S. Rich. 1982. Reduced training duration effects on aerobic power, endurance, and cardiac growth. *Journal of Applied Physiology* 53:225-229.
32. Hickson, R.C., and M.A. Rosenkoetter. 1981. Reduced training frequencies and maintenance of increased aerobic power. *Medicine and Science in Sports and Exercise* 13:13-16.
33. Holloszy, J.O., and E.F. Coyle. 1984. Adaptations of skeletal muscle to endurance exercise and their metabolic consequences. *Journal of Applied Physiology: Respiratory, Environmental and Exercise Physiology* 56:831-838.
34. Howley, E.T. 1980. Effect of altitude on physical performance. In *Encyclopedia of physical education, fitness, and sports: Training, environment, nutrition, and fitness,* ed. G.A. Stull and T.K. Cureton, 177-187. Salt Lake City: Brighton.
35. Howley, E.T., D.R. Bassett Jr., and H.G. Welch. 1995. Criteria for maximal oxygen uptake—Review and commentary. *Medicine and Science in Sports and Exercise* 24:1055-1058.
36. Hultman, E. 1967. Physiological role of muscle glycogen in man, with special reference to exercise. *Circulation Research* 20-21(Suppl. 1): 99-114.
37. Issekutz, B., N.C. Birkhead, and K. Rodahl. 1962. The use of respiratory quotients in assessment of aerobic power capacity. *Journal of Applied Physiology* 17:47-50.
38. Kasch, F.W., J.L. Boyer, S.P. Van Camp, L.S. Verity, and J.P. Wallace. 1990. The effects of physical activity and inactivity on aerobic power in older men (a longitudinal study). *Physician and Sportsmedicine* 18(4): 73-83.
39. Kasch, F.W., J.P. Wallace, and S.P. Van Camp. 1985. Effects of 18 years of endurance exercise on the physical work capacity of older men. *Journal of Cardiopulmonary Rehabilitation* 5:308-312.

40. Kasch, F.W., J.P. Wallace, S.P. Van Camp, and L.S. Verity. 1988. A longitudinal study of cardiovascular stability in active men aged 45 to 65 yrs. *Physician and Sportsmedicine* 16(1): 117-126.
41. Katch, F.I., and W.D. McArdle. 1977. *Nutrition and weight control.* Boston: Houghton Mifflin.
42. Lind, A.R., and G.W. McNicol. 1967. Muscular factors which determine the cardiovascular responses to sustained and rhythmic exercise. *Canadian Medical Association Journal* 96:706-713.
43. MacDougall, J.D., D. Tuxen, D.G. Sale, J.R. Moroz, and J.R. Sutton. 1985. Arterial blood-pressure response to heavy resistance exercise. *Journal of Applied Physiology* 58:785-790.
44. McArdle, W.D., F.I. Katch, and V.L. Katch. 2010. *Exercise physiology, energy, nutrition, and human performance.* 7th ed. Baltimore: Lippincott Williams & Wilkins.
45. McArdle, W.D., F.I. Katch, and G.S. Pechar. 1973. Comparison of continuous and discontinuous treadmill and bicycle tests for max VO_2. *Medicine and Science in Sports* 5(3):156-160.
46. McArdle, W.D., and J.R. Magel. 1970. Physical work capacity and maximum oxygen uptake in treadmill and bicycle exercise. *Medicine and Science in Sports* 2(3): 118-123.
47. Montoye, H.J., T. Ayen, F. Nagle, and E.T. Howley. 1986. The oxygen requirement for horizontal and grade walking on a motor-driven treadmill. *Medicine and Science in Sports and Exercise* 17:640-645.
48. Nagle, F.J., B. Balke, G. Baptista, J. Alleyia, and E. Howley. 1971. Compatibility of progressive treadmill, bicycle, and step tests based on oxygen-uptake responses. *Medicine and Science in Sports* 3:149-154.
49. Plowman, S.A., and D.L. Smith. 2008. *Exercise physiology for health, fitness and performance.* 3rd ed. New York: Benjamin Cummings.
50. Powers, S.K., S. Dodd, and R.E. Beadle. 1985. Oxygen-uptake kinetics in trained athletes differing in VO_2max. *European Journal of Applied Physiology* 54:306-308.
51. Powers, S., S. Dodd, R. Deason, R. Byrd, and T. McKnight. 1983. Ventilatory threshold, running economy, and distance-running performance of trained athletes. *Research Quarterly for Exercise and Sport* 54:179-182.
52. Powers, S.K., and E.T. Howley. 2012. *Exercise physiology.* 8th ed. New York: McGraw-Hill.
53. Powers, S., W. Riley, and E. Howley. 1980. A comparison of fat metabolism in trained men and women during prolonged aerobic work. *Research Quarterly for Exercise and Sport* 52:427-431.
54. Raven, P.B., B.L. Drinkwater, R.O. Ruhling, N. Bolduan, S. Taguchi, J. Gliner, and S.M. Horvath. 1974. Effect of carbon monoxide and peroxyacetyl nitrate on man's maximal aerobic capacity. *Journal of Applied Physiology* 36:288-293.

55. Robergs, R.A., and S.J. Keteyian. 2003. *Fundamentals of exercise physiology: For fitness, performance and health.* 2nd ed. New York: McGraw-Hill.
56. Rowell, L.B. 1969. Circulation. *Medicine and Science in Sports* 1:15-22.
57. Rowell, L.B. 1986. *Human circulation-regulation during physical stress.* New York: Oxford University Press.
58. Sale, D.G. 1987. Influence of exercise and training on motor unit activation. *Exercise and Sport Sciences Reviews* 15:95-151.
59. Saltin, B. 1969. Physiological effects of physical conditioning. *Medicine and Science in Sports* 1:50-56.
60. Saltin, B., and P.D. Gollnick. 1983. Skeletal muscle adaptability: Significance for metabolism and performance. In *Handbook of physiology,* ed. L.D. Peachey, R.H. Adrian, and S.R. Geiger, 555-631. Baltimore: Williams & Wilkins.
61. Saltin, B., J. Henriksson, E. Nygaard, P. Anderson, and E. Jansson. 1977. Fiber types and metabolic potentials of skeletal muscles in sedentary man and endurance runners. *Annals of the New York Academy of Science* 301:3-29.
62. Saltin, B., and L. Hermansen. 1966. Esophageal, rectal, and muscle temperature during exercise. *Journal of Applied Physiology* 21:1757-1762.
63. Schwade, J., C.G. Blomqvist, and W. Shapiro. 1977. A comparison of the response to arm and leg work in patients with ischemic heart disease. *American Heart Journal* 94:203-208.
64. Sherman, W.M. 1983. Carbohydrates, muscle glycogen, and muscle glycogen supercompensation. In *Ergogenic aids in sports,* ed. M.H. Williams, 3-26. Champaign, IL: Human Kinetics.
65. Taylor, H.L., E.R. Buskirk, and A. Henschel. 1955. Maximal oxygen intake as an objective measure of cardiorespiratory performance. *Journal of Applied Physiology* 8:73-80.
66. Vander, A.J., J.H. Sherman, and D.S. Luciano. 1985. *Human physiology.* 4th ed. New York: McGraw-Hill.
67. Wilmore, J.H., D.L. Costill, and W. L. Kenney. 2008. *Physiology of sport and exercise.* 4th ed. Champaign, IL: Human Kinetics.
68. Whittle, M. 2007. *Gait analysis: An introduction.* 4th ed. New York: Butterworth-Heinemann.

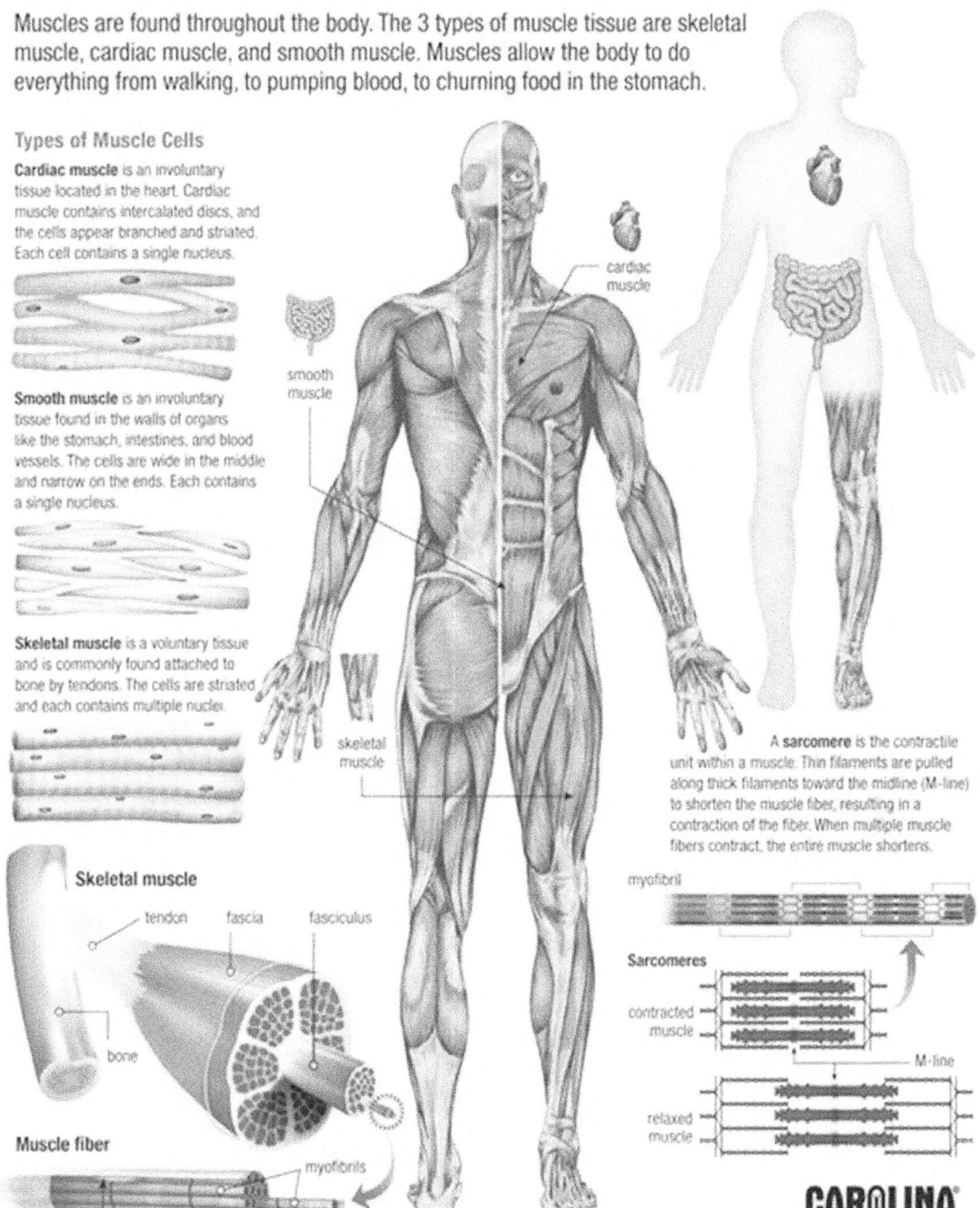

Human Body: Respiratory System

The respiratory system is responsible for gas exchange—the inhalation of oxygen (O_2) and the exhalation of carbon dioxide (CO_2). The lungs, conducting airways, and the diaphragm are key structures of the system.

Lungs and Diaphragm

Human lungs are sponge-like organs found in the thoracic (chest) cavity. The right lung has 3 lobes and is larger than the bilobed left lung, as the heart occupies more space on the left side.

The diaphragm is a domed, sheet-like muscle that separates the thoracic and abdominal cavities.

Breathing

During **inhalation**, the diaphragm contracts, and air is pulled through the conducting airways into the lungs. During **exhalation**, the diaphragm relaxes, and air is pushed from the lungs.

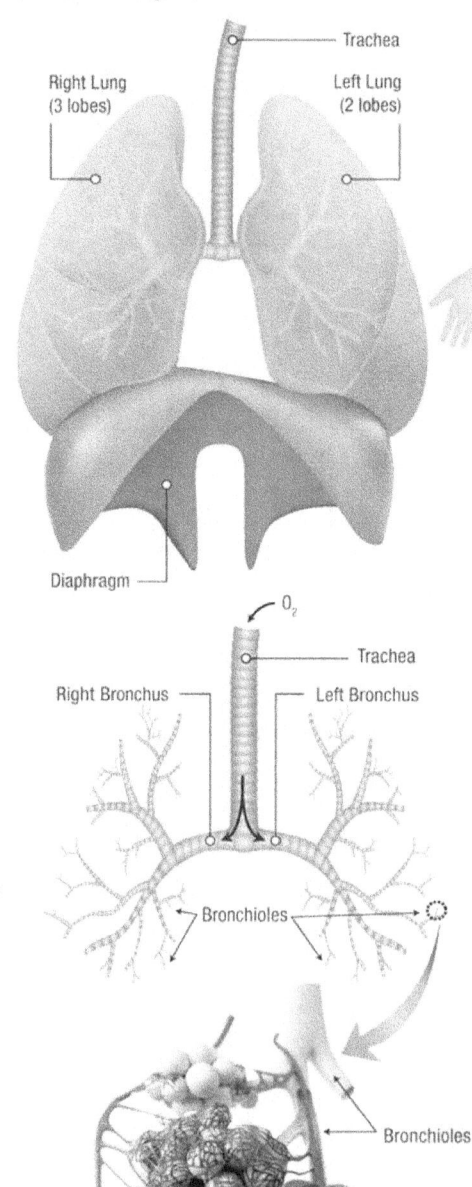

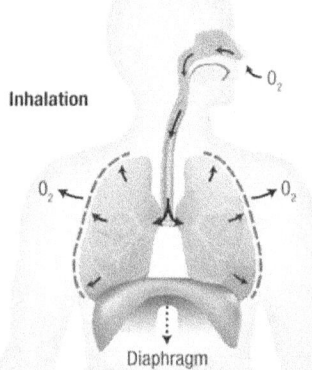

Inhalation

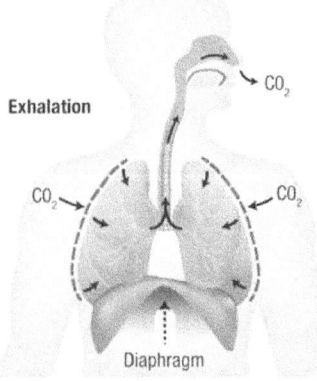

Exhalation

Bronchi, Bronchioles, and Alveoli

Air enters the lungs from the trachea through the right and left bronchus. These branching airways lead to bronchioles and end in microscopic air sacs called alveoli. The alveoli are the sites of gas exchange between the cardiovascular and respiratory systems.

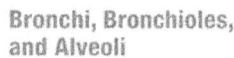

Human Body: Reproductive System

The male and female reproductive systems are controlled by hormones produced by the pituitary gland in the brain, and the reproductive organs themselves.

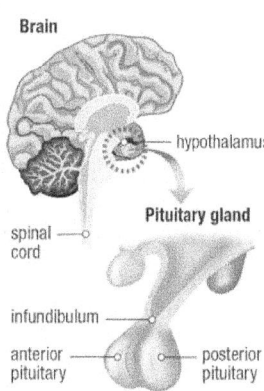

Brain

hypothalamus
spinal cord
Pituitary gland
infundibulum
anterior pituitary
posterior pituitary

The Reproductive Organs

These organs make, mature, and store gametes, or sex cells, in the human body. The male gametes are called sperm and female gametes are called ova or egg cells. Each gamete contributes half of an offspring's DNA, providing genetic variation through sexual reproduction.

Male reproductive system

Sperm is made in the seminiferous tubules and stored in the epididymis. It travels through the vas deferens, where it mixes with seminal fluids and passes through the urethra.

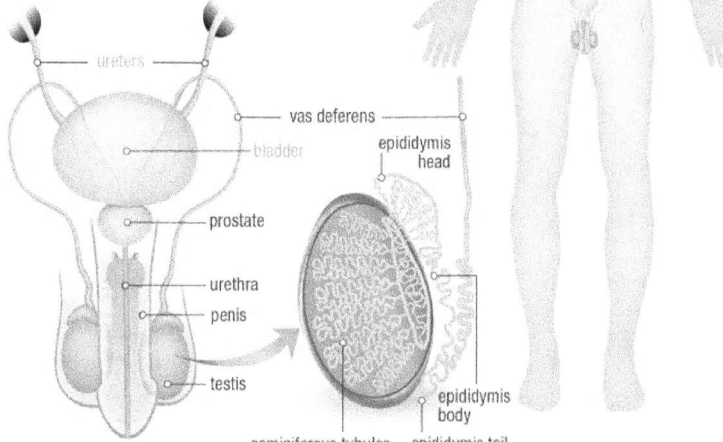

ureters
vas deferens
bladder
epididymis head
prostate
urethra
penis
testis
seminiferous tubules
epididymis body
epididymis tail

Pituitary Gland

The pituitary gland secretes hormones that control the reproductive organs. It signals the production of sex hormones and controls ovulation and the menstrual cycle in women.

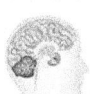

Female reproductive system

Immature eggs are found in the ovaries where they mature and are released into the fallopian tubes. An egg travels down the tube to the uterus, where it either implants and develops into an embryo or is shed with the lining of the uterus at the end of a menstrual cycle.

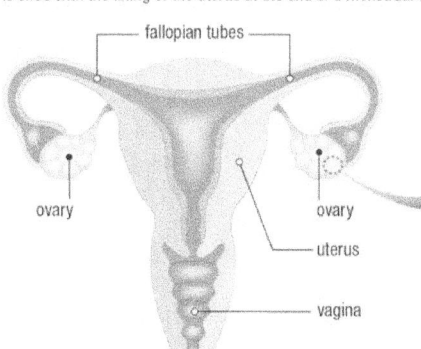

fallopian tubes
ovary
ovary
uterus
vagina

Developing Ovarian Follicle

mature egg

CAROLINA
www.carolina.com

Human Body: Urinary System

The urinary system filters extra water and waste products from the blood to help maintain proper fluid balance inside the body. An elaborate system of tubes and tubules intertwines with arteries and veins within the kidneys to allow for maximum excretion of waste products, such as various salts and proteins. The ureters carry this waste to the bladder, where it is stored until excretion.

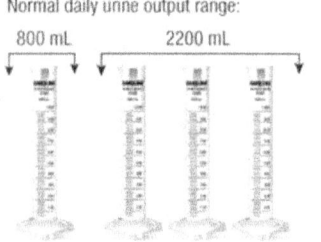

Normal daily urine output range: 800 mL – 2200 mL
1000 mL graduated cylinders

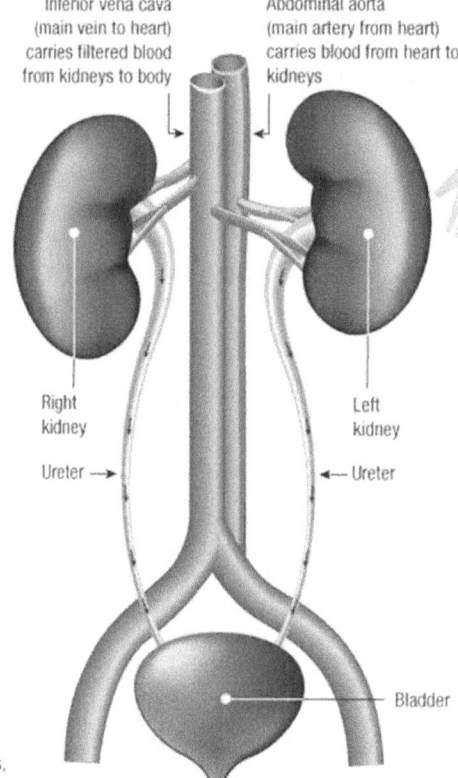

Urinary System

Ureters are long, thin tubes that carry urine from the kidneys (where it is produced) to the bladder.

The **bladder** is a muscular sac that stores urine.

The **urethra** is a narrow tube connected to the bladder that removes urine from the body.

Kidneys
The kidneys are found in the upper abdomen on each side of the spine. These fist-size organs filter waste products out of the bloodstream and produce urine.

Nephrons
Nephrons contain a network of tubes, veins, and arteries that intertwine to exchange salts, wastes, and fluids to remove them from the bloodstream.

Glomerulus
A glomerulus is a small, round pocket within the kidneys that uses concentration gradients to remove nitrogenous waste and salts from the blood vessels that pass through it.

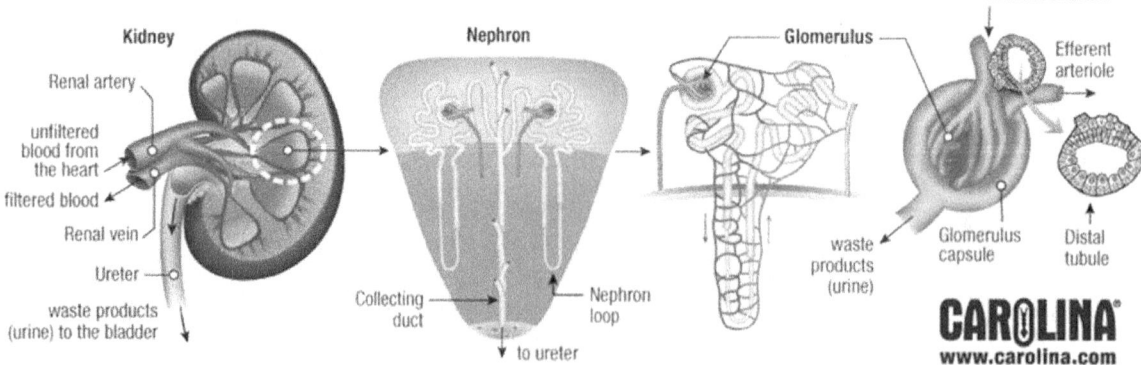

Human Body: Digestive System

The main functions of the digestive system are mechanical and chemical digestion, and absorption. Digestion is the process in which the body breaks food down into smaller molecules so that nutrients can be easily absorbed. The entire digestion process can take anywhere from 24 to 50 hours.

Mouth/Esophagus

Digestion begins in the mouth through the mechanical and chemical breakdown of food. Smooth muscle tissue in the esophagus squeezes the food down toward the stomach in a process called peristalsis.

Stomach

Mechanical and chemical digestion continues in the stomach. Smooth muscle tissue in the stomach wall squeezes and churns the material, while enzymes and chemicals are added to help further break down the food.

Stomach structure

The internal structure of the stomach has ridges and folds called rugae. This increases the surface area within the stomach and allows it to expand to hold more food.

Intestines

The small intestine and large intestine (colon) combined average 25 feet long.

Small Intestine

The majority of absorption takes place in the small intestine, which is about 20 feet long. The small intestine has 3 sections: duodenum, jejunum, and ileum.

Finger-like extensions called villi and microvilli increase the surface area of the small intestine, allowing maximum absorption of nutrients and water.

Large Intestine

The large intestine, about 5 feet long, is responsible for eliminating waste matter.

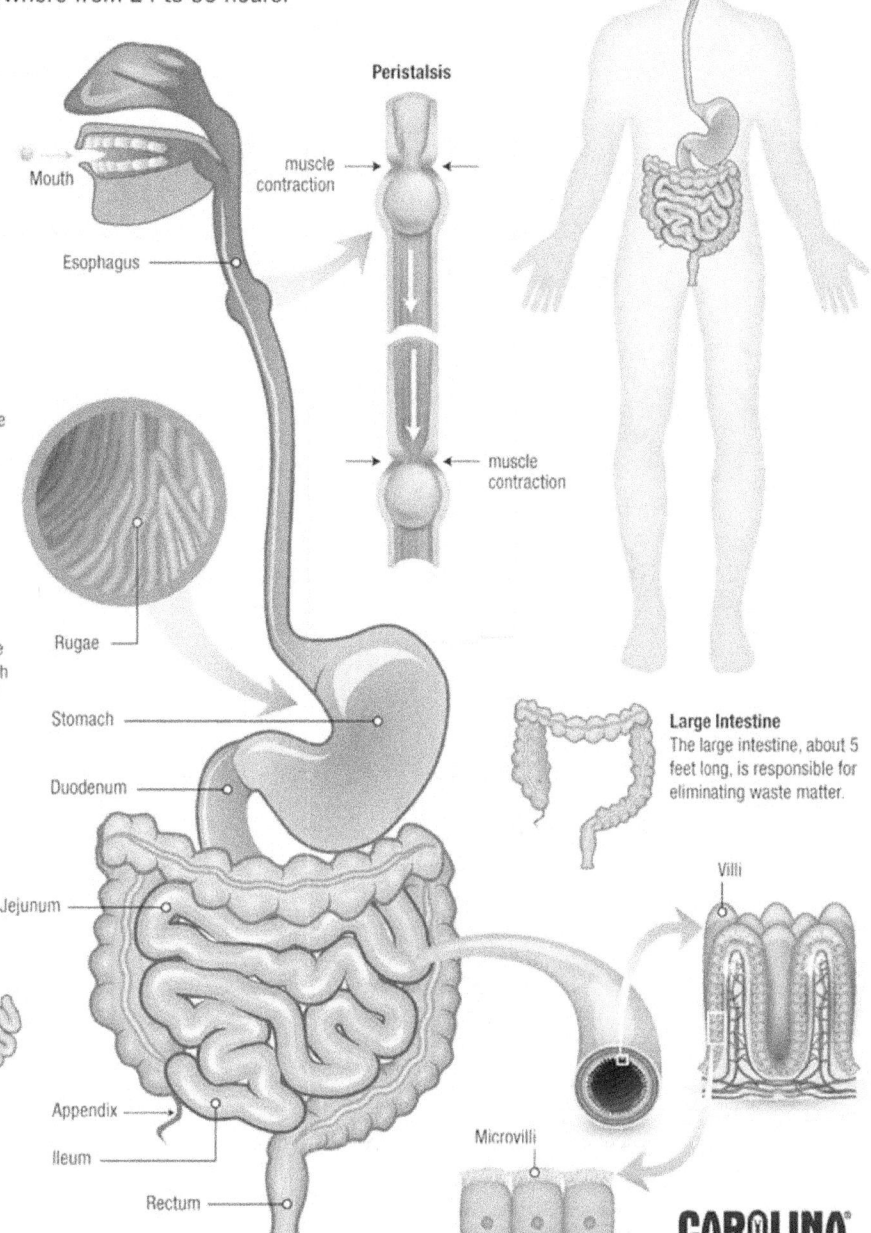

Human Body: Endocrine System

The endocrine system contains 9 major glands and organs that produce, store, and secrete hormones.

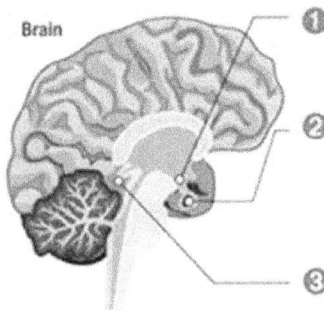
Brain

① Hypothalamus
Maintains the body's homeostasis and regulates body temperature, heart rate, and blood pressure.

② Pituitary Gland
Composed of 2 lobes: the anterior, which secretes hormones involved in the body's growth and development, and the posterior, which secretes hormones that increase the reabsorption of water into the kidneys.

③ Pineal Gland
Responsible for the production of melatonin, which plays a major role in the body's sleep-wake cycle.

④ Thyroid
This butterfly-shaped gland produces 3 major hormones: calcitonin, triiodothyronine (T3), and thyroxine (T4). They help regulate the body's energy and metabolism.

⑤ Parathyroid
The parathyroid secretes hormones necessary for calcium absorption.

⑥ Thymus
The thymus controls production of T-cells (white blood cells) and plays a vital role in the body's ability to fight diseases.

⑦ Ovaries/Testes
The male and female reproductive organs release hormones responsible for blood circulation, mental vigor, and sex drive.

Ovary
Secretes estrogen and progesterone, which play a key role in the health of the female reproductive system.

Testis
Secretes testosterone, which is vital for physical development, bone density, and libido in males.

⑧ Pancreas
Aids in the digestion of proteins, fats, and carbohydrates. Responsible for the production of insulin and glucagon, which regulate the level of glucose in the blood.

⑨ Adrenal Gland
Produces hormones that allow the body to react to stress, such as adrenaline and cortisol.

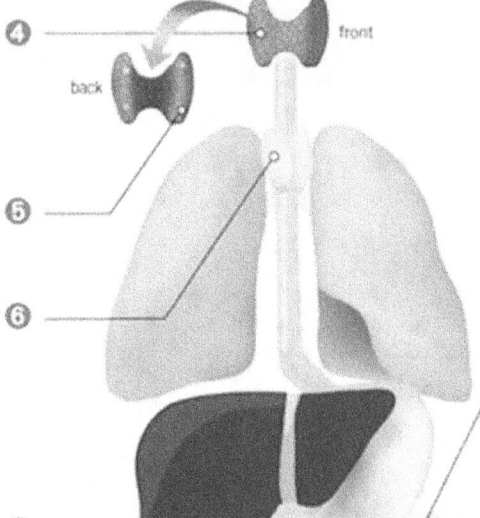

CAROLINA
www.carolina.com

Human Body: Integumentary System

The integumentary system protects the body from the external environment and works with other body systems to regulate internal processes. Major structures include the skin, glands, hair, and nails. The main functions of the integumentary system are protection, regulation, and sensation.

Skin

Skin is the largest and fastest-growing organ in the body. The outermost layer, the **epidermis**, is composed of stratified squamous epithelial tissue. Below this layer is the **dermis**, which contains the cutaneous glands, hair follicles, and most of the skin's nerve endings. The **hypodermis** (subcutaneous layer) consists of loose connective and adipose tissue.

Cutaneous Glands

Cutaneous glands within the dermis include sebaceous and sweat glands. **Sebaceous glands** secrete sebum, an oily substance that waterproofs and lubricates the skin. **Sweat glands** help cool the body through evaporation of sweat.

Fingernails

Fingernails and toenails are made of densely-packed cells covered in keratin. The cuticle, found at the base of the nail, provides a barrier between the skin and the nail. The body of the nail appears pink due to numerous blood vessels in the nail bed underneath. Nails protect the fingers and toes and can be used for scratching.

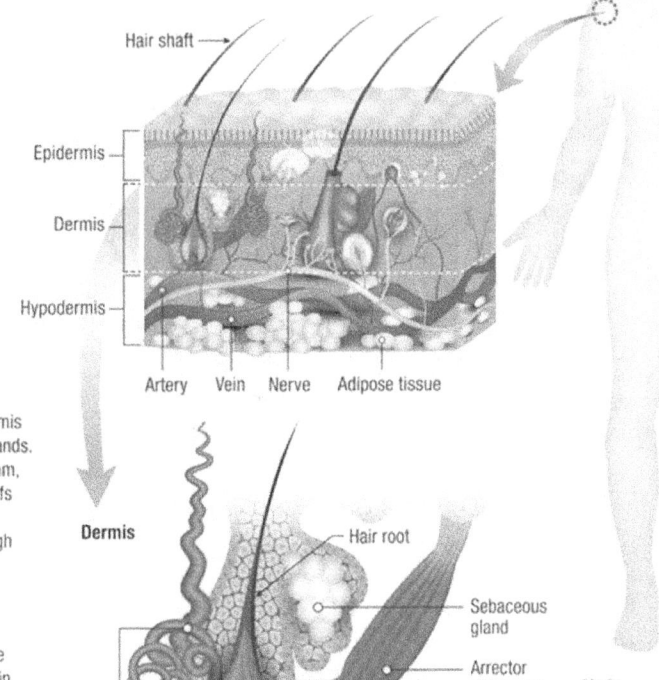

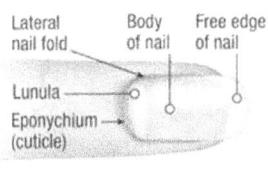

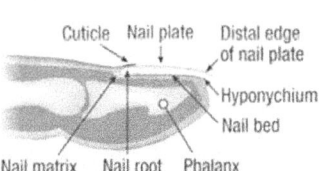

Hair

Hair is a pigmented filament formed by mostly keratinized cells. Human hair follicles can be divided into 3 main segments: the bulb, root, and shaft. The shaft (the visible part of hair) consists of 3 layers: the cuticle, cortex, and medulla. The cortex defines texture and contains the pigment that gives hair its color.

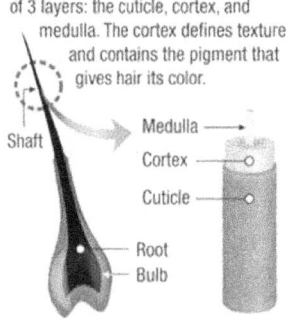

DIGESTIVE TRACT

Absorbtion takes place in the stomach, small intestinal tract and the large colon. You can see the absorbtion veins leading from the tracts and back to the liver. These veins are blue on this diagram.

After food has been filtered by the liver, It move into the hapatic portal which takes it to the heart to feed your blood cells.

After absorption, the food is taken directly to the liver, via the portal vein, to be cleansed.

The waste product from the liver is sent to the gull bladder for disposal by being stored as bile until new food passes from the stomach to the duodenum.
Once food is detected in the duodenum, bile is added to break food down into a liquid, ready for absorption.

The pancreas also secretes enzymes into the duodenum at the same time that bile is added to help break down food.

Soluble fibre absorbs the waste from the liver as well as cholesterol from new food therefore preventing these undesirables from being re-absorbed in the intestinal tracts..

Insoluble fibre does not break down into a paste until it reaches the large intestinal tract. Here is where it encourages the growth of the colon's natural flora..

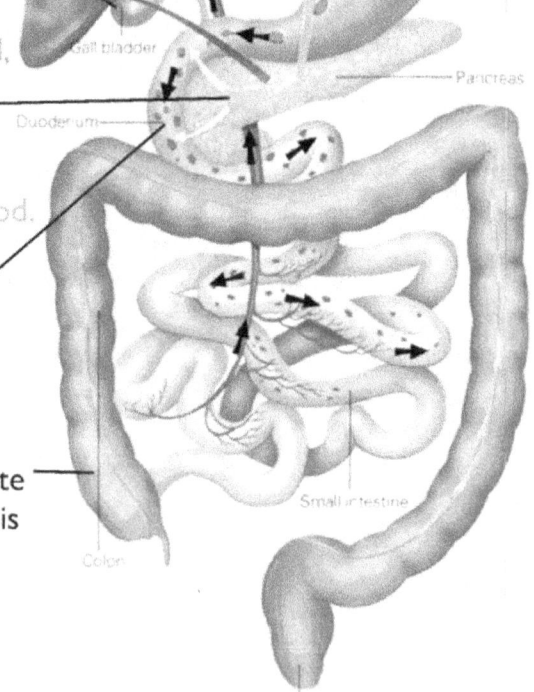

Supreme Health & Fitness! *Health & Wellness Series ... Vol 3!*

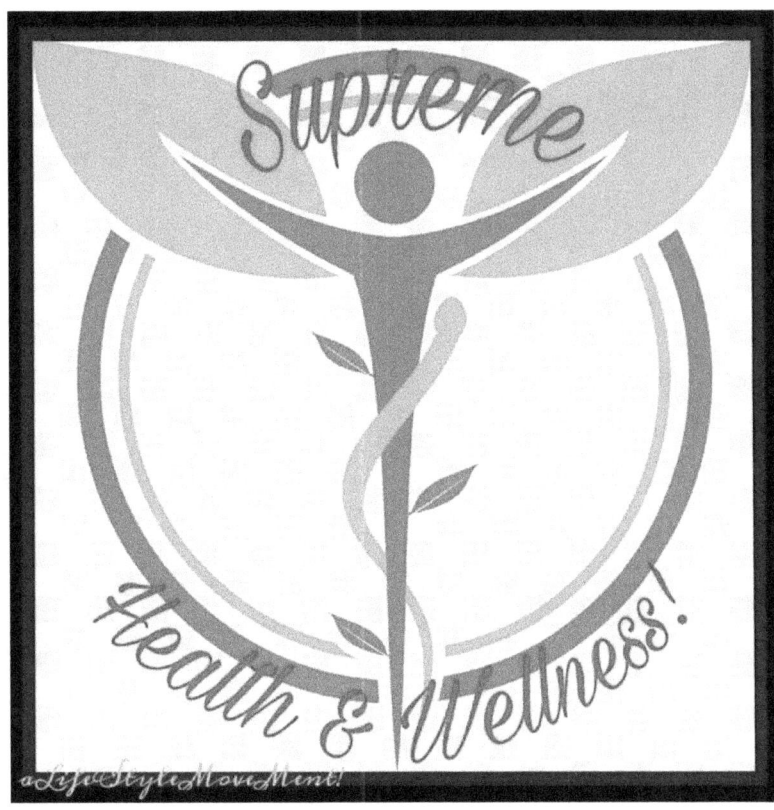

Supreme Health and Fitness by Sean Ali!

Achieving and Maintaining Supreme Health and Wellness by increasing the level of Knowledge and Science of Life!

www.ingramcontent.com/pod-product-compliance
Lightning Source LLC
Chambersburg PA
CBHW082103220526
45472CB00009B/2024